Veterinary
Ethics

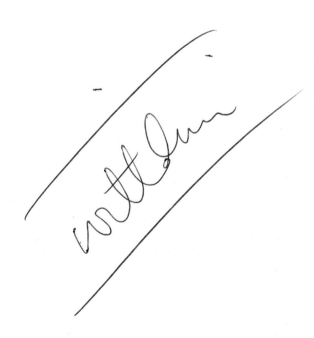

Veterinary
———— Ethics ————

Jerrold Tannenbaum, M.A., J.D.

Clinical Assistant Professor of Environmental Studies
Tufts University School of Veterinary Medicine
Boston, Massachusetts

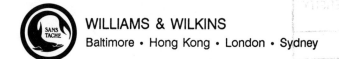

WILLIAMS & WILKINS
Baltimore • Hong Kong • London • Sydney

Editor: Timothy S. Satterfield
Associate Editor: Linda Napora
Copy Editor: Judith Minkove
Design: Alice Sellers/Johnson
Production: Anne G. Seitz

Printed in the United States of America

Library of Congress Cataloging in Publication Data

Tannenbaum, Jerrold.
    Veterinary ethics.

    Includes index.
    1. Veterinary medicine – Ethical aspects.
2.   Veterinarians – Professional ethics. 3. Animals,
Treatment of. I. Title.
SF756.39.T36 1989   174'.9636   88-17351
ISBN 0-683-08102-0

                                                    91   92   93
                      2   3   4   5   6   7   8   9   10

To Nadine and Phillip

The pronouns "he," "him," and "his" as employed at various points in this text are not meant to convey the masculine gender alone. Use of these terms in their generic sense, to denote persons of both sexes, is intended solely to avoid redundancy and awkwardness in expression.

Foreword

Only rarely have I read the manuscript of a new book with the pleasure that accompanied my reading this one. And never have I read a manuscript for a book of which I could predict, as confidently as I can here, that it is only the first edition. For there can be no doubt that Jerrold Tannenbaum has at once defined a now emergent field – veterinary medical ethics – and has literally written the book.

Every one of its crisply reasoned, clearly written, and compassionate chapters can virtually stand alone; yet taken as a whole, the book is greater than the sum of its parts. What Tannenbaum calls the "inescapable" nature of an ethical dimension of veterinary medicine in the late 20th century hits the reader squarely between the brain and the heart. No longer will veterinary medical students, researchers, practicing veterinarians, and their teachers find it difficult to find an ethical signpost in their work. Moreover, no longer can they ignore it, now that we have it.

Professor Tannenbaum has brought a full measure of intelligence, wit, and scholarship to this book and to his teaching at Tufts University. Our first ten classes have benefited from his insights while providing him with the most stimulating feedback a teacher can have. In a sense, this is their book, too.

Long neglected in a formal, recognized way by a profession busily and inherently committed to "doing good," the study of ethics and values as part of veterinary medicine is now finally upon us. Truly, "many that are first shall be last, and the last shall be first."

FRANKLIN M. LOEW, Dean
Tufts University School of Veterinary Medicine
North Grafton, Massachusetts

Preface

THE RELEVANCE OF ETHICS

Some people think that ethics is an esoteric field with little relevance to the real problems of life. Nothing could be further from the truth.

Ethical theories typically have been responses to serious practical problems. Plato's *Republic*, for example, was motivated by the disintegration of the ancient Greek city-states, and was an attempt to find lasting values for a changing world. When 18th century philosophers argued that people have "inalienable rights" to life, liberty, and the pursuit of happiness, they were articulating the demands of the growing middle class against the old monarchies, and were fashioning powerful and exciting ideas that would change the world forever.

Professional ethics, like philosophical ethical theory, thrives on practical issues.

Thirty years ago, medical ethics consisted largely of an official code that few physicians read and an oath dutifully chanted at graduation. The suggestion that all medical students should take courses in ethics would have been greeted with ridicule. The notion that there are issues in medical ethics so complex and far-ranging that professionals from outside of medicine — philosophers, lawyers, and social scientists—might be needed to help address them, would have struck most physicians as preposterous.

Today, all this has changed. Most medical schools now require course work in ethics, and an increasing number boast full-time faculty devoted to the area. Books and journals abound in which representatives of diverse disciplines consider issues in medical ethics. Physicians, ethicists, and society at large are grappling with such questions as whether terminally ill patients should have the right to refuse treatment, whether children with severe birth defects should be treated or left to die, and whether in vitro fertilization and genetic manipulation are good or evil.

This explosion in medical ethics did not occur because some academics found it amusing to think about the subject. Rather, developments (often from within medicine itself) created problems requiring ethical resolution. Physicians and others affected by modern medicine have found that they need a discipline of medical ethics to help them deal with these issues.

A TIME FOR VETERINARY ETHICS

Today, veterinary medicine faces challenges that make a serious field of veterinary ethics imperative.

Many people believe that animals should be accorded a higher value and status than they have thus far enjoyed. Veterinarians are therefore being asked whether *they* have paid sufficient attention to the interests of their animal patients. Should a companion animal doctor oppose a client's requests for procedures that do not benefit the animal? Should a food animal practitioner object if he is asked to be more concerned about the productivity of a herd than the health of individual animals? Is a sports animal practitioner the guardian of the health of his patient or of the profits of his client? Should veterinarians criticize certain uses of animals in industry and research? Have veterinarians been too willing to kill healthy animals because their owners are tired of them or are unwilling to pay for adequate care?

A growing appreciation of the importance of companion animals to the health and well-being of people raises questions about whether veterinarians are sufficiently sensitive to the emotional needs of clients, and about the extent to which practitioners should participate in clients' decisions about medical care for their animals.

Continuing development of more sophisticated and expensive veterinary techniques raises issues about how practitioners should deal with clients who cannot afford the best the profession has to offer, and about whether veterinarians ought to offer low-cost or gratuitous services for the needy.

Economic pressures on private practitioners have produced a host of divisive problems. Should the profession oppose sterilization and vaccination clinics and mobile facilities that can offer clients lower fees than traditional practices? May practitioners advertise, and if so, are there limits to what they may say or do to drum up business? Is it unprofessional for veterinarians to sell nonmedical items? Should nonprofit humane organizations be permitted to compete with private practitioners? Would it be right for the profession to protect established doctors from competition by limiting enrollments in veterinary schools?

The increasing number of veterinary specialists has exacerbated long-standing difficulties regarding competition and collegiality. General practitioners and specialists alike are asking to what extent specialists may appeal to their board certification to promote their practices. Is it unethical for a specialist to assume all future care of a patient once referral treatment is completed? May a specialist, or any subsequent veterinarian, criticize the performance of a previous doctor, and if so, should this criticism be directed to the doctor who may have provided the referral, or to the client who is paying the bill?

These and many other issues in veterinary ethics are troubling the profession. Moreover, veterinarians can no longer count on being left alone to settle these questions among themselves. People outside the profession who want to challenge the ethical values of veterinarians are turning increasingly, and sometimes successfully, to the legal system and to public opinion for assistance. Veterinarians are finding that they need the tools of ethical argument and persuasion to supplement their technical knowledge and skills.

A GUARDED PROGNOSIS FOR VETERINARY ETHICS?

It is far from clear whether a serious field of veterinary ethics will emerge in time to help practitioners deal with these issues.

To the typical veterinarian, who is educated in the sciences and is immersed in the everyday demands of making a living, ethical studies might seem mysterious. Fearful of calls made by some—in the name of morality—for an end to the use of animals in agriculture, industry, and research, some veterinarians may see in ethics itself a direct threat to their livelihoods.

Perhaps because of the perceived foreignness and dangers of ethics, the profession has done little to put in doctors' hands the tools required to articulate and defend positions in veterinary ethics. Few doctors know very much about the profession's official ethical code, and even fewer can recall the Veterinarian's Oath they took at graduation. Serious course work in ethics in veterinary schools is still rare. Nor is there a significant body of scholarly thought to which veterinarians can turn for assistance. Ethical issues concerning the use of animals in research and industry have aroused the interest of the public, and of some in academia. However, the amount of published work concerned with veterinary *professional* ethics—with the moral obligations and ideals of practicing veterinarians—is minuscule.

GETTING STARTED

This book attempts to provide tools that will help veterinary students and practitioners to participate in the ethical debates now confronting their profession.

It is impossible to do ethics without expressing one's own value judgments. Nevertheless, although I feel strongly about many of the moral recommendations developed in the text, it is not the primary purpose of this book to convince the reader of the correctness of these recommendations. My principal aim is to offer a useful structure for approaching veterinary ethics so that veterinarians of all views and orientations can better articulate their own positions on the issues. Those who disagree with my substantive suggestions will be assisted in framing their own positions by the structure developed in the text for classifying the branches and issues of veterinary ethics. When arguments in favor of specific ethical recommendations are made, they are constructed so as to elicit the reader's responses along the way.

Some veterinarians tell me that a course or book in professional ethics should be short and simple. This view makes about as much sense as a demand that a course in pathology or cardiology must not trouble veterinary students with unfamiliar or difficult material because the students are already quite busy. This is an introductory text, and one primarily for present and future veterinarians, not philosophers, lawyers, or social scientists. But because some theoretical background is necessary, and because veterinary ethics presents many challenging issues, too short and simple a book would be worthless. The subject matter requires a certain amount of time and effort.

Considerations of space, however, have necessitated certain limitations in the text. The discussion focuses on ethical issues facing private practitioners, and does not examine in detail several kinds of practice (such as wildlife medicine, academic practice, international veterinary medicine, and government veterinary service) that raise distinctive and important moral issues of their own. I do not provide as extensive argumentation regarding many issues that are considered as would be possible in a longer work. This should not be a problem for the reader, because the primary purpose of the text is to provide a comprehensive introduction to the subject that will stimulate the reader to engage in his own further thought. The text does not discuss laws and official professional standards governing veterinary practice outside the United States. However, veterinarians of other lands will find the bulk of the discussion helpful. I encourage them to consider how the laws and professional codes of their countries and veterinary associations relate to the issues — most of which do, after all, transcend national borders.

Ethics, like medicine or surgery, is best learned by doing. Reading a book cannot substitute for the consideration of real issues in actual clinical settings. Some professional ethics instructors seem to have an irresistible urge to concoct ethics "cases" with fake situations that make them humorous, and irrelevant. Even realistic manufactured cases can foster the view that ethical issues are something that happen to *someone else.*

On the other hand, actual situations accompanied simply by intuitive "gut reactions" will not do either. Responses to real issues must be supported by rational argument. It is the purpose of this book to facilitate such a process.

It would be naive to think that a serious discipline of veterinary ethics will just spring into existence when the world is ready for it. (The world, indeed, has been ready for some time.) Strenuous work must come from within the profession and its schools. If veterinarians permit others to dictate how moral issues affecting their profession and livelihoods will be resolved, they will have no one to blame but themselves.

Acknowledgments

This task could not have been undertaken without the assistance of many who shared with me their perspectives and concerns regarding professional veterinary ethics. To these veterinarians, veterinary students, technicians, scientists, representatives of state veterinary boards, and officers of veterinary medical associations, I offer my heartfelt appreciation. You cannot all be named here. I hope that you are pleased with the results.

Several people can, and must, be mentioned. Dean Franklin Loew gave me the opportunity to learn from as intelligent and spirited a group of veterinary students and faculty as exists anywhere. Andrew Rowan has been a colleague of limitless stimulation and patience. Robert Shomer was an essential source of probing questions and experienced insights. Peter Theran provided a paradigm of the gentle doctor charting the middle course.

Work on this text was supported by grants from the Bristol-Myers Company, the National Science Foundation Program in Ethics and Values in Science and Technology, and the Tufts University Center for Animals.

Permission to reproduce portions of the following works by the author is gratefully acknowledged: "Ethics and Human-Companion Animal Interaction: A Plea for a Veterinary Ethics of the Human-Companion Animal Bond." *Veterinary Clinics of North America Small Animal Practice*, Vol. 15, No. 2, pp. 431-447, 1985. Reprinted with permission from W.B. Saunders Company; "The Human/Companion Animal Bond: Cliché or Challenge?" *Trends*, Vol. 1, No. 5, pp. 45-50, 1985. Reprinted with permission of the American Animal Hospital Association; Tannenbaum J and Rowan AN: "Rethinking the Morality of Animal Research." *The Hastings Center Report*, Vol. 15, No. 5, pp. 32-43, 1985. Reproduced by permission. © The Hastings Center; "Animal rights: Some guideposts for the veterinarian." Originally published in the *Journal of the American Veterinary Medical Association* (June 1, 1986). Reprinted, with minor changes, with permission of the publisher; "Ethics and the Veterinary Technician." *Proceedings of the 17th Annual Seminar for Veterinary Technicians*, pp 206-217. Copyright 1988 by the Western Veterinary Conference. Reproduced with permission.

Permission is also acknowledged to quote from James Herriot, *All Creatures Great and Small*. Bantam Books, St. Martin's Press, Inc., New York, 1973, p 308. Copyright © by James Herriot. Reprinted by permission of St. Martin's Press, Harold Ober Associates, David Higham Associates Ltd., and James Herriot.

Finally, I want to thank my wife, Nadine Osdin, D.V.M., who provided invaluable assistance in the writing of this book and is responsible for my interest in ethical issues involving animals and veterinarians. The book also would not have happened without the influence of another who, though he will never be able to read it, is everywhere throughout it. How blessed a profession to be able to care for such as these!

Contents

Chapter

1

Why Veterinary Ethics Is Inescapable

THE NEED TO MAKE MORAL CHOICES

It would be incorrect to think that because veterinary medicine is a scientific discipline, veterinarians need not make value judgments.

Consider the following example. A client appears in your office for the second time in 4 weeks with her 2-year-old dog. At the first visit, you diagnosed a moderate case of flea allergy dermatitis, dispensed an appropriate medication and flea powder, and advised the client to vacuum and powder her premises thoroughly for several weeks to prevent recurrence of the problem. As the client and the dog enter your examination room, it is apparent that its condition has deteriorated. You believe the medication has not been applied as directed, and you doubt that the client has attempted to remove the fleas and their eggs from her home. She now tells you for the first time that the animal has been impossible to housebreak. She asks you to put it to sleep. What should you do?

In this example, as in many professional decisions, moral choices are unavoidable.

If you would immediately agree to euthanize the dog because the client has requested it, you probably would be expressing your adherence to several ethical views, including the following:

1. A companion animal has no inherent right to live.
2. An animal's owner may have it killed if keeping it has become an inconvenience.
3. The owner of a companion animal with a curable malady or behavioral problem need not take steps to remedy these problems but may just opt for euthanasia.
4. It is proper for a veterinarian to euthanize a companion animal simply because its owner requests that it be killed.

Likewise, if you would decide to persuade the client to try to cure the dog's medical and behavioral problems, you would be expressing your belief in a number of other ethical principles, including, perhaps, the view that an animal like the one in the example ought not simply to be killed, but deserves, at the very least, a "second chance."

Indeed, it is clear that even a routine practice decision can involve a large number of ethical choices. The following are just *some* of the choices that might be made in our example. You might:

1. Euthanize the animal at the client's request.
2. Ask the client whether she has followed your directions and about the housebreaking problem, hoping that this will lead her to conclude on her own that the animal need not be put to sleep.
3. Ask the client whether she has followed your directions and about the housebreaking problem, and actively challenge her decision to euthanize the dog, but agree to euthanasia if she still wants it.
4. Aggressively challenge the client about her failure to treat the dermatitis and insist that she make some serious attempts to do so before you will agree to euthanize the animal.
5. Ask her whether she will board the animal temporarily at your facility and have you treat the skin condition and assess the housebreaking problem.
6. Decline to euthanize the animal and ask for permission to place it with an animal shelter for adoption, or euthanasia if the shelter cannot find a suitable new owner.
7. Decline to euthanize the animal, and ask the client to permit you to place it out for adoption.
8. Tell the client tactfully that although you can understand her desire to euthanize the animal, it is against your personal principles to euthanize pets with curable conditions, and refer her to another practitioner or agency that will put the dog to sleep.
9. Tell her that you think killing a curable animal is morally wrong and criticize her for her indifference about the life of her dog.

Some of these alternatives may well be morally wrong. That is not the point. The point is that, *whatever* your response to this example, you will be choosing only one or some of the possible alternatives. Whether or not you actually think of or consider all the alternatives, the decision you make will reflect your views about what it is morally proper for you to do.

THE DIFFICULTY OF ETHICS

If morally correct decisions in veterinary practice were always obvious, the fact that there are usually many possible alternatives would not be troubling, and would not argue for a serious discipline of veterinary ethics. In almost anything one does, there are many possible alternatives. But most of these alternatives are so obviously unacceptable that one need not consider them seriously. If an acquaintance approaches me on the street and says hello, a proper response is to return the greeting. That I might throw my briefcase in his face, or cry out to a police officer "Thief! Stop him!" or do any of a thousand other awful things does not mean that serious ethical deliberation regarding a proper response is justified.

What makes veterinary ethics important and inescapable is that it is often far from obvious how veterinarians should act.

Several of the possible choices in our example have some plausibility. It appears to be the client's fault that the dog's dermatitis has not improved, and the housetraining problem may be attributable to her as well. If this is so, and if the dog's "problems" can readily be cured, one can argue that it would be unfair to the animal to deprive it of the opportunity to receive care and love from a more suitable owner. This argument may be even stronger the longer the dog has been in the client's possession. For there is some plausibility in suggesting that a companion animal that has been taken care of, and has been a functioning member of a human-companion animal bond for some time deserves extra consideration before it is killed at the whimsy of a now dissatisfied owner.

But saying even just these things raises further questions. Should the client be responsible for treating the dog if doing so would be at significant financial expense? If so, how great an expense can she be expected to bear under these circumstances? Is it unfair not to try to persuade the client, who might, with some education, make a good pet owner, to keep the animal? Should a veterinarian, who has a practice to run, take the time and money to attempt to adopt out curable animals? Even if the dog should not yet be euthanized, why should the veterinarian concern himself with attempting to save it? The client can take the animal elsewhere; by making a nuisance of himself, the practitioner may only risk losing this and other clients as well.

PROTECTING THE PROFESSION

Veterinarians should consider ethical issues because doing so may guide the way to morally correct choices. It is also generally in the profession's self-interest to take ethics seriously.

Between 1981 and 1983 the number of malpractice claims reported to the AVMA Professional Liability Insurance Trust rose by 20 percent (1). By 1985 there were approximately six claims annually for every 100 veterinarians (2, 3). Between 1975 and 1985, the malpractice insurance premiums paid by large animal practitioners rose a staggering 875 percent, almost doubling in the last 2 years of this period alone (4). Equine-exclusive practitioners, who paid $445 for $1 million of coverage in 1985, found themselves paying $1,990 for the same coverage in 1988.

Courts and juries now award veterinary clients large sums of money. According to a 1985 report, "judgments, which once ran from $100-$1,000 in small animal practice, now go as high as $8,000 or $10,000, while awards for suits concerning horses or livestock commonly run to tens or even hundreds of thousands of dollars" (5). One suit alleging a veterinarian's improper inspection of cattle for brucellosis resulted in a total pay-out by the AVMA Professional Liability Insurance Trust of $1.2 million (6). When a practitioner's behavior has been especially bad, in many states he may be forced to pay punitive damages – money not to compensate the client, but to punish the veterinarian. Under certain circumstances, some courts will now award owners of companion animals compensation for pain and suffering caused by a veterinarian's malpractice. Across the country, there are lawyers seeking to expand the grounds on which veterinarians can be sued (7).

If the trend toward increasing legal liability of veterinarians continues, the profession can expect still higher malpractice insurance premiums. There will be more emphasis upon defensive practice: more tests, more written consent forms, more witnesses to important conversations with clients, more attorneys to be consulted more frequently. The costs of such measures must be passed on to clients. An increasing number of animal owners may be unable to pay for veterinary services or may be forced to choose euthanasia as the only affordable alternative.

There is simply no doubt that the dramatic growth in litigation against veterinarians is attributable at least in part to the belief of some clients that their veterinarian has behaved *unethically*.

Thus, the Tennessee Supreme Court recently decided to permit suits for intentional infliction of emotional distress against veterinarians who threaten to kill a pet unless the client pays the bill. The Court reached this conclusion in a case in which a client alleged that she brought her dog to the doctor after it had been hit by a car. The client claimed that she told the doctor she could not pay his $155 bill in full, but was refused permission to pay in installments. According to the client, she was tormented by repeated telephone calls threatening that the hospital would "do away with" the dog as the doctor saw fit unless the bill was paid "in cash and in full." The Court agreed with the client that such conduct (if the client could prove it occurred) would have been "outrageous and extreme and is not tolerable in a civilized society" (8). When a New York judge departed from precedent and awarded a client money for her emotional distress, the veterinarian had promised to deliver the body of her beloved dog to a pet cemetery for burial, but when the client and her sister arrived for the funeral, they found in the casket a dead cat (9). It was a case in which a dog was severely burned after being left on a heating pad, in the Court's words, "for a day and the better part of a second day with an absence of care or attention," in which a Florida court declared that a veterinary client can collect damages for his emotional distress where his animal is injured by negligence amounting to "great indifference" (10).

Nor are malpractice suits by clients the only manifestation of the law's increasing concern about unethical behavior by veterinarians. As we shall see, veterinarians are suing each other in record numbers over the allegedly unethical conduct of colleagues. The profession has also been gravely embarrassed by the many criminal prosecutions and administrative investigations of doctors who have falsified interstate transportation documents and have been derelict in their duty to conscientiously inspect animals for dangerous communicable diseases (11, 12). (See Chapter 21.)

Heinous or grossly unethical behavior on the part of veterinarians may well be rare. However, it takes only one legal case – one outraged jury, judge, or appellate court – to break new legal ground and subject the entire profession to dramatically increased liability. Attorneys tell me that many clients who sue their veterinarian for malpractice are not bothered primarily by alleged incompetence. Rather, they feel more aggrieved by a fee perceived to be excessive, by a doctor's failure to understand the importance they attach to an animal, or by being treated like children who are incapable of making important decisions for themselves. Some observers believe that such criticisms of veterinarians are not uncommon (13, 14).

The medical profession understands the dangers of insensitivity to ethics. Its recent recurring malpractice crises cannot be explained by sudden outbreaks of incompetence, or by "lawyer greed." Attorneys do not prosecute lawsuits unless their clients want them to. Many people who years earlier would not have dreamed of suing a physician began to take their complaints to court because they believed that they were being treated arrogantly, uncaringly, and unfairly. Today, ethics has been brought into the medical school curriculum, the hospital setting, and medical policy discussions, not just as a matter of morality, but as a matter of self-protection.

Veterinarians, too, may find that the most effective defense against litigation from clients and government is greater attention to ethics.

REFERENCES

1. Williams L: Malpractice Suits Escalating. *DVM* 14(10):1, 1983.
2. Insurance Note. *J Am Vet Med Assoc* 189:642, 1986 (reporting 7.01 claims per 100 participants in the AVMA insurance program in 1983, 6.03 per 100 in 1984, and 6.02 per 100 in 1985).
3. Katz K: Letter dated March, 1988 to recent veterinary school graduates on behalf of the AVMA Professional Liability Insurance Trust (indicating a rate of 5.79 claims per 100 participants in 1987).
4. 1985 AVMA activities summary. *J Am Vet Med Assoc* 188:347, 1986.

5. Benson, M: Malpractice Suits on the Rise. *DVM* 16(10):24, 1985.
6. Dinsmore JR: Anatomy of AVMA's largest insurance malpractice claim. *J Am Vet Med Assoc* 188:26-27, 1986.
7. Benson M: East Coast Malpractice Attorney Rebuffs "Quick Buck" Theory. *DVM* 16(10):30, 1985.
8. Lawrence v. Stanford, 665 S.W.2d 927 (Tenn. 1983).
9. Corso v. Crawford Dog and Cat Hospital, Inc., 97 Misc. 2d 530 (Civ. Ct., Queens Cty. 1979) (awarding plaintiff $700).
10. Knowles Animal Hospital, Inc. v. Wills, 360 So.2d 37 (Fla. 3d DCA 1978) (holding the professional corporation, but not the practitioner-owner, liable for $1,000 compensatory and $12,000 punitive damages).
11. E.g., Veterinarian Receives Stiff Fine for Falsifying Records. *J Am Vet Med Assoc* 188:670, 1986 (reporting four incidents of falsification, including one in which a veterinarian pleaded guilty to a criminal charge after submitting blood samples from one animal to represent an entire shipment of 187); and September Suspensions. *J Am Vet Med Assoc* 188:16, 1986) (reporting nine suspensions of federal accreditation licenses, including one in which a veterinarian was charged with removing official eartags from cattle and retagging the same cattle to prevent traceback, and another in which health certificates were presigned).
12. Glosser JW: Advancing compliance in the accredited veterinarian program. *J Am Vet Med Assoc* 188:1147-1149, 1986.
13. Caras R: Public Viewpoint of Veterinary Medicine. *Journal of Veterinary Medical Education* 9:110-112, 1983.
14. Pusateri FG: Letter. *J Am Vet Med Assoc* 188: 1111, 1986.

Chapter

2

The Four Branches of Veterinary Ethics

VETERINARY ETHICS AND ANIMAL ETHICS

Ethics concerns itself with what is morally good and bad, right and wrong, just and unjust.

As a kind or branch of ethics, veterinary ethics shares these concerns. However, the words "veterinary ethics" do not have a single accepted usage, and, indeed, seem open to two quite different interpretations.

By "veterinary ethics" one might mean ethics as it relates to animals, just as veterinary medicine is medicine relating to animals. In this sense, any ethical issue concerning animals – whether or not it involves veterinarians – would be an issue of veterinary ethics. In this sense, whether people have a moral obligation to protect endangered wildlife, or whether it is morally proper to wear animal fur, are questions of veterinary ethics, because these are questions concerning what it is morally right to do with or to animals.

On the other hand, by "veterinary ethics" one might mean ethics as it relates to veterinarians and others (e.g., veterinary technicians) directly involved in the provision of veterinary care. This is how veterinarians appear to understand the term. For example, the American Veterinary Medical Association *Principles of Veterinary Medical Ethics* is a document about ethical issues in veterinary practice.

In this book, "veterinary ethics" will be understood in the second or restricted, professional sense. The term "animal ethics" will be used to refer to the broader range of moral issues relating to animals, including those relating to veterinarians.ʷʷʷʷʷʷʷʷʷʷ

ʷʷʷʷʷʷʷʷʷʷʷIn this text, the terms "ethics" and "morality" are used synonymously. Some writers attempt to distinguish the two. They sometimes base their distinctions on the fact that the word "ethics" can be traced back to the ancient Greek term *ethikos*, which emphasized the character of the individual, while the word "morality" derived from the Latin *mores*, which connoted rules that larger groups of people applied to each other. However these terms may have been employed in the past, today, differentiations between the "ethical" and the "moral" seem forced and unnatural. Indeed, among those who think that there is a commonly recognized difference, there frequently is disagreement about what this difference is supposed

The focus of this text is veterinary ethics in the professional sense. However, there are important issues in veterinary ethics that cannot be tackled without venturing into the broader, and sometimes extremely difficult, realm of animal ethics. For example, if, as some people assert, animals and human beings have equal moral value (a claim in animal ethics), it would be wrong for people to eat or experiment on animals, and veterinarians who engage in food or laboratory animal practice would therefore be acting immorally (a claim in veterinary ethics). Likewise, how strong a role one thinks a veterinarian should play in advocating the interests of animals will depend, in part, on how one ranks animals and people in the moral spectrum. The less value one accords to an animal patient, for example, the less one might oppose a client's wish to kill a healthy but no longer wanted pet.

Because a number of questions in veterinary ethics involve underlying issues in animal ethics, it is impossible for any text or course in veterinary ethics to provide complete and definitive answers to all questions in professional veterinary ethics. As we shall see, a fundamental question of animal ethics that touches many issues in veterinary ethics is precisely the issue of how much value animals have relative to people. However, as philosopher Robert Nozick has noted, there has been very little persuasive thinking, even by academic philosophers, about this question (1). This does not mean that veterinarians (or society in general) should be racked by wholesale doubt about whether animals are being treated morally. As Nozick observes, many of our long-standing intuitions and attitudes concerning animals (for example, that they are not equal in value to human beings) are surely correct. What is needed, however, is more sophisticated philosophical and empirical underpinning of these attitudes. The implication for veterinary ethics is that while one will sometimes know that certain positions are correct, one may lack all the principles of animal ethics required to support these positions. There may also be times when one will be unable to answer a question in veterinary ethics because an underlying question in animal ethics is still unsettled. We must expect that discussions and conclusions in veterinary ethics will need to be revised and refined as we develop greater sophistication in animal ethics.

THE FOUR BRANCHES OF VETERINARY ETHICS

Even when one conceives of veterinary ethics as ethics relating to veterinary medicine, there are four different things one might have in mind.

Descriptive Veterinary Ethics

By the "ethics" of a profession like veterinary medicine, one might mean the actual values or standards of the profession, that is, what members of the profession in fact think is right and wrong in professional behavior and attitudes. In this sense, understanding the ethics of a profession is a matter of describing the profession's actual values, and does not involve making value judgments about what is moral or immoral in that profession's behavior. (One can study the "ethics," in this sense, of

---

to be (2, 3). Today, the overwhelming majority of speakers of the language, as well as most theorists (2), use the words "ethical" and "moral" interchangeably. There seems little point in attempting to resurrect a distinction between the two, provided that the legitimate considerations these terms might have suggested in the past are not overlooked.

a profession one believes to be utterly evil.) I shall call the study of the actual ethical views of members of the veterinary profession regarding professional behavior and attitudes *descriptive veterinary ethics*.

Official Veterinary Ethics

In speaking of the professional ethics of veterinarians or other professionals, one might also mean the official ethical standards formally adopted by organizations composed of these professionals and which these organizations impose upon their members. In this sense, too, one can understand (or appeal to) part of a profession's "ethics" without believing that the standard involved is in fact right. For example, some attorneys believe that they should sometimes be able to speak directly to the person suing their client, instead of dealing only with the opposing attorney, but would never do so because "legal ethics," the official bar association ethical rules, forbid it. I shall call the process of the articulation and application of ethical standards for veterinarians by the organized profession *official veterinary ethics*.

Administrative Veterinary Ethics

Another important source of moral standards for veterinarians are administrative governmental bodies that regulate veterinary practice and various activities in which veterinarians engage. What distinguishes the moral standards of such bodies from those of professional organizations is that only the former can carry the force of law. If a practitioner violates the ethical standards of the AVMA, the most severe penalty he can face from the AVMA is expulsion from this organization. However, violation of administrative standards can result in criminal or civil penalties or, if the administrative body is one's state board of registration, revocation or suspension of one's license to practice. I shall call the process of the application of ethical standards to veterinarians by administrative governmental bodies *administrative veterinary ethics*.

Normative Veterinary Ethics

Finally, in speaking of veterinary ethics, one can mean the attempt to discover correct moral standards for veterinarians and others involved in providing veterinary care. I shall call the activity of looking for correct norms for veterinary professional behavior and attitudes *normative veterinary ethics*.

THE IMPORTANCE OF ALL FOUR BRANCHES
OF VETERINARY ETHICS

Clearly, the standards of descriptive, official, administrative, and normative ethics can differ. Practitioners' actual values can deviate from official or administratively imposed standards, and any of these can, in turn, differ from what is objectively right.

Some students (and some ethics teachers as well) tend to equate professional ethics with normative professional ethics. They believe, for example, that the official standards of their profession, are "just" what in fact happens to be accepted at the time, and they are eager to get to what is *really* right and wrong. Each year, several students in my course in veterinary ethics initially protest that it is a waste of time to study the AVMA *Principles of Veterinary Medical Ethics*. They suppose that once one determines what is actually right in veterinary practice, one need only make the official, administrative, and actual standards coincide with these correct moral principles.

Certainly, normative veterinary ethics is the most important of the four branches of veterinary ethics. Most veterinarians become interested in ethics because they want to determine how they really should behave, and not just how their fellow professionals, official rules, or governmental bodies say they should.

However, it would be a terrible mistake to underestimate the importance of the other branches of veterinary ethics.

For reasons that shall be explained in later chapters, there will always be differences between official and administrative rules on the one hand, and the principles of normative ethics on the other. This means that even the most moral of practitioners must study official and administrative standards to understand what they say. One reason any practitioner should *want* to understand what they say is that he can get himself into various kinds of trouble if he violates these standards. To be sure, it might not always be morally right to follow official or administrative standards. But it is a foolhardy practitioner indeed who does not know that in choosing to follow the dictates of his conscience he might be exposing himself to the censure of his colleagues, or worse.

Another reason it is important to study official and administrative veterinary ethics is that there will always be such standards, and one cannot improve them without knowing what they are and how they have or have not worked.

Official veterinary ethics is especially useful in approaching normative veterinary ethics. The official rules indicate what ethical questions the profession has found most pressing, and they contain specific answers to many of these questions. Descriptive veterinary ethics, too, will reveal the concerns of the profession, and can help the drafters of official and administrative rules understand what standards might be necessary, and whether proposed rules are likely to be accepted or resisted.

THE TASKS AHEAD

This book concentrates primarily on normative veterinary ethics and secondarily on official veterinary ethics. The latter is worth considering in some detail because it is of such great practical importance to the profession and because currently it is the most developed branch of veterinary ethics.

Much less can be said, at least at present, about administrative and descriptive veterinary ethics. As shall be explained in Chapter 7, the most important potential source of administrative veterinary ethical standards are the state boards of registration. However, some of the boards do not yet take an active role in enforcing ethical (as opposed to technical) standards. Moreover, because few boards share their deliberations about individual cases with the public, it is extremely difficult to obtain a clear general picture of the nature and extent of the activity of the boards in the arena of ethics. Likewise, no treatment of veterinary ethics can yet give descriptive ethics the treatment it deserves. There has been very little empirical work describing the values of veterinarians. However, as activity in the other branches of veterinary ethics increases, interest in understanding how practitioners actually think about and deal with ethical issues should grow as well.

REFERENCES

1. Nozick R: About Mammals and People. *New York Times Book Review* November 27, 1983:11.

2. Beauchamp TL and Childress JF: *Principles of Biomedical Ethics*. ed 2. New York: Oxford University Press, p 18 (stating that "'ethics' often refers to theoretical and reflective perspectives, while 'morality' often refers to actual conduct and practice").
3. Williams B: *Ethics and the Limits of Philosophy*. Cambridge: Harvard University Press, 1985, pp 6, 177 (holding that morality is a narrower subsystem within ethics that emphasizes the notion of obligation and whose characteristic reaction is "blame between persons").

Chapter

————— 3 —————

Veterinary Ethics and Religion

Veterinary ethics can be made difficult by more than just animal ethics. This chapter will consider how religious beliefs can affect views about how veterinarians ought to act. Chapter 4 will examine the complicating force of the law.

RELIGIOUS AND METAPHYSICAL VIEWS ABOUT ANIMALS

There can be little doubt that many people, including a good many veterinarians, hold views about animals that are based at least in part on religious beliefs. According to Dr. Robert M. Miller, for example, "man has a right to utilize animals for his own welfare [because] the Bible says [so]" (1). Dr. Harry Rowsell contends that "the Bible not only establishes man's dominion over animals, but urges us not to waste our resources, among which animals must be listed" (2). Dr. John Mulder argues that the Bible declares

All animals . . . subject to the uses and bounds established by human beings. However, sufficient instructions are provided suggesting compassionate as well as proper and humane use and care of animals. Although the Biblical position does not recognize animal rights it strongly advocates respect for animal life (3).

People sometimes also make similar metaphysical claims (statements not directly or indirectly verifiable by experience or observation) about animals, claims which seem to be based on religious belief. One veterinarian, for example, states that animals have the right "to live their intended lives, which for some is to serve man"(4). A former AVMA president holds that "animals are here for man to use but not abuse ... Animals are here on earth to better the life of human beings which are more important in the overall than animal life" (5).

THE RELIGIOUS PROBLEM

The fact that claims about our ethical obligations concerning animals are sometimes based on religious belief can cause problems for normative veterinary ethics.

11

Different people can appeal to religion – indeed, sometimes to the very same religious texts – to reach diametrically opposing views. For example, one Jewish theologian denies that God granted any rights to animals and concludes that His prohibition against cruelty to animals is based on a "concern for the moral welfare of the human agent rather than concern for the physical welfare of the animals, i.e., the underlying concern is the need to purge inclinations of cruelty and to develop compassion in human beings" (6). Another Jewish scholar, however, insists that God did give animals their own "status and rights," and that He demands that "man obligate himself toward them, to consider their welfare and treat them with kindness and benevolence" (7). Among Christian thinkers, too, there is a wide divergence of views about what God decrees regarding animals. These range from Cardinal Newman's statement that "(w)e have no duties toward the brute creation; there is no relation of justice between them and us... they can claim nothing at our hands; into our hands they are absolutely delivered" (8), to the view of Anglican animal rights advocate Andrew Linzey that certain animals have moral rights because when they suffer they "share in the effects of the crucifixion of Christ and his victory over evil and negative forces" (9).

Religious differences can produce differences in views about the obligations of veterinarians. Someone who believes that God made animals to serve people may have no problem killing a pet no longer of interest to its owner, while someone who does not share this religious belief, or who believes that God gave animals a right to live, may come to a very different conclusion. Few veterinarians would object to the sterilization of animals to prevent breeding, but to the Orthodox Jew, this practice violates religious law. Hindus who believe eating meat to be a heinous sin cannot but find much of food animal practice morally abhorrent.

It is extremely difficult to know what to do when people disagree on religious grounds about moral obligations concerning animals. If they are of the same religion, it might be possible for them to reach agreement about the meaning of a certain text or doctrine, but this may not always be possible. If they are of different religions, they might be faced with the prospect of convicing each other that one of their religions is correct, and if some of them have no religious beliefs, the task may be even more difficult. Even if they reach agreement about the correct course of action regarding animals, the *reasons* they give for their conclusions, if based on conflicting religious doctrine, may be incompatible.

A SECULAR SOLUTION?

The way many academic ethicists deal with these problems is to put them aside as avoidable. They take the approach that, whether or not there is a God or whatever He may or may not decree about moral matters, normative ethical issues can always be considered without the need to resort to religious doctrine.

Different reasons have been given for the possibility of a purely secular normative ethics.

According to one argument, it cannot be the case that something is good because God wills it. Rather, God wills something *because* it is good. If things were otherwise, there would be no excellence in God's actions, for anything He willed would automatically be good. Therefore, it is argued, what is right and wrong is independent of, and can be understood without reference to, God's will (10).

In *The Case for Annual Rights*, philosopher Tom Regan provides the following argument for dispensing with appeals to a moral authority (like God) who might be the source of all right and wrong. Those of us who are not such authorities, Regan states, can have no reason for thinking that there is one unless the judgments of this supposed authority can be checked for their truth or reasonableness, and it is not possible to check for this unless what is true or reasonable can be known independently of reliance on what the supposed authority says. If, however, there must be some independent way of knowing what moral judgments are true or reasonable, the introduction of a moral authority will not succeed in providing a method for answering moral questions (11).

The problem with these and other arguments for dispensing with religion in normative ethics is that they do not work against all religious attitudes about ethics. Many people believe that God's reasons are ultimately unknowable to man, who must receive them by faith (12). Thus, for many believers, it would not follow from God's choosing something because it is good that we mortals can fully understand why what is good is good. Likewise, an insistence that one must have independent, nonreligious reasons for knowing whether God is right will strike many believers as false, again, because they hold that people cannot fully appreciate God's ways. In order to refute the claim that only God knows why His ethical commandments are correct, one must engage in religious argument.

Those who maintain that ethical deliberation need never include consideration of religious claims have a special problem regarding religious beliefs about animals. For some of these beliefs go beyond mere claims about what is right and wrong in our treatment of animals. Some religious views concerning animals are claims about what animals *in fact are*. One such belief is that animals were made by God for the purpose of serving human needs and desires. Another is that animals, unlike human beings, do not have immortal souls. If there is a secular, or purely empirical or scientific, way of proving or disproving such claims, it is hard to imagine what it would be.

THE POSSIBILITY OF SECULAR NORMATIVE VETERINARY ETHICS

It is impossible, then, to engage in normative veterinary ethics and suppose that one will *never* have to confront religious arguments or beliefs. This does not mean that one must accept any or all religious justifications for ethical positions. But it does mean that differences in ethical views may sometimes reflect fundamental and irreconcilable differences in religious belief.

On the other hand, it is certainly beyond the scope of this book (or a veterinary school course in professional ethics) to engage in theological argument, or to assess the validity of religious beliefs about the nature of animals and our moral obligations regarding them.

All, however, is not lost. There are several reasons why nonreligious normative veterinary ethics seems possible.

First, a great many believers do think that what is good is independent of God's will and that moral issues can therefore be resolved without appeal to religion. Rabbi J. David Bleich, for example, contends that although a Jew committed to following religious laws will not look to secular ethics for guidance, secular ethics is possible.

> The Sages clearly recognized that the ethical moment of [Jewish law] consists of commandments which, "Had they not been written, it would have been proper that they be written." Thus [one Rabbi] states that in the absence of a revealed Torah "we would have learned modesty from the cat, aversion to robbery from the ant, marital faithfulness from the dove, and conjugal deportment from the rooster." Basic moral values are universal and not contingent on sectarian claims (13).

Speaking of animal ethics, Protestant theologian John B. Cobb, Jr. states that

> Ethical questions can be discussed apart from questions relating to beliefs about
> God. In a time when all talk of God is problematic, this is fortunate. Broadening the
> scope of ethics to include serious consideration of the welfare and rights of other
> animals can and should be urged on its own merits (14).

Second, people of differing religious belief (including those with no religious
belief) quite often approach ethical argument with the same basic moral principles,
even though these principles may have different religious (or nonreligious) sources.
When this happens, the religious differences can drop out – not because they are
unimportant to the disputants, but because they are unnecessary to the process of
discussion.   Thus, as Rabbi Bleich notes, the basic virtues, such as honesty,
compassion, loyalty, and modesty are accepted at least in theory by almost everyone,
of whatever religious belief and of whatever view about the need to ground ethics in
religion. Because most people start with these and other moral building blocks, and
because it is these building blocks (and not specific religious commandments) on
which argument can often turn, ethical discussion is usually possible.

Indeed, it may well be easier for people of differing religious convictions to
engage in normative *veterinary* ethics than in other kinds of ethical disputes, such as,
for example, issues concerning abortion and euthanasia of terminally ill people.
Every religion has much to say about these fundamental issues of life and death. But
no religion provides voluminous specific guidance to those who give medical care to
animals.   Thus, regarding veterinary ethics, we seem forced to rely on basic moral
principles that all good people, whatever their theological persuasion, may be able to
accept.

In fact, those who have differing religious beliefs that relate directly to animals
often do approach ethical issues concerning animals with the same basic general
moral principles. Most people believe that although animals have less value than
human beings, and can therefore often be used for legitimate human purposes, they
should not be caused unnecessary pain.[a] People who share this principle can talk
to each other and argue about what it requires. Yet, this same principle finds direct
support in Jewish (15), Christian (16), and Hindu[b] doctrine. And the principle can
be endorsed by someone who believes that God made the animals for man's
purposes as well as by someone who does not. In fact, many people with deeply held
religious beliefs do think that normative veterinary ethics can proceed without appeal
to religious doctrine. Thus, Drs. Miller and Rowsell, whose Biblical arguments are
quoted above, both proceed in their discussions to give nonreligious support for their
views.   Dr. Mulder, too, asserts that the Biblical perspective on humane care and

---

[a]For example, even Cardinal Newman, quoted at page 12 above, believed that although
we have no duties to animals, "we are bound not to treat them ill, for cruelty is an offense
against that holy Law which our maker has written in our hearts, and is displeasing to him"(8).

[b]According to one Hindu scholar, man's life "is a privilege because it is superior to the
lives of animals and plants" (17). One school of Hinduism therefore permits the use of animals
in biomedical science, "if and only if (1) the benefits humans receive far outweigh the pain
animals endure, and (2) the use of animals is necessary (that is, the benefits are not otherwise
obtainable)" (18).

animal rights[c] is "really quite rational" and "does not differ from most other current options" (3).

Nevertheless, anyone engaged in normative veterinary ethics must remember that differences in ethical positions may sometimes come down to fundamental differences in religious conviction. If this happens, our ability to pursue purely secular moral argument will end.

Ultimately, the best way to prove that one can engage in normative veterinary ethics without appealing to religious belief is to attempt to do so in a way that is helpful and satisfying.

REFERENCES

1. Miller RM: Animal welfare-yes! Human laws-sure! Animal rights-no! *California Veterinarian* 37:21, 1983.
2. Rowsell HC and McWilliam AA: The animal in research: domination or stewardship. *Animal Regulation Studies* 2:238, 1979/1980.
3. Mulder JB: Letter. Who is right about animal rights? *Lab Anim Sci* 29(4):436, 1979.
4. Marshall RT: Animal Welfare, Animal Rights, Expectations. *California Veterinarian* 37:18, 1983.
5. Rigdon CR: Interview. *Intervet* 21:14, 1985.
6. Bleich JD: Judaism and Animal Experimentation. In Regan T (ed): *Animal Sacrifices*. Philadelphia: Temple University Press, 1986, p 67.
7. Cohen, NJ: *Tsa'ar Ba'ale Hayim: The Prevention of Cruelty to Animals, Its Bases, Development and Legislation in Hebrew Literature*. Jerusalem: Feldheim Publishers, 1976, p 105.
8. Newman JH: *Sermons Preached on Various Occasions*. 2nd ed., quoted in Passmore J: The Treatment of Animals. *Journal of the History of Ideas* 36:203, 1979.
9. Linzey, A: *Animal Rights*. London: SCM Press, 1976, p 76.
10. E.g., Plato: Euthyphro. In Hamilton E and Cairns H (eds): *Plato. The Collected Dialogues*. Princeton: Princeton University Press, 1961, pp 169-185.
11. Regan T: *The Case for Animal Rights*. Berkeley: University of California Press, 1983, p 126.
12. Baillie J: *Our Knowledge of God*. New York: Scribners, 1959.
13. Bleich JD: The A Priori Component of Bioethics. In Rossner F and Bleich JD (eds): *Jewish Bioethics*. Brooklyn: Hebrew Publishing Co., 1985, p xix.
14. Cobb JB: Beyond Anthropocentrism in Ethics and Religion. In Morris RK and Fox MW (eds): *On the Fifth Day*. Washington, DC: Acropolis Books, 1978, p 148.
15. Bleich JD: Judaism and Animal Experimentation. In Regan T (ed): *Animal Sacrifices*. Philadelphia: Temple University Press, 1986, pp 89-90.

---

[c]Dr. Mulder's conclusion that the Bible does not recognize any animal rights may not follow from his statements about the text. Mulder asserts that although the Bible gives man "full authority over the animal kingdom," animals must be given "compassionate care and proper treatment" and "righteous people are admonished to show concern for the lives of their animals" (3). As shall be explained in Chapter 12, such views are not necessarily incompatible with the attribution of moral rights to animals, although they need not reflect a belief in animal rights.

16. See, e.g., Gaffney J: The Relevance of Animal Experimentation to Roman Catholic Ethical Methodology. In Regan T (ed): *Animal Sacrifices*. Philadelphia: Temple University Press, 1986, pp 161-169.
17. Lal BK: Hindu Perspectives on the Use of Animals in Science. In Regan T (ed): *Animal Sacrifices*. Philadelphia: Temple University Press, 1986, p 209.
18. *Id.*, 208.

Chapter

—— 4 ——

How the Law Affects
Veterinary Ethics

One thing that makes ethics of great practical importance to veterinarians is the relationship between veterinary ethics and the law. A person may be able to choose (without penalty in this life at least) to ignore the dictates of any particular religion. But we often have no such choice regarding the requirements of the law. Indeed, what characterizes standards as rules of law is that the government can use its substantial power to force people to comply with these standards, and can subject us to some punishment or deprivation if we do not.

THE LAW AND VETERINARY ETHICS: A TWO-WAY RELATIONSHIP

Ethical principles can influence legal standards that apply to veterinarians. This can happen in several ways. As we have already seen, perceived violations of ethical norms can lead to lawsuits against veterinarians. Moreover, courts can sometimes turn the standards of official, administrative, or normative veterinary ethics into legal standards that apply in suits against veterinarians. State licensing boards can also appeal to principles of official or normative veterinary ethics to regulate and discipline practitioners.

Conversely, the law can influence veterinary ethics, by affecting veterinarians' decisions about how they ought to act in given circumstances.

We will have many occasions in this book to examine various ways in which ethical attitudes of veterinarians influence how the law deals with them. This chapter will discuss how the law can affect the process of determining how one should act.

THE DIFFERENCE BETWEEN ETHICAL AND LEGAL STANDARDS

In considering how the law can affect ethical deliberation, there is an important fact one must always keep in mind: that something is required by law does not necessarily make it morally right or desirable. Laws are made by people, and they can be as morally bad as the people who make them. Therefore, it is conceivable that there be situations in which the law would require a veterinarian to do something, but his moral conscience might tell him something quite different.

17

WHY ONE CANNOT ALWAYS FOLLOW THE LAW

If one could always follow the dictates of the law when faced with an ethical problem, one would only have to determine what the law says and one's questions would be answered. Unfortunately, this approach will not work.

The law is often ethically neutral. First, there are many instances in which the law is consistent with a number of different approaches. For example, it is perfectly legal for a veterinarian to euthanize a healthy animal no longer wanted by its owner, but it is also just as lawful for him to refuse to do this on ethical grounds. The law does not attempt to decide whether the veterinarian should refuse on ethical grounds, or what ethical grounds might or might not justify such a refusal.

The law can differ from correct normative standards. A second reason why one cannot just follow the law in answering ethical problems is that sometimes the dictates of normative veterinary ethics might be morally preferable to legal standards. For example, assuming he has not held himself out to the public as willing to accept certain kinds of cases and does not turn away a client because of racial or some other kind of legally prohibited discrimination, a veterinarian has no legal obligation to accept a patient.[a] He can refuse to begin treating any animal simply because he does not feel like it. It seems clear, however, that it is sometimes *morally* wrong for a veterinarian to turn away an animal in need of care simply because he feels like it. Official ethics also condemns such an attitude, at least regarding emergencies; the AVMA *Principles of Veterinary Medical Ethics* hold that "every practitioner has a moral and ethical responsibility to provide service when because of accidents or other emergencies involving animals it is necessary to save life or relieve suffering" (1).

WHY ONE CANNOT IGNORE THE LAW

Although following the law will not always provide satisfactory guidance for approaching moral questions, it would also be wrong for veterinarians to ignore the law.

It can sometimes be morally wrong to disobey a bad law. First, a strong argument can often be made that it is morally correct to obey a law which, in its restricted application, may be a morally bad law. For violation of a particular bad law

---

[a]There may be an exception to this long-standing legal principle. In 1987, the Massachusetts Board of Registration in Veterinary Medicine adopted regulations stating that "a veterinarian shall not refuse to provide treatment to an animal unless such refusal is based on reasons such as the inadequacy of the facilities then available or the unavailability of all-night veterinary medical care for the animal" (2). The only other approved reasons for refusing a case specifically enumerated in the regulations are the failure of an animal to be currently vaccinated (3), or a client's engaging in "physical or verbal abuse" towards the veterinarian or one of his employees (4). These regulations (which apply only in Massachusetts) appear to prohibit, among other things, declining a case because a client cannot afford to pay the fee or refuses to leave a deposit. Such an approach is objectionable on moral grounds because it sometimes is justifiable to decline or withdraw from a case when a client cannot or will not pay (see Chapter 19). It is also highly doubtful whether a state veterinary board has the legal authority to issue a regulation compelling practitioners to provide services for *all* potential or current clients who cannot or will not pay for them, a requirement that appears to be implied by the Massachusetts regulations.

can sometimes lead to more general disregard for the law, which can, in turn, result in great harm.

For example, in all states it is illegal for private citizens to possess, and for veterinarians to treat, certain designated species of wildlife without permission from state government. Yet there are veterinarians who ignore such laws. In Massachusetts, for example, as in some other states, ferrets cannot be kept as pets, and veterinarians are prohibited from giving routine, nonemergency care to these animals. However, there are veterinarians in Massachusetts who accept pet ferrets as patients. They argue that ferrets can make wonderful pets. They protest that it makes no sense to prohibit ferrets in Massachusetts when they are permitted just across the border in Connecticut.

Supposing only for the purpose of argument that a legal prohibition against treating ferrets is, taken by itself, unjustified, one must still consider the potential wider effects of disobeying such a law. Someone who feels justified in keeping or treating one kind of prohibited species may feel justified in judging for himself which species are appropriate to keep or treat. This may in turn result in some very bad decisions by veterinarians and clients to possess species which the law is indisputably correct in prohibiting. Thus, there are already in Massachusetts (and doubtless in other states) veterinarians who treat not only ferrets, but also skunks and raccoons, and who already seem to have a general disregard for the right of the state to restrict possession of wild animals. If a general practice of keeping skunks and raccoons contributes to a rabies epidemic, or results in injuries to people who do not know how dangerous these animals can be, those veterinarians who consider themselves above the law may have to share part of the blame.

It can be imprudent to ignore the law. A second reason veterinarians engaged in ethical deliberation cannot ignore what the law might say about a particular issue is that it can be exceedingly imprudent to disobey the law. Disobeying the criminal law can result in a criminal prosecution, imprisonment, or fine. Disobeying the civil law can result in a malpractice or other kind of lawsuit. Disobeying either the criminal or civil law can sometimes result in revocation or suspension of one's license to practice veterinary medicine by one's state board of registration. In short, ignoring the law can ruin one's professional and personal life. One may, of course, still decide that it is better to disobey the law. However, given the potential consequences of violating the law, one at least ought to know whether a certain course of action would be unlawful.

The Legitimacy of Self-interest in Veterinary Ethics

Some veterinarians tell me that veterinary ethics should not concern itself with whether a given course of action would be dangerous from a practitioner's point of view because it might be illegal. Such a consideration, these doctors assert, is "merely" one of self-interest, not of ethics.

Such a conception of ethics is mistaken. It is difficult to find many normative ethical theories that have not recognized the legitimacy of self-interest in moral deliberation. To think otherwise would be to say that *other* people count enough to deserve my moral consideration, but that *I* do not – a position which makes no sense. If a course of action will cause one or one's family pain or ruin, that is, surely, a fact he may take into account in deciding what it is morally right for him to do. If disobeying the law might damage a veterinarian's professional or personal life, that fact is relevant to a decision about how he ought to act.

To be sure, the dictates of self-interest and of morality can conflict, and there may be times when even the most conscientious person will allow self-interest to win out. But it does not follow from the fact that self-interest may sometimes cause one to follow a bad law instead of morality, that an understanding of what the law requires is irrelevant. In such a case, one should still know that one is choosing to follow a bad law, so that one can try to change the law. Also, if the prospect of disadvantage at the hands of the law is so strong that it can supplant one's conscience, one should know about it, so that one can properly assess the goodness of one's character.

HOW TO WEIGH THE LAW IN NORMATIVE VETERINARY ETHICS

There are many ways in which the law can affect veterinary practice, and there are many different ethical issues involving veterinarians about which the law can voice an opinion. It is thus extremely difficult to state in general terms how much weight one should give to legal standards in normative ethical deliberations. I have found it useful to ask the following questions in thinking through a problem in normative veterinary ethics:

1. *Is there a law that speaks to the ethical issue under discussion?*

Although much of what we do in life is affected in some way by the law, quite often the law does not attempt to guide or restrict one's choices in ethical decision-making. For example, it has been noted that the law permits a veterinarian to euthanize, or not to euthanize, a healthy animal (or to try to attempt to change the client's mind, or accept the animal and try to place it himself, and so on). Where the law does not attempt to guide one toward a particular decision, ethical deliberation can proceed on its own without legal interference.

2. *If the law does speak, does it state a permission or an imperative?*

Sometimes, the law might appear to suggest a course of action that seems to offend normative ethical standards, but in reality only sets forth a permission which cannot result in legal reprisal. When this occurs, ethical deliberation can also proceed without fear of legal interference. For example, the law that a veterinarian may generally choose his clients states a permission and not an imperative. It says that a veterinarian *may*, if he likes, turn away whatever cases he wants, but he *need not* do so, and he is equally free to treat all animals lawfully presented to him.

On the other hand many laws (e.g., those prohibiting routine treatment of designated species of wildlife) set forth imperatives – requirements or prohibitions – violation of which can result in criminal or civil liability.

3. *If the law states an imperative, does it conflict with the requirements of normative ethics?*

That there is a law requiring or forbidding a veterinarian to undertake some course of action does not, of course, mean there *must* be a conflict between this law and the correct standards of morality. Indeed, in the great majority of cases one can expect no conflict whatever, and one can proceed with moral deliberation without having to balance the demands of ethics against those of the law.

4. *If the law states an imperative and does conflict with the standards of normative ethics, what are the potential costs of violating the law, and how strong are the moral arguments in favor of violating the legal requirements?*

Among the relevant considerations here are the likelihood that the law will be enforced, the severity of any potential punishment if it is enforced, the possible wider effects of disobeying the law whether or not it is enforced, and the strength of the moral arguments against the law. If, for example, there is a moral obligation that is of great importance which is opposed by a law that is never enforced and violation of which is unlikely to have wider bad effects, there may well be a strong argument for ignoring the law.

5. *Does the rationale for a law affecting a decision in veterinary practice suggest factors one should want to consider in determining the morally best course of action?*

Because laws are often responses to ethical and social problems, examining the purpose of a law can reveal considerations that are important to even a purely ethical discussion, considerations one might ignore had one not asked why this law exists in the first place. For example, the legal rule that veterinarians may choose whom they serve expresses the ethical principle that people should generally be free to decide with whom they will enter into economic, professional, and personal relations. This is an important moral principle which must be taken into account in considering, for example, when veterinarians might be obligated to accept patients or to offer low-cost or gratuitous services to the needy.

LEARNING ABOUT THE LAW

Because the law can be relevant to veterinary ethics, veterinarians must make themselves familiar with legal principles affecting ethical issues. Some doctors may find this just one too many burden to bear and may be tempted to forsake the study of veterinary ethics entirely. However, the law applies to veterinarians' professional activities, whether or not they take veterinary ethics seriously. Thus, learning about the law is not an additional task imposed by ethics.

It is beyond the scope of this text to describe all laws relevant to veterinary ethics. As ethical issues are raised, certain laws important to the consideration of these issues will be discussed. It is useful to note at this point that the following are among the kinds of laws relevant to normative veterinary ethics: 1) statutes enacted by federal and state legislatures (e.g., the federal Animal Welfare Act and state anticruelty to animals statutes); 2) general rules or particular determinations made by regulatory bodies (e.g., the Animal and Plant Health Inspection Service of the United States Department of Agriculture and state veterinary boards of registration); and 3) common law rules of legal precedent developed by courts (e.g., the rule that a veterinarian is free to choose whom he wishes to serve).

REFERENCES

1. *Principles of Veterinary Medical Ethics.* "Emergency Service." *1988 AVMA Directory,* p 477.
2. 256 *Code of Massachusetts Regulations* § 7.01(22) (1987).
3. *Id.,* § 7.01(29).
4. *Id.,* § 7.01(31).

Chapter

5

Veterinary Ethics and Moral Theory

One remaining area of thought must be considered before the four branches of veterinary ethics can be discussed in detail. This chapter will examine several concepts and principles of philosophical moral theory essential to the study of veterinary ethics.[a]

THREE APPROACHES TO ETHICS

The history of ethics reveals many different kinds of ethical theories. However, there are three major approaches to understanding how people ought to live and act that the student of veterinary ethics will find it useful to distinguish. These approaches are not mutually exclusive. Indeed, as shall become apparent, elements of each will play a role in any satisfactory account of descriptive, official, administrative, and normative veterinary ethics. But by considering these kinds of theory as if they existed in their "pure" state (as they sometimes have), one can best perceive what each has to offer.

Virtue-oriented Ethical Theories

One approach to ethics concentrates on examining and promoting the moral virtues. A virtue is a character trait or disposition which manifests itself over a wide range of situations and which can be said to contribute to, or, indeed, be part of what is meant by, a good and moral life. Among the character traits that have been explored by virtue-oriented ethicists (who include the great philosophers Socrates and Aristotle) are honesty, kindness, generosity, courage, loyalty, modesty, compassion, and fairness.

---

[a]This introductory text cannot consider all these concepts and principles, nor can it discuss all topics in moral theory relevant to veterinary ethics. Philosophical ethics is a challenging field of study, with its own professional practitioners, its own long history, and its own specialized vocabulary and competing points of view. This does not mean that veterinarians must become philosophers before they can study professional ethics. There is, however, much in philosophy that is of use to veterinarians.

A virtue-oriented approach to morality does not reject actions as irrelevant. Indeed, one could not speak of the virtues (or their opposite, the vices) apart from actions. One could not, for example, say that a person is courageous unless, when faced with certain kinds of challenges, he acts in certain ways. However, virtue-oriented ethics is suspicious of attempts to formulate a set of rules or recipes for how one ought to behave in particular situations. According to virtue-oriented ethics, simply attempting to encourage people to act morally in various kinds of situations is putting the cart before the horse. People will only act well, according to this approach, if they *already* have those dispositions of character that are good and can be counted on over the long haul to motivate good behavior. Virtue-oriented ethical theories characteristically place a great deal of emphasis on education. They attempt to inculcate attitudes, feelings, and states of mind central to the virtuous dispositions. As shall be discussed in Chapter 9, a virtue-oriented approach has long played a major role in official veterinary ethics.

Action-oriented Ethical Theories

In contrast, action-oriented ethical theories are less concerned with how we should be than with how we should act. While virtue-oriented approaches focus upon what it is to live a good and virtuous life, action-oriented theories ask what people ought to do. They tend to search for rules or decision-procedures that can be applied to particular moral issues to determine the correct course of behavior. Action-oriented ethical theories tend to stress the concepts of duty and obligation.

Value-oriented Ethics

Finally, there are ethical theories that concentrate not on dispositions or actions but on values, states of affairs, or ways of being which are good and therefore should be sought after. These values tend to be very general and are seen as following from very basic kinds of considerations. A value-oriented approach seeks to establish a structure or hierarchy of basic values and will appeal to such a structure in determining how people should behave and what character traits should be considered virtuous. A recent influential text provides a good example of one important value in the context of a theory of medical ethics. It proposes four very general "principles" as the foundation of biomedical ethics: autonomy, nonmaleficence, beneficence, and justice. Duties of nonmaleficence (not harming someone), beneficence, and justice are interpreted in light of autonomy, which is defined as "self-governance: being one's own person, without constraints either by another's action or by psychological or physical limitations" (1). It is argued that autonomy can require that competent adults be left alone to make their own informed decisions about their medical treatment. Autonomy is viewed in part as a value, a fundamental good, that makes people distinctively human.

THE IMPORTANCE OF VIRTUES, ACTIONS, AND VALUES

It seems intuitively clear that any satisfactory approach to normative veterinary ethics must give attention to virtues, actions, and values. There can, for example, be no doubt that such virtues as honesty and compassion are to be prized in a veterinarian. However, there are times when these virtues can lead to conflicting tendencies and when the practitioner will need a way of deciding between them.

Thus, it may be honest to tell a client who wants to know about his pet's prognosis the complete and unvarnished truth, but compassion may suggest giving a less truthful and less upsetting account. Here, it would seem, one needs some kind of rule for action to resolve the conflict, or perhaps a theory of values which would indicate the proper approach. Likewise, views about the moral duties of veterinarians in certain kinds of situations will sometimes turn on very general principles concerning the value of animal life.

UTILITARIAN AND DEONTOLOGICAL ETHICAL THEORIES

Philosophers distinguish two fundamental kinds of action-oriented ethical theories: utilitarian and deontological. Utilitarian (sometimes called consequentialist) theories look to the *consequences* of actions or kinds of actions to determine whether they are right or wrong. These theories begin with a conception of what is good in itself, and hold that actions or kinds of actions are right insofar, and only insofar, as they will, *in the future*, produce this good.

For some utilitarians, the "good" that right actions must produce is conceived as pleasure in the sense of a primal feeling of contentment. Other utilitarians hold that certain pleasures are better than others, and that these "higher" pleasures are the good people should seek. But for all utilitarians, it is the total *quantity* of this good (however conceived) that determines one's moral obligations. Thus, according to one leading utilitarian, "the only reason for performing an action A rather than an alternative B is that doing A will make mankind (or, perhaps, all sentient beings) happier than will doing B" (2). In other words, a utilitarian asks people to total up the consequences of each alternative act (or, if he is what is called a "rule-utilitarian," of each alternative general rule for behavior) and to choose that which, on balance, will produce no less good than any other.[b]

Deontological ethical theories, in contrast, hold that there are some moral obligations that are independent of how much good will be produced in the future. Deontologists can recognize that how much good one might produce is sometimes relevant to how one ought to act. However, a deontologist denies that future consequences are the *only* source of moral duties. As with utilitarianism, there have been many varieties of deontological ethics. Some deontologists, like the 18th Century German philosopher Immanuel Kant, attempt to derive all moral obligation from a

---

[b]The view that people should always choose an action that will produce no less good than any alternative is called "act-utilitarianism." Rule-utilitarianism has been proposed to avoid some of the counterintuitive results of act-utilitarianism. For example, act-utilitarianism requires that people break any individual promise if doing so would produce more utility (pleasure, happiness, etc.) than would keeping it – an implication many people find unacceptable. A rule-utilitarian, however, can urge people to keep an individual promise even though breaking it would produce more good, on the grounds that a *general rule* requiring people to keep promises would produce more good than a rule that permits people to break promises. Rule-utilitarianism is controversial. Some act-utilitarians claim it makes no sense; they point out that although rule-utilitarians advocate their theory because they are supposedly concerned with promoting good, at the same they time settle for an approach that does not maximize good (3).

single unified principle or rule.[c]   Others, like the English philosopher W.D. Ross, advocate a number of fundamental moral principles (such as the duty to tell the truth and the duty to help others), each of which is generally obligatory but can on occasion be overridden by one of its fellow fundamental principles (4).

A famous example illustrating the difference between utilitarianism and deontology is provided by Protestant theologian Joseph Fletcher. He asks us to imagine that one has come upon a burning building, in which there are two people. The first is one's father. The second is "a medical genius who has discovered a cure for a common fatal disease" (5). One can rescue either the genius or the parent, but not both. Whom should one choose?

For the utilitarian like Fletcher, who demands that we ask which of the alternatives would produce, on balance, the greatest good for the greatest number, the answer is obvious: the genius must be saved. A deontologist, however, will hold that there is a strong obligation to save one's parent in virtue of one's distinctive relationship with that person in the past – an obligation that must also be taken into account and exists independently of considerations of utility.

As will be apparent when the subject of animal rights is considered (see Chapter 12), it is impossible to explore a number of major issues in veterinary ethics without understanding the difference between utilitarian and deontological approaches to these issues. Moreover, there are questions in veterinary ethics whose solution does depend in large measure on comparing the benefits and detriments resulting from alternative actions. It is no secret, however, that the overwhelming majority of people reject utilitarianism as an exhaustive normative ethical theory. Most people believe, for example, that promises ought generally to be kept not because (or not just because) doing so will cause more happiness than unhappiness, but because someone who makes a promise has *already* thereby obligated himself to keep it. Most people believe that it is generally wrong to lie, not just because lying may create distrust and unhappiness in the future, but because there is something fundamentally disrespectful and dishonorable in telling falsehoods.

IDEALS AND FAILINGS

Utilitarians who seek to maximize good consequences also reject another concept that most people find self-evident. To such utilitarians, every alternative is either obligatory (if it produces no less utility than any other alternative) or prohibited (if it does not).

Most people, however, believe there are actions that are morally valuable and ought to be encouraged but are not obligatory. Failure to do them means that one has not acted as well as one might, but not that one has acted wrongly. For example, many people consider giving to charity under circumstances in which one does not have much money to spare a morally desirable thing to do, but would not say that someone who fails to give under these circumstances has acted wrongly. Philosophers

---

[c]According to Kant's "categorical imperative," one must always ask whether a proposed alternative is universalizable, whether everyone could will the same principle. Thus, for Kant, one must keep one's promises because "the universality of a law that everyone believing himself to be in need can make any promise he pleases with the intention of not keeping it would make promising, and the very purpose of promising, itself impossible, since no one would believe he was being promised anything, but would laugh at utterances of this kind as empty shams" (6). Kant's position is not utilitarian. His objection to promise-breaking is not that it would lead to unhappiness but that it is inherently incoherent.

call these nonobligatory but desirable acts "supererogatory," a term which means "above and beyond the call of duty."

Just as most of us believe that there are supererogatory actions, we also believe that there are ways of behavior which are morally undesirable but at the same time cannot be said to be prohibited. Many would argue, for example, that people who abuse themselves with drugs are acting in a morally unseemly and undesirable manner, but are not morally prohibited from behaving in this way so long as they harm only themselves.

Nonobligatory moral ideals and nonprohibited moral failings have played a major role in veterinary codes of ethics, as they have in the ethical codes of other professions. It has been a large part of official professional ethics to urge, but not require, adherence to certain ideals and to discourage, but not prohibit, the commission of certain disapproved actions.

CAN MORAL STANDARDS BE OBJECTIVELY RIGHT OR WRONG?

Sooner or later, in any discussion of ethics among a group of veterinary students or practitioners, someone will voice the opinion that moral claims are really not objectively right or wrong but just express the personal preferences of those who make them. This opinion may take the form of what philosophers call ethical skepticism, the view that no moral claim can be right or wrong. Or, the troublemaker may be an adherent of ethical relativism, the view that each person's (or each society's) ethical opinions are as right and correct as any other's.

Some veterinarians, like others who have a scientific background, appear to be attracted to skepticism or relativism. For scientists are trained to demand that statements and theories be tested by empirical observation. And there can be no doubt that while one can, for example, determine with one's eyes whether a given disease involves certain physiological processes, there is nothing out there in the observable world that can be held up next to a moral claim to verify whether it is true. No photograph or videotape of an assault upon an elderly person itself demonstrates that such an action is wrong. The claim that such behavior is wrong is a proposition not about how the world is, but how it *ought* to be.

If right and wrong were merely a matter of personal preference, descriptive, administrative, and official veterinary ethics would still be possible, but highly unsatisfying. One need not believe that there are objective moral truths to discover what veterinarians actually believe is right and wrong, or what moral views administrative bodies and professional veterinary associations impose on practitioners. However, most veterinarians want their actual moral attitudes to be morally *correct*. And most veterinarians, surely, think that the purpose of having administrative and official ethical standards is to encourage professional behavior that is really right, not just behavior that happens to fit the preferences of government administrators or professional associations.

If skepticism or relativism were correct, normative veterinary ethics would be impossible, because there would be no objectively correct moral standards to discover and apply.

The overwhelming majority of people reject skepticism and relativism. We believe that moral claims can indeed be right or wrong. It is, however, beyond the scope of this book to attempt a philosophical refutation of skepticism and relativism. Moreover, in my discussions with veterinary students and practitioners who do express these views, I have found almost invariably that any such refutation is unnecessary.

Rather, it has proven just as effective to point out that skepticism and relativism are abstract notions about the nature of ethics which tend to be voiced in hypothetical discussions, but which virtually no one accepts in everyday life. When a professed relativist, for example, is confronted with a real challenge to his moral values, such as a burglary of his home or the mugging of an elderly relative, he will almost certainly protest that such actions are wrong and immoral. He will not insist that the burglar or mugger is also right, and that anyone who thinks otherwise (including himself) is just expressing a personal preference which is as good as any other personal preference. Even in classroom discussions about hypothetical cases, the skeptic or relativist will soon find himself talking like the rest of us. He will insist that certain things are right and wrong. He will not claim that these things are right (for him) because he happens to prefer them, but he will ask others to prefer them *because* these things are right.

HOW DOES ONE DECIDE NORMATIVE MORAL ISSUES?

Granted that moral preferences and opinions can be correct or incorrect, how *does* one determine the correct approaches to moral issues in normative veterinary ethics?

This is the central question for normative veterinary ethics. It is also a question that cannot possibly be answered at the beginning of an exploration of veterinary ethics. Indeed, if normative veterinary ethics proves even remotely as complex and challenging as medical ethics, one might never have a complete answer, because there will always be new issues to resolve and new insights to learn.

However, even at this point there are several demands we can reasonably make of any acceptable approach to normative veterinary ethics.

There must first of all be an interplay between our moral intuitions – what people, on reflection, think is right or wrong about a particular alternative or general moral position – and more general principles that can be used to justify and correct such intuitions. Mere intuitions are not enough. If all one could say is that some view is right because one *feels* that it is, there will be no objective standard, no reasoning, which can be measured against an intuition to justify it or to judge that it is correct or incorrect. This is why one is unhappy with the child who, when asked to explain the rock he just tossed through a neighbor's window, answers "Because." One wants to know why, one wants a *reason* or justification.

On the other hand, general rules, principles, and theories must sometimes be tested against basic moral experiences and intuitions. Just as one would reject a scientific theory that implies the Earth is flat, because we all know it is not flat, so would one reject a moral theory that offends one's most basic views about right and wrong. This is why utilitarianism, which is intended as a general and complete theory to guide all our moral intuitions, is accepted by very few people; its recommendations simply contradict too many moral intuitions people *know* must be correct.

Recognizing this essential interplay between moral experience and moral theories, biomedical ethicists Tom L. Beauchamp and James F. Childress (7) suggest five tests for judging whether approaches to determining correct moral behavior and attitude are acceptable. First, a proposed approach must be as clear as possible, so that one can understand what it says and how it is supposed to be applied. Second, it should be internally consistent and coherent. Third, it should be as comprehensive as possible and should leave no major gaps or holes. Fourth, it should be as simple as possible; like a good scientific theory, it should have no more principles than necessary, and people should be able to apply it without confusion. Finally, a theory or general approach must be able to account for the whole range of moral experience. "Ethical theories must build on, systematize, and criticize our ordinary concepts and beliefs" (7).

These tests do not attempt to determine what is right and wrong in ethics generally or in normative veterinary ethics in particular. Moreover, at present, normative veterinary ethics is very far from anything like a general approach that can systematize all issues. However, the five tests are useful in reminding us that normative veterinary ethics should at least attempt to bring order to the moral issues facing veterinarians, and must find reasoned arguments for ethical recommendations.

REFERENCES

1. Beauchamp TL and Childress JF: *Principles of Biomedical Ethics.* ed 2. New York: Oxford University Press, 1983, p 59.
2. Smart JJC: *An Outline of a System of Utilitarian Ethics.* Reprinted in Smart JJC and Williams B: *Utilitarianism, For and Against.* Cambridge: Cambridge University Press, 1987, p 30.
3. Smart, *Id.,* 5.
4. Ross WD: *The Right and the Good.* Oxford: Clarendon Press, 1930, p 21.
5. Fletcher J: *Situation Ethics.* Philadelphia: Westminster Press, 1966, p 115.
6. Kant I: *Groundwork of the Metaphysic of Morals.* Paton HJ (trans.) New York: Harper and Row, 1964, p 90.
7. Beauchamp TL and Childress JF: *Principles of Biomedical Ethics.* ed 2. New York: Oxford University Press, 1983, pp 12-13.

Chapter

—————— 6 ——————

Descriptive Veterinary Ethics: Mapping the Moral Values of Veterinarians

EMPIRICAL AND INTROSPECTIVE DESCRIPTIVE VETERINARY ETHICS

Descriptive veterinary ethics is the study of the actual ethical views of members of the veterinary profession regarding professional behavior and attitudes.

One might be tempted to think that descriptive veterinary ethics should be viewed as a branch of social science, consisting of empirical surveys of the moral attitudes of veterinarians. As we shall see, studying the actual professional moral views of veterinarians is clearly useful. Moreover, if one wants a reliable picture of the attitudes of veterinarians, one must engage in empirical research and use the most accurate available tools of sociological and statistical analysis.

There is, however, another way of conceiving of the study of veterinarians' actual professional moral attitudes that is quite different from, and at least as valuable as, conducting empirical surveys. Descriptive veterinary ethics can consist of an *individual* doctor or student seeking to understand his own professional moral values. Such an enterprise cannot proceed by empirical surveys or statistical analysis. It involves a process of self-understanding and evaluation. This kind of inquiry may sometimes involve asking the same questions a social scientist would put to numbers of practitioners. However, someone engaged in introspective understanding of his own professional moral values will often ask different questions from those raised by someone doing sociological research, and he will typically ask these questions for quite different purposes.

I shall call the factual study of the professional moral attitudes of numbers of veterinarians (as well as those training to become veterinarians) *empirical descriptive veterinary ethics*. I shall call the personal description by any such person of his own professional moral values *introspective descriptive veterinary ethics*.

GENERAL AND SPECIFIC ATTITUDES

Whether one is trying to understand the ethical attitudes of oneself or of one's profession, one must have a way of classifying or categorizing such attitudes.

Ethical attitudes can be classified according to their degree of generality or specificity. Some attitudes are extremely general, as is, for example, the pronouncement of the AVMA *Principles of Veterinary Medical Ethics* that "the responsibilities of the veterinary profession extend not only to the patient but also to society" (1). Such general attitudes can lie behind a wide range of quite different professional activities. Doctors who inspect meat, or conduct spay and neuter clinics for local humane societies, or who are engaged in biomedical research can all say, legitimately, that they are motivated at least in part by the desire to render service to society.

Ethical attitudes can also be extremely specific and can assert detailed answers to very focused questions. An example of such an attitude is the statement of the AVMA *Principles* that "a commercial boarding kennel may be owned by a veterinarian but should not be operated under the veterinarian's name, and the telephone number should be separate from that used by the veterinarian in the conduct of the practice" (2).

Between the most abstract ethical principle and the most specific ethical opinion, there is a wide range of possible degrees of specificity.

Those engaged in empirical or introspective descriptive veterinary ethics must be extremely careful to include in their descriptions a proper mix of general and specific attitudes. A useful account of professional attitudes cannot consist only of statements of very specific attitudes. Veterinarians are faced with many situations about which they have specific views; a list of all such opinions (of a single practitioner much less of the entire profession) would be unreadable if not endless. Moreover, one's specific ethical attitudes are often generated by more general values that apply across a range of situations. It might not be inaccurate to say that Dr. Jones believes that it is wrong to sell pet toys and that he believes it is wrong to take out newspaper advertisements containing coupons entitling clients to discounts on fees. However, both of these ethical beliefs might better be seen as flowing from a more general view about what is permissible for someone who is not an ordinary businessperson but is a practitioner of one of the healing arts (see Chapter 16).

On the other hand, members of the profession must also beware of classifying their ethical attitudes in too general a manner. General attitudes can be consistent with quite different (and sometimes hostile) points of view. For example, two practitioners might agree that doctors should not be overly competitive, but may disagree about whether operating low-overhead mobile clinics is being overly competitive. Likewise, we would not say enough about the ethical values of two veterinarians by simply describing both as devoted to rendering "service to society" if for one such service means earning less than he might otherwise earn by working for his state public health department while for the other it means spending free time at local schools and community organizations talking about pet care.

Because they can be so vague, and can sound quite nice, *very* general statements of ethical values can also lull people into not thinking carefully about ethical issues and into not looking objectively at their own attitudes. Some of my students assert that a major ethical attitude in their value system is a "love for animals." Yet many of them support the euthanasia of stray animals in shelters or the culling of healthy but unproductive farm animals. I am *not* saying here that such euthanasia or culling is wrong. What is unfortunate is that the person who professes a general "love for animals" may not be thinking clearly about the fact that he believes certain animals are entitled to protection and care that is properly described as love, while other animals are not. If he in fact believes that certain animals are not entitled to love, he ought to be clear that he has such a belief and about why he thinks such a belief is proper – a clarity that professing a generalized "love for animals" is likely to hinder rather than encourage.

CENTRAL AND PERIPHERAL VALUES

Any useful description of one's own or of one's profession's ethical attitudes must also recognize that some attitudes and values are more central – they are held more strongly and insisted upon more firmly – than others.

Some attitudes are so central to a profession or person that they define that profession or person, in the sense that if these attitudes were abandoned or changed, we would have to say that we would be dealing with a different profession or personality. For example, if the legal profession abandoned its centrally held view that it is right to try to convince judges and juries by argument, and began using the old custom of trial by drowning (in which someone won a dispute if he survived being tied up and thrown into water), we would say that the legal profession as we now define it would have disappeared.

Other attitudes, on the other hand, are less central to a profession or personality. Thus, some lawyers see criminals they represent as victims of society, while other lawyers prosecute these same people, believing that they are evil and ought to be punished. There are lawyers who like to sue big corporations, feeling that these businesses are greedy and immoral, and other lawyers who are happy to represent them. All these (and many more) different ethical attitudes can be encompassed within the profession of law. And part of what differentiates, for example, a corporate lawyer from a public prosecutor is how they *rank* their values; for the latter, earning money is likely to be less important than service to society.

Like lawyers, veterinarians have some ethical attitudes that are more and others that are less central to their profession. Like law, veterinary medicine contains within it subgroups, and individual practitioners, who rank certain values differently. Thus, it is impossible to be a private veterinary clinical practitioner and believe that animal suffering is not worth human concern. On the other hand, some veterinarians and groups of veterinarians can have different ethical views and still remain within the profession. Veterinarians can (and do) disagree about, for example, whether laboratory practitioners should participate in the use of animals to test cosmetics, or whether it is right to crop dogs' ears or dock their tails so that they can meet breed standards, or whether it is morally appropriate for veterinarians to treat individual wild animals that are not members of endangered or threatened species.

SELF- AND OTHER-REGARDING MORAL VALUES

Some philosophers believe that ethics or morality relates to one's behavior or attitudes toward other people. These philosophers assert that values or attitudes that pertain primarily to oneself (such as the value one places on art, contemplation, or research) are essentially aesthetic or intellectual in nature and are not the concern of ethics. This distinction between the ethical and the personal or aesthetic is a departure from traditional philosophical ethical theory, and has been criticized by a number of contemporary philosophers (3). These latter thinkers subscribe to Aristotle's view that ethics must concern itself with the good life. They remind us that living the good life includes not just behaving well toward others but also behaving well towards oneself – acquiring knowledge about the world, enjoying art and music, appreciating nature, and so on. Therefore, these philosophers insist, ethics must consider values that relate to one's personality and personal lifestyle as well as to one's obligations toward others.

Whatever conclusion philosophers may reach about including self-regarding values in the study of ethics, there can be no doubt that descriptive veterinary ethics must concern itself with such values. Part of the purpose of descriptive veterinary ethics is to help practitioners understand what really underlies value judgments they make in their professional lives, so that they can understand what value issues are important to them and their profession and what solutions to these issues may be realistic. But it is clear that personal attitudes do play an important role in the value judgments of many veterinarians. Many bovine practitioners, for example, tell me that they receive intense personal satisfaction from working outdoors with large animals, associating with farmers, and participating in a rural and agricultural lifestyle, and that these things are more important to them than a lavish standard of living. No one can understand the value judgments such practitioners make about how they ought to treat their clients and patients without understanding that they have these personal attitudes.

MAPPING THE VALUES OF VETERINARIANS

Descriptive veterinary ethics is in its infancy. Therefore, any suggested way of studying the ethical attitudes of veterinarians will doubtless require revision and modification as we learn more about how to describe these attitudes.

Table 6.1 offers a schematic for describing the ethical values of practitioners and students. The table distinguishes several very general attitudes and several subcategories within these attitudes. For example, there are what can be called "self-oriented" attitudes of veterinarians and "society-oriented" attitudes. A doctor for whom self-oriented values are of great importance may choose a career in private practice, while another for whom society-oriented values are important may join government service. One veterinarian for whom profession-oriented values are important may become active in his state veterinary association; another, for whom scientific research is a consuming interest, may have little to do with fellow veterinarians. For one doctor, private practice may be the only possible vocation because he wants to help individual animals (a "patient-oriented" value); another may choose private practice because he wants to assist clients in achieving their desires regarding their animals (a "client-oriented" value). One veterinarian may be less interested in animals in the hospital or clinic setting than in promoting the welfare of animals in general (an "animal-oriented" value); while another may spend his life in the public health area protecting people from animal-transmitted diseases (a "society-oriented" value).

Within a general kind of value, there can be different and sometimes conflicting values. Among veterinarians legitimately described as patient-oriented, some may see the alleviation and prevention of animal suffering as an overriding goal and will have no problem with the slaughter of animals for food, provided they are not caused to suffer; other veterinarians may object to the termination of an animal's life for any reason other than benefiting that animal.

Many of the general and more specific values I have distinguished need not conflict with each other, may exist comfortably within the value structure of an individual practitioner, and indeed can be intimately connected. Thus, a veterinarian may build a prosperous practice and join his state veterinary association, motivated to do both by an interest in monetary gain and a desire to be recognized as a valued member of his community. A veterinarian engaged in research may be committed to helping people as well as animals, and believe that the acquisition of knowledge about biological processes is valuable in its own right.

Table 6.1

Selected Values in Veterinary Medicine

Self-oriented
   Monetary gain
   Personal satisfaction
      e.g., working outdoors
      e.g., interacting with pet owners
      e.g., competitive lifestyle
      e.g., participation in running a profitable business
      e.g., freedom from business pressures
   Recognition
Client-oriented
   Clients' monetary gain
   Clients' personal satisfaction

Patient-oriented
   Alleviation of pain/suffering
   Promotion of patient health
   Protection of lives of patients

Animal-oriented
   Protection of animal interests in general
   Protection of certain species/kinds of animals

Profession-oriented
   Enjoyment of professional associations/activities
   Protection of profession from external challenges
   Education of future veterinarians or technicians

Knowledge/Science/Theory-oriented
   Scientific aspects of animals/animal disease
   Scientific aspects of human disease
   Promotion of basic animal research
   Promotion of basic scientific research

Society-oriented
   Public (human) health
   Individual human health and well-being
   Human-directed environmental concerns
   Human-directed industry/agriculture
   Animal control

A DIVERSE PROFESSION

Doubtless many further subdivisions and refinements of the values listed in Table 6.1 are possible. However, the table and this brief discussion already make it plain that veterinary medicine is an extraordinarily diverse profession, not just in terms of what its members can do, but by virtue of their different ethical attitudes and priorities. Veterinarians traditionally have been associated with human as well as animal concerns. They have worked in areas ranging from agribusiness to wildlife management to the pharmaceutical industry to the military. Therefore, the ethical "map" of veterinary medicine may well be far more diverse and complex than that of human medicine or any of the other learned professions.

The rich diversity of the ethical attitudes of veterinarians refutes those who, like Professor Rollin, speak about "the essential *raison d'être* for the veterinarian" (4), *the* necessary and overriding value by which all veterinarians supposedly guide their professional lives. Although all veterinarians may share certain values, if descriptive veterinary ethics stops at such universal values and fails to recognize all the complex different possibilities, it will fail to describe accurately the attitudes either of the profession as a whole or of very many of its members.

THE VALUE OF EMPIRICAL DESCRIPTIVE VETERINARY ETHICS

Virtually any problem or issue in official, administrative, or normative veterinary ethics can be illuminated by an empirical description of the actual views of practitioners or students. The following are only some of the things a study of the actual values of such persons might reveal:

1. What ethical issues are most troubling to the profession (or to different components of the profession) and therefore might require prompt discussion or resolution;
2. Whether an important ethical issue is appreciated as such by the profession and whether the profession might therefore require sensitization to the issue;
3. Whether an ethical problem important to the profession is appreciated sufficiently by clients or society and whether the profession should therefore educate them concerning its significance;
4. Whether an ethical issue assumed to be in need of urgent resolution is not sufficiently troubling to those affected to justify significant allocation of the profession's time and resources;
5. What proposed solutions to ethical issues are likely to be accepted by the profession and might therefore be attractive to drafters of official or administrative ethical standards;
6. What ethical issues are likely to concern the profession in the future and the profession might therefore want to consider before these issues become divisive.

The value of empirical descriptive ethics is demonstrated by a 1983 study of the ethical attitudes of first- and fourth-year students at 16 United States veterinary schools (5).

Some of the survey's findings indicated that there are issues the profession is not addressing adequately. For example, although at the time of the study only one veterinary school had a required course in ethics, 67% of the students believed that such courses should be required of all students, and fewer than half felt that their education prepared them adequately to form opinions on ethical issues. (Seniors found their exposure to ethical issues less satisfactory than did freshmen.) The study also concluded that "female students supported the interests of animals to a greater degree than male students." If correct, this finding may forecast the issues of the future, because the majority of veterinary students are now women (6).

On the other hand, the survey appeared to indicate that the profession need not be as worried about certain matters as some have supposed. Some practitioners and veterinary educators are concerned about students who might refuse on ethical grounds to participate in surgery laboratories involving the use and subsequent euthanasia of healthy animals. More than a few academic veterinarians are wary of exposing students to the views of animal rights activists. The survey, however, indicated that although 88% of the students wanted controversial issues like animal rights addressed in the curriculum, only 5% disagreed with the proposition that the death of animals as a result of animal research is justified if people will benefit from the research.

SOME PITFALLS OF EMPIRICAL DESCRIPTIVE VETERINARY ETHICS

It is beyond the scope of this book to propose a set of guidelines for empirical studies of the ethical attitudes of veterinarians. However, there are clearly several considerations that empirical descriptive veterinary ethics must address.

Asking the Right Questions

How one phrases a question in a survey can elicit either an answer one is hoping to obtain, or one that does not reflect accurately the views of a respondent. In ethics, we must be especially careful because there is often a range of different possible responses that a single question can obscure. For example, 9% of the students in the 1983 study agreed with the statement that "the number of live animals used in teaching surgery in veterinary schools should be reduced." However, agreement with this statement is consistent with many different attitudes, ranging from the position that such use of animals should be eliminated, to the view that surgery on live animals is crucial, although there might be room for minor reduction in their numbers.

Subtlety in asking about ethical attitudes is important because our ethical concepts are themselves subtle and precise. As was discussed in Chapter 5, there is a difference between the morally obligatory and the ideal, and between moral prohibitions and moral failings. The study of student attitudes emphasized moral obligations and prohibitions, asking, for example whether "the veterinarian has an obligation to provide services such as ear cropping or debarking when requested by a client." Some people may interpret the fact that fewer than 25% of the students agreed with this statement as general condemnation of ear cropping or debarking (or perhaps even of automatic assent to clients' requests). However, the statement that "the" veterinarian has an "obligation" to provide a service – that any doctor will *always* fail in his moral *duty* if he does not provide the service – is very strong, and one about which some of the students might have felt uncomfortable. It would be interesting to learn how the students would have reacted had they been asked the following questions: 1) whether *under certain circumstances* a veterinarian is morally obligated to provide a requested service such as ear cropping or debarking; 2) whether it would be morally *commendable*, but not morally required, for a veterinarian to refuse to provide certain services; and 3) whether a veterinarian asked to do ear cropping or debarking ought to do something *other* than just agree or disagree with the client's request, such as discussing with the client the pros and cons of the requested procedure with the aim of giving the client all the relevant information.

Attitudes and Actions

Another pitfall that empirical descriptive veterinary ethics must avoid is excessive reliance on questionnaires as indicators of actual attitudes. Sometimes, people report not the attitudes they really exhibit in their daily or professional lives, but the attitudes they would like to think (or would like others to think) they have. Moreover, it is sometimes much easier to express an ethical view than to act in accordance with it. For example, it costs little to assert, as 88% of the students in the 1983 survey did, that "the veterinarian has an obligation to educate the public concerning public health, such as by speaking before community groups." This seems a fine thing to say. However, it is unlikely that such a high proportion of these people, or of any group of busy practitioners, will have the inclination or time to speak before community groups.

Facts and Values

Although empirical descriptive veterinary ethics seeks to understand the moral attitudes of veterinarians, it would be a mistake to limit investigation to ethical attitudes in the strict sense. Sometimes moral values and priorities are illuminated by asking certain questions about factual beliefs that play a role in moral discussions.

The usefulness of inquiry into factual beliefs is demonstrated by a survey of 600 practitioners conducted by the journal *Veterinary Economics*. After a 1985 AVMA manpower study predicted an oversupply of veterinarians, some practitioners began to demand that fewer students be permitted to attend veterinary schools. In March 1986, *Veterinary Economics* published an article characterizing the controversy over enrollments as a "fire raging over the manpower problem" (7), and reporting substantial support for reducing veterinary school enrollments. This article (and other published studies and views of the matter) appeared to indicate that the difficult moral issues raised by the enrollment debate needed immediate and decisive resolution. However, in its next issue, the journal reported that its own survey found that 53% of practitioners did not believe there was a surplus of veterinarians. Moreover, many practitioners who did believe there was an oversupply based this opinion primarily on the AVMA manpower study and other published articles and not on their own personal knowledge of a surplus. The journal's editor asked "(w)hy hasn't anyone asked rank and file veterinarians about practitioner overload?" He warned that "(b)efore we rush to hammer our educational and practice system into a different and unknown mold, we'd better do our homework first and find out if the system really needs changing" (8). The journal subsequently undertook an extensive study that found substantial, though differing, concerns about the supply of veterinarians in different areas of the country and various kinds of practice (9).

The factual questions posed by the *Veterinary Economics* surveys concerned whether practitioners believed in the existence of a state of affairs that would trigger a moral problem or demand its prompt resolution. Another kind of factual belief of importance to empirical descriptive ethics are those that, *together* with certain value judgments, can draw practitioners to differing conclusions about what ought or ought not to be done. For example, some veterinarians criticize the raising of calves in confinement crates for "milk-fed" veal as immoral while others disagree. But many of these veterinarians appear to share the same general *ethical* principle: that animals should not be caused unnecessary pain and suffering. What separates them is a disagreement about whether such animals in fact suffer or are experiencing unnecessary pain or suffering. It is this difference in their factual beliefs that is responsible for their reaching opposite conclusions about the morality of raising calves in this way. It would be inaccurate to characterize these doctors simply as having different ethical views about milk-fed veal.

Recognizing that people may have an ethical disagreement that is based upon on differing views about the facts often facilitates resolution of an ethical dispute, because it can direct the parties to the real issue that may be separating them. On the other hand, ethical disputes do not always turn on differences about facts. People who believe that raising animals for food is inherently immoral, whether or not it causes animal suffering, will not withdraw their opposition to animal agriculture if it could be demonstrated that certain food animals do not experience suffering or distress. They have a fundamental ethical disagreement with those who believe that animals may be used for food so long as they do not suffer. This is a disagreement that no appeal to facts alone can resolve.

THE VALUE OF INTROSPECTIVE DESCRIPTIVE VETERINARY ETHICS

The Choice of a Practice Style

Because veterinary medicine can encompass such a diversity of values and attitudes, it is extremely important for each practitioner and student to understand his own value structure. Failure to do so can have disastrous results.

For example, veterinary schools tend to encourage students who earn high grades to enter academic veterinary medicine. Indeed, because such a career is often perceived as the highest award a veterinary school can bestow, the path to academic practice – including an internship, residency, board certification in a specialty, and teaching – is seen by many students as the ideal in professional life.

The problem is that such a path involves values and attitudes that are not shared by all who are thrust toward it. Internships and residencies require long hours and intense competition for the smaller number of openings on each successive rung of the academic ladder. Those who make it into academic practice may find that because of the need to publish new research, they must ignore everyday kinds of cases and gravitate toward the unusual, the unexplained, the "interesting." Moreover, the academic veterinarian may sometimes be less concerned about assisting a particular animal than in learning about and ultimately being able to help larger numbers of animals. He may try a certain procedure on a research subject, knowing that someone who wanted to do everything possible to help that particular animal might act differently.

Each year there embark upon the academic trail some young veterinarians for whom enjoyment of leisure time is an important value, who abhor competition, who are so touched by the needs of each individual animal that they feel they must always do everything possible to help it, or who enjoy dealing with everyday clients more than teaching students. Likewise, there are some academic veterinarians who yearn for the hubbub of private practice, and doctors for whom the daily pressures of running a practice are intolerable and who might be happier and more productive in academic medicine.

Veterinarians whose temperaments and ethical values are not suited to the way they find themselves practicing may fail in their chosen area, or, if "successful," may be miserable for the rest of their lives. They may blame their misfortune on their chosen field and may even come to see it as morally wrong. They may think that *they* are somehow deficient. They may even abandon the practice of veterinary medicine.

We are not always able to choose the career or practice style we would prefer. Moreover, the field of psychology would be out of business if it were a simple matter for people to always understand the forces that motivate their personalities. Nevertheless, the profession and the schools can do a great deal more than they are now doing to help individual doctors and students to clarify their own values and to understand the values and attitudes of the various areas of veterinary medicine.

REFERENCES

1. "Principles of Veterinary Medical Ethics," Part 6. *1988 AVMA Directory,* p 474.
2. "Boarding Kennels." *1988 AVMA Directory,* p 476.
3. See, e.g., MacIntyre A: *After Virtue.* ed 2. Notre Dame, Indiana: University of Notre Dame Press, 1984, pp 154-155.
4. Rollin BE: *Animal Rights and Human Morality.* Buffalo, Prometheus Books, 1981, p 173. According to Rollin, this is "the health and welfare of animals."
5. Shurtleff RS, Grant P, Zeglen ME, McCulloch WF, and Bustad LK: A nationwide survey of veterinary students' values and attitudes on ethical issues. *Journal of Veterinary Medical Education* 9:93-96, 1983.
6. Enrollment Declines in DVM-Degree Programs. *J Am Vet Med Assoc* 192:1028, 1988 (reporting that women comprised 50.8% of the total student body of U.S. veterinary colleges in 1985-1986, 53% in 1986-1987, and 55.03% in 1987-1988).
7. Enrollment Under the Knife. *Veterinary Economics* Mar 1986:28-39.
8. Sollars M: Memo from the Editor. *Veterinary Economics* Apr 1986:2.
9. DVM Glut: Is the Squeeze on You? *Veterinary Economics* Jul 1987:26 *et seq.*

Chapter

7

Administrative Veterinary Ethics: The Governmental Application of Ethical Standards

Administrative veterinary ethics is the process of the application of ethical standards to veterinarians by administrative governmental agencies. It is important to recognize administrative veterinary ethics as a separate branch of veterinary ethics. Almost every aspect of veterinary practice can be affected by administrative application of ethical standards. Moreover, because administrative agencies are branches of government, they can use the substantial force of the law to compel adherence to these standards. In recent years, administrative bodies such as state boards of registration have exhibited a marked increase in activity in the regulation of physicians and attorneys. If this trend extends to veterinarians – and evidence that this is already happening is provided by the increased activity of some of the state veterinary boards and of federal agencies such as the Food and Drug Administration (FDA) and United States Department of Agriculture (USDA) in regulating veterinary practice – administrative veterinary ethics may become a major concern of all practitioners.[a]

THE NATURE AND FUNCTIONS OF ADMINISTRATIVE AGENCIES

An administrative agency can be defined as "a governmental authority, other than a court and other than a legislative body, which affects the rights of private parties through either adjudication, rulemaking, investigating, prosecuting, negotiating, settling, or informally acting" (1). Administrative agencies can consist of varying numbers of

---

[a]This book may be the first to present administrative ethics as a separate branch of professional ethics. In light of the growing role of governmental bodies in applying moral standards to the professions, this approach seems mandatory. Administrative bodies will more likely engage in serious, reflective moral deliberation if their *ethical* activity is recognized as such – and is studied as a distinct kind of endeavor by members of these bodies, scholars, and practitioners. Another important topic that is usually ignored in discussions of professional ethics is employee relations (see Chapter 22).

persons (including one). They go by various names, which usually have no special significance in defining their activities.

It is not the courts or legislatures, but administrative agencies that perform the overwhelming majority of governmental functions. From the USDA to state departments of public health, from the FDA to the National Institutes of Health (NIH), from the Federal Bureau of Investigation (FBI) to county district attorneys offices, from the Internal Revenue Service (IRS) to municipal zoning boards, administrative agencies affect virtually every aspect of the lives of everyone.

Administrative bodies exist because there is too much for legislative and executive officeholders to do by themselves, and because certain areas of government require expertise these officeholders do not possess. No administrative agency is entirely free to do what it wants. Statutes usually define the functions and proper activities of an agency; decisions that violate these boundaries or that are in error can often be appealed in the courts. Administrative bodies differ widely in the amount of independence they possess. Sometimes, as in the case of the Federal Trade Commission (FTC), or state boards of veterinary medicine, agencies are relatively independent; their members are appointed for fixed terms and they can adopt policies or make decisions that the current legislature, President, or Governor may oppose. Sometimes, as in the case of the USDA or state departments of agriculture, agencies are subdivisions of a branch of government (usually, the executive); such agencies often take orders directly from, or are ultimately accountable to, an elected official.

Although the powers of administrative bodies differ, the following are among the kinds of activities they can perform. They typically:

1. Enforce specific standards or requirements written into a statute;
2. Interpret statutory provisions that were not made entirely clear by the legislature;
3. Write their own regulations to assist them in carrying out their functions;
4. Grant licenses or permissions based on statutory standards or their own regulations;
5. Investigate suspected violations of statutory or regulatory standards;
6. Determine for themselves in adjudicatory proceedings whether violations have occurred;
7. Impose penalties (e.g., a fine or suspension of a license) upon those found to be in violation;
8. Refer a matter to another agency (e.g., the state Attorney General) for criminal or civil action;
9. Issue specific rulings or opinions determining that a certain kind of activity or a specific private party is or is not in compliance with the agency's standards;
10. Engage in a wide range of informal actions not normally subject to public scrutiny or review by the courts, including pressuring those under their jurisdiction to meet their standards, assisting parties privately, publicizing their standards and policies, negotiating agreements and settlements, and deciding whether to investigate, negotiate, or prosecute.

ADMINISTRATIVE AGENCIES AND ETHICAL STANDARDS

There are several ways in which administrative agencies impose or apply ethical standards.

First, they may apply statutes or regulations that are *purely* ethical in nature. For example, many veterinary practice acts direct the state board of veterinary medicine to grant licenses only to those who are of good moral character, and permit the board to discipline licensed practitioners who engage in fraud or in false and misleading advertising. These can be purely ethical issues that need not relate to competence or technical ability.

Second, administrative agencies sometimes make decisions applying ethical *and* technical standards. The USDA's regulations under the Animal Welfare Act governing the housing and care of laboratory animals draw heavily on the Department's technical knowledge about the needs of different laboratory species and the nature of laboratory facilities. But the underlying aim of these regulations is to assure due regard for the animals' welfare. This is an *ethical* goal that is applied in light of technical knowledge to generate what is hoped are morally appropriate standards. Likewise, when the FDA proposes policies governing the extra-label use of drugs in food animals, it must consider empirical data about the effects and elimination times of these drugs in light of ethical concerns – including how the moral right of the public to safe products is to be balanced against the need of farmers and veterinarians to earn a living. It is sometimes easy to forget the extent to which administrative bodies are motivated by ethical concerns. The rules they adopt can be technical in appearance and do not always make explicit reference to their underlying ethical motivation. As they do their jobs, the meat inspector, customs agent, racing commission veterinarian, or state health department toxicologist may not be engaging in ethical deliberation. Nevertheless, many of the technical standards they apply have resulted from decisions that certain interests *ought* to be protected and that certain kinds of behavior (such as selling adulterated meat or overworking race horses) are morally intolerable.

Third, ethical considerations can play an important role in an administrative body's exercise of what lawyers call its "discretionary power," its ability to make decisions (such as whom to investigate or prosecute and when not to investigate, negotiate, or prosecute) that are generally not open to challenge by the public or the courts. A state board of veterinary medicine, for example, may decide to give friendly, and private, guidance to a practitioner who has committed an act of incompetence if he exhibits an appropriate attitude of remorse. On the other hand, the board may suspend the license of another veterinarian who has done the same thing but who is disrespectful and unrepentant. One cannot overestimate the extent to which administrative bodies can be affected in their discretionary decisions by perceptions of whether they are dealing with a morally good person who merits sympathy, or with a morally bad one who deserves punishment.

THE RANGE OF ADMINISTRATIVE VETERINARY ETHICAL STANDARDS

It is beyond the scope of this book to discuss all the administrative agencies that apply ethical standards to veterinarians. Subsequent chapters will consider the ethical activity of several of the more visible agencies. Table 7.1 lists some of the administrative bodies that apply ethical standards to veterinarians. The table is illustrative only. It does not list all ethical issues relating to veterinarians in which administrative agencies are involved, all the administrative bodies applying ethical standards to veterinarians, or all the areas of ethical involvement of the listed agencies.

Table 7.1

Ethical Areas of Concern of Administrative Agencies Other than the State Veterinary Boards

AREA OF CONCERN	FEDERAL AGENCIES	STATE AND LOCAL AGENCIES
Animal diseases, protection, animals from contagious	USDA	State departments of agriculture, public health
Animal food products, protection of public from impure and adulterated	FDA	State departments of agriculture, public health
Competition among doctors, assurance of fair	Federal Trade Commission (FTC)	State attorneys general
Controlled substances, use by veterinarians	Drug Enforcement Administration (DEA)	State public health departments, district attorneys, and attorneys general
Cruelty to animals (general)		District attorneys Special animal protection agencies
Deceptive commercial and trade practices by veterinarians	FTC	State attorneys general
Discrimination against employees on the basis of race, religion, age, sex	Equal Opportunity Employment Commission (EEOC)	State and local anti-discrimination agencies
Drugs, use by veterinarians	FDA	State public health departments
Food animals, humane slaughter of	USDA	State agriculture departments
Insecticides and pesticides, use by veterinarians	Environmental Protection Agency (EPA)	
Laboratory animal welfare	USDA (Animal and Plant Health Inspection Service – APHIS); EPA; FDA; NIH; Public Health Service (PHS)	State public health departments (in some states)
Meat and poultry, protection of public from impure	USDA (Food Safety and Inspection Service – FSIS)	State meat inspection agencies

Table 7.1 – *continued*

AREA OF CONCERN	FEDERAL AGENCIES	STATE AND LOCAL AGENCIES
Pets, commercial raising and transportation of	USDA (APHIS)	
Racing animals, regulation of drug use in and conditions of		State racing commissions
Safety of veterinary premises for the public ·		Local building, fire, and health departments
Safety of working conditions for veterinary employees	Occupational Safety and Health Administration (OSHA)	State departments of labor and public health
Show horses, protection of from certain inhumane practices	USDA (APHIS)	
Unfair labor practices	Department of Labor; National Labor Relations Board	State labor departments
Wildlife, protection of; veterinary care by private doctors	Department of Interior (Fish and Wildlife Service)	State departments of fisheries and wildlife
Veterinary facilities, proper location and use of		Local zoning boards and planning commissions
Zoonoses	Department of Health and Human Services (Centers for Disease Control; NIH)	State and local public health departments

ADMINISTRATIVE VETERINARY ETHICS ON THE FRONT LINE: THE STATE VETERINARY BOARDS

By far the most important potential source of administrative veterinary ethical judgments are the state boards of veterinary medicine. This is so because the boards, unlike other administrative bodies that regulate veterinarians, deal exclusively with providers of veterinary services and their relations with patients, clients, and the public. Moreover, the boards have at their disposal a far larger number of rules that are purely ethical in nature than do other kinds of administrative agencies whose activities affect veterinarians.

The Veterinary Boards

The law begins with the principle that veterinary practice is not a right but a privilege, and that it is the state (not the federal government) that has the responsibility of deciding upon whom this privilege will be conferred. Each state goes about making this decision by enacting a statute (usually called the veterinary practice act) that sets forth the legislature's decisions about who will be permitted to practice and under what conditions. The act creates an administrative agency (usually called the board of registration or board of examiners in veterinary medicine) that grants licenses to practice and has the authority to regulate licensees and to discipline them for failure to meet required standards. Typically, some of these standards are specified in the practice act. Sometimes, the board will adopt standards it writes itself, pursuant to its authority to make rules and regulations to assist it in implementing the practice act.

There are significant differences among the veterinary boards. The veterinary practice act of each jurisdiction is different, so that a standard imposed in one state may not exist in another. In some jurisdictions, the legislature has placed all its requirements (both technical and ethical) in the veterinary practice act; other states have statutes and regulations governing all licensed professionals that apply standards to veterinarians in addition to those found in the veterinary practice act. In some states, it is the board itself that disciplines practitioners; in others, the board makes a recommendation that is reviewed and can be modified by a supervisory administrative agency before becoming final. The procedures used in investigating and adjudicating cases differ from state to state. Some boards have nonveterinarian members, and among those with public members, some boards have a larger number of public members than others. The boards also vary widely in how actively and vigorously they make regulations and investigate and discipline infractions, both technical and ethical.

Ethical Standards of the Veterinary Boards

The following are some of the more common ethical standards set forth in the veterinary practice acts and regulations of the states. The typical practice act or regulations will contain several of the provisions listed below. The precise wording of these standards can vary from state to state.[b]

Good moral character. Many states permit the licensing only of persons of good moral character. Practice acts with this requirement sometimes specify criteria the board may use in defining good moral character. For example, the Illinois act states that "any felony conviction may be taken into consideration" (2) in determining an applicant's good moral character. However, most practice acts do not define good

---

[b]The following discussion lists practice act provisions as they are typically phrased. References in brackets are to states that have the listed provisions, though not necessarily in these precise words. State listings are illustrative only; when a state is listed, there may be other states with the same or similar provisions. State references are given only for provisions that are noteworthy or must be distinguished carefully from other listed provisions. References to states are not given for provisions that are shared by many states. The reader should consult his own practice act or regulations for the precise wording of the standards currently applicable in his jurisdiction.

moral character, and appear to leave it to the board to decide who might and who might not have such character. At least one state requires good moral character "as it relates to the functions and duties of a licensed veterinarian" (3). However, there usually is no such restriction. Some practice acts list absence of good moral character among the grounds for disciplining present licensees, while the statutes of other states specify that new applicants can be denied a license if they lack good moral character. It seems clear, however, that if a board can deny a new license because of bad moral character, it can revoke or suspend an already existing license for this reason as well (4).

The theory behind the good moral character requirement − and indeed of many of the ethical standards imposed by the practice acts − is that society has a right to expect that its veterinarians be more than technically proficient. A veterinarian must also be a good and decent person. He must be worthy of the great trust placed in him by his clients, and he must be sensitive to the great power he has over the health and lives of his patients.

Conviction of a felony or of a crime involving moral turpitude. The underlying rationale for these disciplinary grounds is that a conviction of a felony or of a crime involving moral turpitude can itself provide evidence of bad moral character and lack of trustworthiness.

In most jurisdictions, a felony is any crime punishable by more than 1 year imprisonment. A judgment based upon a guilty plea is a conviction, and a person can be convicted of a felony even if he in fact serves less than a year in jail or is ordered to pay a fine instead of being incarcerated. The reason that moral turpitude is not added as an extra requirement to felonies is that the law considers a felony conviction as itself evidence of bad moral character.

A crime involving moral turpitude is one that by its very nature always reflects bad moral character. Sometimes, this definition leads to odd results. For example, in a California court case, a chiropractor had been charged with owning and operating a bordello, but pleaded guilty only to the lesser charge of willfully residing in a house of ill repute. The court ruled that he could not be disciplined by the board of chiropractic for conviction of a crime involving moral turpitude because he was only convicted of *living* in a house of ill repute, and a chiropractor could conceivably live in such a place and not contribute other than peripherally to the enterprise of prostitution (5). Among the crimes that are generally regarded as involving moral turpitude are theft, fraud, tax evasion, homicide, violent crimes, indecent exposure (6), and, increasingly, crimes involving abuse of alcoholic beverages or drugs (7).

Conviction of a crime directly relating to the practice of veterinary medicine or the ability to practice veterinary medicine [CA, FL, IN] (8). Some states permit the board to discipline a practitioner who has been convicted of any crime (felony or misdemeanor), provided the crime related directly to the practice of veterinary medicine or is evidence of a lack of ability to practice veterinary medicine. In fact, such a provision probably will not protect most veterinarians convicted of any crime, and certainly does not always require a board to find that a criminal conviction is evidence of technical incompetence. As one court has observed, any crime that reflects poorly on a practitioner's *honesty, truthfulness,* and *good reputation* is a crime related to the practice of veterinary medicine. For a veterinarian not only takes possession of and promises to protect the valued property of others; he engages to help beings that are "often as deeply revered as members of the family" (9). The Supreme Judicial Court of Massachusetts, upholding the revocation of the license of a physician who had been convicted of illegal possession of unregistered submachine guns, stated that any crime that provides evidence of bad moral character or "undermines public confidence in the integrity of the profession" calls into question a practitioner's "ability to practice" (10). The Court reiterated the traditional legal doctrine that

> Mere intellectual power and scientific achievement without uprightness of character may be more harmful than ignorance. Highly trained intelligence combined with disregard of the fundamental virtues is a menace (11).

The great majority of criminal offenses involve dishonesty or disrespect for the rights of others, traits that a board could easily find are inconsistent with the high moral standards essential to veterinary practice.

Conviction of any crime [MA, NY] (12). Some states permit the board to discipline a veterinarian on the grounds that he has been convicted of committing any crime, whether or not the crime is a felony or misdemeanor, involves moral turpitude, or can be said to relate directly to veterinary practice. Courts have upheld such provisions as a legitimate exercise of the state's strong interest in licensing only those with high moral character (13).

Conviction of the federal Controlled Substances Act or state controlled substances or drug laws. Although such crimes would almost always be either felonies, crimes of moral turpitude, or crimes evidencing an inability to practice veterinary medicine, many practice acts make specific reference to conviction of drug offenses. Again, there is usually no requirement that the act giving rise to the drug conviction be related to the licensee's ability to practice competently. In one case, the license of a California veterinarian was revoked in part because of his conviction of conspiracy to smuggle 12,000 pounds of marijuana into the country. The court reviewing the board's action stated that this act "would constitute a crime involving moral turpitude as far as a veterinarian is concerned" (14). Veterinarians should not be misled into thinking that conviction of only "serious" infractions of drug laws will endanger their licenses. Because of the special trust the law places upon veterinarians regarding possession and dispensing of controlled substances, any conviction relating to misuse of such drugs is likely – and rightly – to result in quick discipline by the state board.

Chronic inebriety or habitual use of drugs. The practice acts of some states, e.g., Alaska (15) Colorado (16), and Utah (17), specify as a ground for discipline inebriety or drug use that has affected the veterinarian's ability to practice competently. However, most states do not impose such a restriction; they permit the board to suspend or revoke a license simply on the grounds that the practitioner is chronically affected by alcohol or drugs.

Traditionally, the alcoholic or drug-dependent practitioner was viewed as fundamentally bad, as someone of obviously deficient moral character. As a growing number of states adopt programs to assist the rehabilitation of alcoholic or drug-impaired veterinarians, it can be argued that inebriety and drug dependency are coming to be viewed by the practice acts as signs of illness rather than of badness. However, even where such programs exist, the boards are still permitted a good deal of ethical deliberation. Impaired veterinarians can engage in outright immoral behavior. They can resort to illicit or illegal means to support their dependency. They can stubbornly deny their impairment and recklessly subject clients and animals to inferior care. Thus, even where a board can divert an impaired practitioner into a rehabilitation program, it usually still has the discretion to decide that he has acted so immorally that he merits punishment instead of, or in addition to, rehabilitation.

Moreover, even where a board suspends or revokes the license of an impaired practitioner and considers him to be ill rather than evil, the board is still applying the fundamental *ethical* principle that underlies the inebriety and drug dependency standard: the public has the right to expect veterinarians to function in a competent and trustworthy manner that is beyond reproach.

Use of false, misleading, or deceptive advertising. Although the First Amendment to the United States Constitution prohibits the government from banning advertising by professionals (see Chapter 17), administrative bodies are empowered to protect the public against such abuses as false, deceptive, or misleading advertising, and in-person solicitations by professionals (18). Whether a board can constitutionally discipline a veterinarian for such things as "sensational or flamboyant" (19) advertising or "demonstrations, dramatizations, or other portrayals of professional practice on radio or television" (20) remains to be decided by the courts.

Conviction of cruelty to animals [IL, NC] (21)
Practice of cruelty to animals [ID, IN, ME] (22)
Treating a patient inhumanely [MO, OK, OR] (23). Although most practice acts mention cruelty to animals as a ground for discipline, in some states the standard specifies that the veterinarian actually have been convicted of the crime of cruelty. Convictions under state cruelty statutes are rare. All criminal convictions require proof beyond a reasonable doubt and adherence to strict rules of evidence and court procedure. Moreover, animal cruelty cases are seldom a high priority in overburdened prosecutors' offices. States that specify the *practice* of cruelty to animals or inhumane treatment of patients as grounds for discipline permit the board itself to make an administrative determination of whether a practitioner has engaged in such behavior.

The employment of fraud, misrepresentation, or deception in obtaining a license to practice
Fraud or dishonesty in the application of or reporting of any test for disease in animals
Fraudulent issuance or use of any health certificate, vaccination certificate, test chart, or blank forms used in the practice of veterinary medicine to prevent the dissemination of animal disease, transportation of diseased animals, or the sale of inedible products of animal origin for human consumption [CO] (24)
Willful misrepresentation in the inspection of food for human consumption [CO] (25)
Fraud, deception, misrepresentation, dishonest, or illegal practices in or connected with the practice of veterinary medicine [CO] (26)
Failure to conduct one's practice on the highest plain of honesty, integrity, and fair dealing with one's clients in time and services rendered, and in the amount charged for services, facilities, appliances, and drugs [OK, TX, WA] (27)
Using the term "specialist" without being board certified and/or registered as a specialist with the state board [OH] (28). Provisions prohibiting deliberate fraud and misrepresentation have long been present in practice acts. The problem of fraudulent issuance of health and transportation documents will be discussed more fully in Chapter 21. However, it should be noted here that the boards can deal swiftly and effectively with this continuing problem that has embarrassed the entire profession. Most veterinarians caught issuing fraudulent documents are given temporary suspensions (usually a few months in duration) of their federal accreditation. Such a "penalty" need not seriously disrupt one's practice.

A state veterinary board, however, can temporarily – or permanently – remove one's ability to practice at all. And a state board can do this by either relying on an administrative determination of fraud by the USDA or by making its own determination that there has been fraud or misrepresentation. Likewise, the profession's increasing concern with nonboard-certified practitioners who call themselves specialists could be addressed quickly and decisively by boards that are authorized to discipline doctors for misrepresentation.

Permitting, aiding, or abetting an unlicensed person to perform activities requiring a license
Permitting another to use one's license for the purpose of treating or offering to treat sick, injured, or afflicted animals [CO] (29)
Knowingly maintaining a professional connection or association with any person who is in violation of provisions of the practice act or regulations of the board [FL] (30). There have been a number of court decisions upholding board discipline of doctors who have aided or abetted unlicensed persons to engage in the practice of veterinary medicine (31).

Guaranteeing a cure or result
Violating the professional confidences of a client
Exercising undue influence on the patient or client, including the promotion of the sale of services, goods, appliances, or drugs in such a manner as to exploit the patient or client for the financial gain of the practitioner or of a third party [NY] (32)
Paying or receiving kickbacks, rebates, bonuses, or other remuneration for receiving a patient or client or for referring a patient or client to another provider of veterinary services or goods [FL, NY] (33)
Attempting to restrict competition in the field of veterinary medicine other than for the protection of the public [FL] (34)
Knowingly engaging in an act of consumer fraud or engaging in the restraint of competition or participating in price-fixing activities [DE] (35)
Belittling or injuring the professional standing of another member of the profession or unnecessarily condemning the character of his professional acts [AR] (36)
Belittling the knowledge of another veterinarian for the purposes of monetary gain [AR] (37). These standards are intended to curtail unfair or anticompetitive business practices in which veterinarians can promote their own interests at the expense of individual clients, the public at large, or other practitioners. Although some veterinarians appear to be aware of federal laws prohibiting unfair competition and restraint of trade (see Chapter 18), few may realize that such activities are also within the purview of quite a few state boards. These boards may be able to act more swiftly and decisively than federal authorities to curb such abuses.

Engaging in lewd or immoral conduct in connection with the provision of veterinary services [AK, IN] (38). This standard appears intended to permit discipline for immoral behavior that does not necessarily reflect an inability to practice competently, but nevertheless occurs during the provision of veterinary services. It can be argued that this protects the practitioner against questionable charges about his personality and character. On the other hand, the phrase "lewd or immoral" is no less vague than "bad moral character." Moreover, requiring lewd or immoral behavior during the providing of veterinary services might sometimes subject *clients* to unfair risks by precluding discipline until an egregious act has actually occurred during the practitioner's activities as a veterinarian.

Unprofessional conduct. This may be the most important ethical standard that can be applied by the boards. In some states, the practice act or regulations list the kinds of kinds of conduct considered to be unprofessional. (Typically, these lists include such things as making fraudulent statements in one's application for a license, and false and deceptive advertising.) However, many practice acts provide no definition or examples of unprofessional conduct. In these states, the board must decide either on a case-by-case basis or after promulgation of its own regulations, what is unprofessional. Even those practice acts that do provide examples of unprofessional conduct usually do not preclude the board from finding other, nonlisted kinds of conduct to be unprofessional.

The courts have held that the phrases "unprofessional conduct" or "professional misconduct" are not impermissibly vague and can be used liberally by the boards in disciplining practitioners (39). As one court has stated, unprofessional conduct "of necessity involve(s) conduct in the common judgment dishonorable;" moreover, a profession "so long established and regulated" as veterinary medicine has developed a storehouse of shared judgments about what is professionally dishonorable (40).

A prohibition against unprofessional conduct can permit a board to discipline a veterinarian for something that may not come within the strict letter of a practice act provision or regulation but is nevertheless fundamentally incompatible with honorable practice. For example, there can be no doubt that cruelty to a patient is unprofessional conduct for a veterinarian. Therefore, it seems clear that a board could revoke or suspend a practitioner's license for engaging in behavior the board determines was cruel or inhumane, even if the practice act lists *conviction* of cruelty to animals as a ground for discipline. Likewise, even if a practice act does not explicitly mention charging clients for services not actually rendered, or putting undue pressure on clients to agree to certain procedures, or fraudulent completion of health certificates as grounds for discipline, a board could clearly find such conduct – and many other kinds of behavior as well – to be fundamentally unprofessional.

Several states have incorporated the AVMA *Principles of Veterinary Medical Ethics* into their definitions of unprofessional conduct (41). An argument can be made in favor of this approach. As shall be explained in Chapter 9, the *Principles* do reflect the profession's most fundamental judgments about what it finds "in the common judgment dishonorable." A board that adopts the *Principles* can quickly have at its disposal, and in the hands of all doctors in the state, a lengthy and familiar set of ethical guidelines.

However, there are two strong arguments against wholesale incorporation of the *Principles* into state board definitions of professional conduct.

First, as shall be explained in Chapter 9, the *Principles* are a text of official veterinary ethics, and among the most important functions of official veterinary ethics is promotion and protection of the profession. In contrast, the primary function of the state boards, and indeed of all administrative veterinary ethical activity, is protection of the public and its animals. These interests are not always consistent with those of the profession or, as we shall see, with the requirements of the *Principles*.

Second, in many states there is a legal impediment to wholesale incorporation of the *Principles* into administrative ethical standards. The constitutions of most states prohibit administrative agencies from delegating their responsibilities to others. It can be argued that blanket adoption of the entire *Principles* by a state board would violate its obligation to determine on its own what constitutes professional or ethical conduct. This argument seems quite reasonable given the fact that official ethical standards do tend by their nature to concentrate on the interests of members of the profession.

There seems no reason why the state boards should be prohibited from consulting the *Principles* as one source of standards of professional conduct, provided the boards exercise their own discretion and adopt rules that will truly protect the interests of the public and its animals.

How Active Are the Boards in Applying Ethical Standards?

It does not follow from the fact that the practice act or regulations of a state board contain ethical standards for veterinarians that the board actively enforces these standards. Therefore, in preparation of this text, I sent a questionnaire to the boards inquiring about the extent to which they enforce ethical standards. Approximately three-fourths of the boards responded.

Almost all the boards acknowledged their authority to discipline veterinarians on ethical grounds. They cited the practice act provisions setting forth ethical standards as evidence of their activity in this area. Several of the boards that responded in detail about their activities reported that the great majority of complaints filed with them allege that a veterinarian has committed an act of malpractice. Most disciplinary actions center around a finding of technical incompetence. Nevertheless, when a complaint is made that falls within the ethical standards of the practice act or regulations, it is handled procedurally as would any complaint filed with the board.

Although malpractice is the primary focus of the boards, several boards reported that the most egregious cases reported to them, those that result in license suspension or revocation, do commonly raise both technical and ethical issues. For example, in Oregon, some 97% of complaints involve purely technical matters, 2% purely ethical complaints, and 1% both technical and ethical misdeeds; but the last 3 cases resulting in revocation presented important ethical problems (A. Ehelebe, personal communication).

A few board representatives were wary of characterizing their activities as ethical, until reminded by the author that provisions of their practice acts that they do enforce (such as those prohibiting false advertising) are indisputably ethical in nature. Representatives of two boards declined to characterize any of their rules as "ethical," even though some are clearly such and do appear to be enforced by the board. One stated that ethical matters are "more appropriately the responsibility of the professional association, unless the alleged conduct appears to relate to the competent practice of veterinary medicine. ... For example, advertising is only a matter of Board consideration if it is fraudulent" (B.J. Sargent, Indiana Board of Veterinary Medical Examiners, personal communication). But fraud, of course, is not necessarily a matter of competence. Another board, whose state statutes and regulations contain a large number of ethical standards, reported that "by omission, statute and regulations do not address ethics therefore precluding involvement of the board" (P.A. Ferguson, New York State Board for Veterinary Medicine, personal communication).

My impression from such remarks is that these boards are indeed applying ethical standards – their practice acts direct them to – but are uncomfortable about using the term "ethics." This is understandable. Members of veterinary boards are likely to see themselves as experts in good medicine and not in morality. Many undoubtedly feel more comfortable deciding whether a surgical procedure was performed competently than whether a doctor acted immorally. Nevertheless, the practice acts do call upon the boards to apply and enforce ethical standards. This process may not in fact be hindered by a refusal to characterize these standards as "ethical." But the process can only be helped by so characterizing them.

Several of the boards singled out ethical issues that recently have been of special concern to them, including misleading advertising [NH] (J.B. Rausch, personal communication); claims by general practitioners that they are "specialists" [OR] (A. Ehelebe, personal communication); appropriate names for veterinary facilities [OR]

(A. Ehelebe, personal communication), [PA] (A.J. Matthews, personal communication); fraudulent alteration of patient records [OR] (A. Ehelebe, personal communication); dispensing of caution legend prescription drugs to purchasers without a doctor-patient relationship [PA] (A.J. Matthews, personal communication); and failure of some doctors to inform patients of the availability of tests and other treatment options in a caring and considerate manner [VA] (M. Lux, personal communication).

BENEFITS OF THE ADMINISTRATIVE APPLICATION
OF ETHICAL STANDARDS

There are many potential benefits of the administrative application of ethical standards. It is usually much easier for a client to make a complaint of an ethical nature to an administrative agency than in a court of law. Veterinarians cannot be sued simply because they have acted unethically or unprofessionally; their actions must also have resulted in some compensable injury or damage to the client. Even where a client could prove such damage, it may cost him more to prosecute the case than he could ever win in a trial. In contrast, administrative agencies typically permit a simple written complaint or telephone call to initiate an investigation, the costs of which are then borne by the agency.

Court trials and appeals can also stretch on for years, leaving both accused and accuser on tenterhooks. Most administrative agencies are not encumbered by rigid court procedures or rules of evidence and can resolve complaints and disputes relatively quickly. To the veterinarian, an administrative agency can also provide an audience that is more sensitive to the realities of veterinary practice than a civil court jury. Veterinary boards are composed largely (and in some states entirely) of fellow practitioners. Such people may be able quickly to see through unjust complaints. An administrative agency may also be able to settle a dispute or remedy a problem with a minimum of publicity.

Of course, the most significant potential advantage of the administrative application of ethical standards is that administrative bodies can *compel* adherence to moral norms. The AVMA or state veterinary association, for example, may suspend or revoke the membership of someone who behaves unethically. However, the veterinary board can suspend or revoke his license to practice, or impose a wide spectrum of other incentives, ranging from censure to continuing supervision to (in some states) a fine.

PROBLEMS IN THE ADMINISTRATIVE APPLICATION
OF ETHICAL STANDARDS

Unfortunately, some of the advantages of administrative application of ethical standards pose potential problems as well. Where people can complain against veterinarians with minimal trouble and expense, practitioners may find themselves easily exposed to frivolous or malicious complaints. Rigid rules of court procedure and evidence may sometimes delay discovery of the truth or resolution of a complaint. But these rules also protect the accused against allegations that cannot be substantiated or against accusers who cannot be cross-examined. The ability of a government agency to bear the costs of its investigation may assist complaining clients. However, this can be a disaster to a veterinarian, whose malpractice insurance does not cover legal fees for representation before an administrative agency or before a court to which the agency's decision may be appealed.

Application of ethical standards by the veterinary boards can pose special problems. A board's power to take away the ability to earn a living in one's chosen profession is frightening enough. But in addition, the boards can do this by appealing to a number of standards that are exceptionally vague, or that give them virtually unbridled discretion to apply their own moral values.

What, after all, *is* bad moral character or unprofessional conduct? People can disagree about these things. Some may find bad moral character in a veterinarian who demonstrates against nuclear power by trespassing on the property of a nuclear plant, while others may see in the same behavior a brave moral act. For some, homosexuality is a vice utterly inconsistent with good moral character, while for others it is a disease, and for still others merely a different lifestyle. For some, a veterinarian who advertises on radio or television is behaving unprofessionally; others find such a criticism preposterous. Opinions about good moral character and professional conduct also change over time. In the 1950s, several physicians had their licenses suspended by their medical board after they were found in contempt of Congress for refusing to cooperate with the House Committee on Un-American Activities (42). Such a response would be highly unlikely today. In the 1940s, the AVMA denounced *all* advertising aimed at obtaining patronage "as unethical and unprofessional" (43), and in 1954 condemned the use of professional envelopes and stationery containing portraits or drawings of animals as "unprofessional and unethical" (44). Today these views seem extreme.

A veterinarian accused of bad moral character or unprofessional conduct, or threatened with revocation of his license on the grounds that he has been convicted of a felony, a crime involving moral turpitude, or any crime, may wonder whether he is being subjected to standards that simply reflect the moral tastes of his place and time.

A TASK FOR ADMINISTRATIVE VETERINARY ETHICS

The answer to these potential difficulties is not for administrative agencies to turn their backs on ethics and to restrict themselves to purely technical concerns. The public has a right not only to technically competent veterinarians but also to doctors who are honest, trustworthy, and compassionate. The public and its animals must rely on some governmental intervention to promote these ideals. Good moral character and professional conduct are *not* irrelevant or outdated concepts because there have been some disagreements about how these concepts should be applied.[c] Many of the ethical standards enforced by administrative bodies, such as prohibitions against theft, fraud, and illegal use of dangerous drugs, are unambiguous and clearly legitimate.

Careful study of current and proposed administrative ethical standards may help governmental bodies to articulate moral standards that reflect the legitimate interests of the public and its animals, without infringing unduly upon veterinarians' personal taste and lifestyles.

REFERENCES

1. Davis KC: *Administrative Law Text.* ed 3. St. Paul, MN: West Publishing Co., 1972, p 1.

---

[c]At the time of this writing, Oregon and Virginia were in the process of removing the good moral character requirement from their practice act or regulations.

2. Ill. Rev. Stat. 1983. Veterinary Medicine and Surgery Practice Act of 1983, § 7008.
3. UTAH CODE ANN. § 58-28-4(1) (1981).
4. Raymond v. Board of Registration in Medicine, 443 N.E.2d 391 (Mass. 1982).
5. Cartwright v. Board of Chiropractic Examiners, 548 P.2d 1134 (Cal. 1976).
6. Annotation: Physician's conviction of offense not directly related to medical practice as ground of disciplinary action. 12 ALR3d 1213, 1216-1219.
7. Annotation: Alcoholism, narcotics addiction, or misconduct with respect to alcoholic beverages, as ground for revocation or suspension of license to practice medicine or dentistry. 93 ALR2d 1398.
8. CAL. BUS. & PROF. CODE § 4883(a) (West 1987); FLA. STAT. § 474.214(c) (1986); IND. CODE § 15-5-1.1-22.1(b)(2) (1985).
9. Thorpe v. Board of Examiners in Veterinary Medicine, 163 Cal.Rptr. 382, 385 (Cal. App. 1980).
10. Raymond v. Board of Registration in Medicine, 443 N.E.2d 391, 395 (Mass. 1982).
11. Id. at 394, quoting Lawrence v. Board of Registration in Medicine, 132 N.E. 174 (Mass. 1921).
12. Raymond v. Board of Registration in Medicine, 443 N.E.2d 391 (Mass. 1982); N.Y. EDUCATION LAW, tit. VIII, Art. 130, Subart. 3, § 6509(5)(a).
13. See, e.g., Barsky v. Board of Regents of the University of New York, 11 N.E.2d 222, 226 (N.Y. 1953), aff'd 347 U.S. 442, 452 (1954); Matter of Erdman v. Board of Regents of the State of New York, 24 A.D.2d 698 (3d Dept. 1965); Raymond v. Board of Registration in Medicine, 443 N.E.2d 391 (Mass. 1982).
14. Thorpe v. Board of Board of Examiners in Veterinary Medicine, 163 Cal.Rptr. 382, 385 (Cal. App. 1980).
15. ALASKA STAT. § 08.98.235(7)(B) (1980).
16. COLO. REV. STAT. § 12-64-111(v) (1983).
17. UTAH CODE ANN. § 58-28-2(6)(b) (1981).
18. Bates v. State Bar of Arizona, 433 U.S. 350 (1977).
19. Rules of The New York State Board of Regents Relating to Definitions of Unprofessional Conduct, 1985. § 29.1(b)(12)(i)(a).
20. Id. § 29.1(12)(iv).
21. ILL. REV. STAT. 1986. Veterinary Medicine and Surgery Act of 1983. § 7025(V); N.C. GEN. STAT., Art. II, Chapt. 90 § .0205(b)(12) (1982-83).
22. IDAHO CODE tit. 54, Chapt. 21, § 54-2112(12) (1984); IND. CODE § 15-5-1.1-22.1(b)(7) (1985); ME. REV. STAT. ANN tit. 32, Chapt. 71-A, § 4864 (9) 1983.
23. MO. REV. STAT. § 340.145(17)(1981); Rules of Professional Conduct of the Oklahoma Veterinary Practice Act (59 OS 1981 § 698.7), § 17 (1986); Veterinary Medical Examining Board, Oregon Administrative Rules, § 875-10-060(10)(1986).
24. COLO. REV. STAT. § 12-64-111(f) (1983).
25. COLO. REV. STAT. § 12-64-111(e) (1983).
26. COLO. REV. STAT. § 12-64-111(d) (1983).
27. Rules of Professional Conduct of the Oklahoma Veterinary Practice Act (59 OS 1981 § 698.7), § 18 (1986); Rules of Professional Conduct of the Texas State Board of Veterinary Medical Examiners, § 19 (1986); Chapt. 308-150 WAC. Washington Veterinary Board of Governors – Veterinary Code of Professional Conduct/Ethics. § 014 (1986).
28. 1984 Ohio Administrative Rules § 4741-1-02(C).
29. COLO. REV. STAT. § 12-64-111(s) (1983).
30. FLA. STAT. § 474.214(k) (1986).

31. See, e.g., In re Walker's License, 300 N.W. 800 (Minn. 1941); Hannah H:
    Professional association with unlicensed persons. *J Am Vet Med Assoc* 189:510-
    511, 1986.
32. *Rules of The New York State Board of Regents Relating to Definitions of
    Unprofessional Conduct*, 1981. § 29.1(b)(2).
33. FLA. STAT. § 474.214(l) (1986); *Rules of The New York State Board of Regents
    Relating to Definitions of Unprofessional Conduct*, 1981. § 29.1(b)(3).
34. FLA. STAT. § 474.214(o) (1986).
35. 24 Del. Laws § 3313(a)(6) (1984).
36. Arkansas Veterinary Medical Practice Act. Act 650 of 1975. Unprofessional
    Conduct. § H.
37. Arkansas Veterinary Medical Practice Act. Act 650 of 1975. Unprofessional
    Conduct. § I.
38. ALASKA STAT. § 08.98.235(8) (1980); IND. CODE § 15-5-1.1-22.1(b)(5) (1985).
39. E.g., Megdal v. Oregon State Board of Dental Examiners, 586 P.2d 816 (Or.App.
    1978); Matter of Bell v. Board of Regents, 65 N.E.2d 184 (N.Y. 1946).
40. In re Walker's License, 300 N.W. 800 at 802 (Minn. 1941).
41. E.g., *Rules and Regulations of the Idaho Board of Veterinary Medicine*, § E.1,
    ¶ 10; *Pennsylvania Veterinary Medicine Practice Act and Regulations*, 63 P.S.
    § 485.5(2) and 49 Pa. Code § 31.21.
42. Barsky *et al.* v. Board of Regents of The University of New York, 111 N.E.2d
    222 (N.Y. 1953).
43. *Code of Ethics of the American Veterinary Medical Association. J Am Vet Med
    Assoc* 96:92, 1940.
44. Proceedings of the Business Sessions and Preconvention Conference. *J Am Vet
    Med Assoc* 126:63, 1955.

Chapter

8

The Nature and Functions of Official Veterinary Ethics

Official veterinary ethics is the process of the articulation and application of ethical standards for practitioners by organized veterinary medicine.

Official veterinary ethics is a rich and complex enterprise. This chapter presents an overview of its substantive standards, its functions, and the structure in which national, state, local, and practice associations contribute to the process. Chapter 9 will focus on the most important texts of official veterinary ethics, the Veterinarian's Oath and the *Principles of Veterinary Medical Ethics*.

THE NATURE OF OFFICIAL PROFESSIONAL ETHICS

It is no accident that professions such as veterinary medicine, law, and medicine have developed procedures by which members articulate and enforce ethical standards for themselves. It is the process of self-imposed regulation, both ethical and technical, that distinguishes what we call the learned professions from occupations. The engineer or business executive may learn his trade at an accredited school, may be regulated by governmental bodies, and may join associations that promote his interests. But his training and supervision differ markedly from that of the veterinarian, lawyer, or physician. The latter attended a school the curriculum of which must meet the expectations of the respective organized professions, and indeed are unlikely to be approved by licensing authorities unless they meet these expectations. Although professionals must be licensed to practice and are regulated by governmental bodies, these bodies give great deference to what the organized professions deem to be appropriate behavior – from the choice of acceptable schools and training programs, to the standards of competence expected of practitioners, to the values that define acceptable professional behavior.

Most important, fields traditionally recognized as professions have a long history of officially agreeing upon ethical codes expressing their most central moral ideals.[a] And they have invested these codes with dignity and importance by creating and enforcing them much as the law creates and enforces: code standards are adopted by formal vote of representatives of the profession, and they are applied by quasi-judicial bodies that resemble courts of law. The ethical self-regulation of a profession like veterinary medicine is so central to the definition of an individual as a *veterinarian* that even a practitioner who does not choose to belong to the AVMA (like a lawyer who does not join the American Bar Association) will have great difficulty convincing a court of law or administrative body that the official ethical standards do not apply to him.

WHAT OFFICIAL VETERINARY ETHICS IS NOT

Although official veterinary ethics by its very nature involves veterinarians deciding upon and applying ethical standards for veterinarians, there are several things that official ethics does not entail.

First, an official decision that some kind of behavior is right or wrong does not make that conduct right or wrong. Veterinarians, like other human beings, can be mistaken in their moral judgments and therefore can be mistaken in their official ethical pronouncements.

Second, neither veterinarians nor the public need view the official ethical apparatus as the sole or the final judge of ethical issues involving practitioners. Administrative bodies, for example, must come to their own conclusions about the propriety of certain kinds of behavior by veterinarians. Veterinarians can also regard official standards as open to debate in forums in which veterinarians do not control the outcome. But such discussions cannot be considered part of the process of official veterinary ethics, although changes in official standards made *by veterinarians* motivated by discussion with nonveterinarians can be part of official professional ethics.

Third, although decisions regarding official ethics must be controlled by veterinarians, there is nothing that prevents nonveterinarians from observing or participating in the process of developing and applying official standards. Ethicists, lawyers, and members of the public and the other learned professions can be consulted about (and might even be given limited voting power regarding) official norms.

WHO NEEDS OFFICIAL VETERINARY ETHICS?

Because official standards need not coincide with moral truth, several philosophers have questioned the wisdom of allowing the professions to engage in official ethics. Medical ethicist Robert Veatch, for example, concludes that official

---

[a]The significance of formal ethical codes is illustrated by the fact that such groups as real estate brokers (1), social workers (2), and librarians (3), which are not traditionally included among the learned professions, have adopted official ethical codes to enhance their own self-image and the regard of the public for their technical and ethical virtues.

professional ethics "can have *no* ethical bite" (4). "The fact that a professional or his or her group believes that a confidence should be kept, a patient killed, or an advertisement proscribed cannot definitively resolve the issue of whether each of these acts is ethically or legally right" (5). Veatch finds it "strange that lay people and professionals alike assume that it is correct for professions to form their own codes of ethics and then adjudicate ethical disputes arising out of the application of these codes" (6). Issues of professional ethics, Veatch insists, should be the business not only of professionals, but of the clients they serve and indeed of anyone who is affected by their actions.

Veatch is surely correct that official decisions cannot be the sole means of resolving ethical questions regarding professionals. It is also possible that, in the past, some in the professions and the public have granted official ethics too much authority in the moral arena. However, official ethics still has a useful role in addressing ethical concerns.

One important benefit of official ethics is its ability to address moral issues effectively and efficiently. Neither government nor the populace has the time or resources to constantly monitor the ethical values of any of the professions. The public may take an interest in certain flashy issues (such as animal experimentation). But its attention to such matters can be fleeting, and it may never focus sustained attention on some of the less conspicuous ethical issues arising from everyday professional practice.

Official veterinary ethics offers an apparatus that is continuously in place, raising questions and suggesting solutions. Often, the apparatus can effectively compel adherence to ethical norms without expenditure of resources by government or by disgruntled clients or members of the public. If government or the public likes what they see, they can leave the process of official ethics alone. If society has questions about the official ethical positions of the profession, it can ask the profession to justify its standards. By demanding reasons or justifications from the profession as a whole, the public can expect informed and carefully-presented responses prepared with the resources available to the official apparatus.

The following are just two examples that illustrate the value of official veterinary ethics.

In 1977, the United States Supreme Court held for the first time that professionals have a constitutionally protected right to advertise (7). The Court also stated that certain kinds of inappropriate advertising could be prohibited by government or the professions. However, the Court deliberately refrained from defining or listing all kinds of advertising that could be proscribed, leaving suggestions for new legal standards to future cases and emerging attitudes. Like other professions, veterinary medicine had to reconsider many of its previous disapprovals of advertising and had to search for new ethical rules that would meet yet undefined constitutional requirements. By allowing veterinary medicine to discover new advertising standards, the law gained several benefits. First, it could count on the official apparatus to assure that the old blanket prohibitions against advertising were not enforced. Second, the law could call on the official apparatus to do something courts are rarely good at, the process of changing entrenched values and nurturing over time new attitudes consistent with new freedoms. Finally, the law could ask the profession to begin looking for ethical standards that reflect not just the legal right to advertise but the specific ethical needs and concerns of veterinarians. In the decade since the decision permitting professional advertising, this process of probing the limits of professionally acceptable marketing by the official ethical apparatus has continued. Should the courts have to decide how far the profession can go in limiting professional marketing, they will have at their disposal a substantial body of official ethical deliberations, contained both in the Advertising Regulations of the *Principles of Veterinary Medical Ethics* and in pronouncements of the AVMA Judicial Council, to assist them.

A second valuable use of official veterinary ethics involves its ability to resolve disputes before they result in lawsuits or government action. As we have seen, malpractice cases against veterinarians are sometimes brought because clients believe their veterinarian has acted unethically. By settling some of these complaints, state ethics and grievance committees and the AVMA Judicial Council can spare veterinarians and clients unnecessary and costly litigation. Resolution of ethical issues by the official professional apparatus can sometimes also make intervention by the state veterinary board unnecessary.

In addition to its effectiveness in addressing moral disputes, official veterinary ethics plays a crucial role in binding together doctors as a unified profession that can speak forcefully both to members and the public. This cohesiveness enables the profession to improve the competence of practitioners, by helping it to promote strong veterinary school curricula, effective continuing education programs, dissemination of knowledge, and veterinary research. As part of the cement that strengthens the profession, official veterinary ethics contributes to *better medicine* for patients and clients.

OVERVIEW OF THE SUBSTANTIVE STANDARDS
OF OFFICIAL VETERINARY ETHICS

The following are the more important substantive standards that are utilized by official veterinary ethics.

The Veterinarian's Oath

The Veterinarian's Oath expresses the most general values of the profession. Professional oaths are not intended to provide a decision-procedure for the solution of all ethical issues. They are offered to inspire a sensitivity to key goals and values.

Principles of Veterinary Medical Ethics

This is the definitive statement of the profession's official ethical standards. Like the codes of other professions, the *Principles* are an amalgam of general ideals and specific requirements and prohibitions.

Adjudications, Advisory Opinions, and Statements
of Official Judicial Bodies

Those bodies that apply the official code and other standards to particular cases make different kinds of judgments, which can take on independent significance in the enunciation of official standards.

An *adjudication* is an official response to an actual complaint against a member of the professional association. Adjudications are often accompanied by an expression of a general principle justifying the decision. When reports of adjudications are disseminated to the profession, they can serve as general warnings about (or approvals of) the kinds of behavior involved in the particular case.

An *advisory opinion* is a pronouncement by a judicial body, not part of an adjudication of an actual complaint, regarding a matter about which ethical guidance has been requested. Advisory opinions can be prompted by the request of a practitioner or association about the appropriateness of some activity in which they would like to engage. An advisory opinion can also be sought after some conduct has occurred, but which is raised hypothetically to the judicial body with the hope of bringing a practitioner into line before a formal complaint must be brought. Advisory opinions can apply to specific individual practitioners or to very general kinds of behavior. Like adjudications, advisory opinions can put practitioners on notice about what the judicial body is likely to do if confronted with a certain kind of situation.

A judicial body can also issue statements at its own instigation expressing its concern about certain kinds of behavior that have come to its attention.

Official Policies and Guidelines

Veterinary associations can also adopt official policies, approved by the representative body, on ethical issues. A policy can contain recommendations that practitioners are strongly urged to follow, or may contain definitive prohibitions that can be applied in official disciplinary proceedings. The AVMA has adopted a lengthy set of policies and guidelines that provide supplementation to the *Principles* and stand in their own right as important standards of official veterinary ethics.[b]

Official Positions and Recommendations

These are statements made on behalf of the organization that may, but are not required to be, adopted by vote of the representative body. The AVMA has issued a number of positions and recommendations, including several contained in its booklets, *The Veterinarian's Role in Companion Animal Welfare* and *The Veterinarian's Role in Food Animal Welfare*. Official positions and recommendations can be as specific as the statement of the former publication that "AVMA declares that declawing of domestic cats is justifiable when the cat cannot be trained to refrain from using its claws destructively" (8). Positions can also express very general ethical values such as the declaration of the booklet on food animal welfare that veterinarians are

---

[b]These are reprinted in the AVMA *Directory* and include the Guidelines on Acupuncture, Guidelines on Emergency Veterinary Service, AVMA Guidelines for Horseshow Veterinarians, Guidelines on Pet Health Insurance and Other Third Party Animal Health Plans, Guidelines for Referrals, AVMA Position on Animal Health Certificates, AVMA Position on Presigned Health Certificates, AVMA Position on Animal Population Control and Ovariohysterectomy Clinics, Wild or Exotic Animals as Pets, AVMA Guidelines for Veterinary Associations and Veterinarians Working with Humane Associations, and Guidelines for Animal-Facilitated Therapy Programs.

"obligated morally, ethically, and philosophically to utilize the sciences in every form to encourage the best possible attitudes and practices toward the welfare of all creatures of the animal kingdom" (9).[c]

Reports and Statements of Delegated Bodies

Veterinary associations such as the AVMA also have standing councils or committees and specially designated bodies or panels that can issue statements and recommendations of an ethical nature. Because these bodies can be delegated the responsibility to issue such statements by the association, their opinions can represent the views of a portion of the official organizational apparatus. Statements of delegated bodies can be proposed to the representative body for inclusion into the ethical code or an official policy statement.

THE ACTIVITIES OF OFFICIAL VETERINARY ETHICS

Self-regulation

Self-regulation is the process by which veterinary associations encourage adherence to official norms. There are many different ways self-regulation can occur, including the formal disciplining of a particular practitioner, putting informal (and sometimes friendly) pressure on a member to behave properly, and the issuance of official policy statements or additions to the AVMA *Principles*. Self-regulation can be initiated by request of a fellow professional, a client, a member of the public, or by a unit of government such as a state board of veterinary medicine.

Education

Among the most important functions of official veterinary ethics is educating veterinary students and practitioners about official standards. Education prevents future violations and makes the process of self-regulation, which can deal effectively only with a limited number of cases, possible. Like self-regulation, ethical education can proceed in many ways, ranging from formal courses in the veterinary schools, to lectures on ethics sponsored by state associations or veterinary conventions, to statements on ethical issues by officers or representatives of professional associations.

Because the veterinary schools are charged with the task not only of servicing the needs of the organized profession, but also of advancing knowledge in all areas relating to veterinary practice, the schools have a two-fold role in the ethical arena. They must inform students about the official ethical standards. But they must also

---

[c]In a section entitled "Guiding Principles," both publications make the curious statement that "AVMA positions are concerned primarily with the scientific aspects of the medical well-being of animals. It is also recognized that certain ethical, philosophical, and moral values must be considered." In fact, there is at least as much ethics as science in the positions articulated in these booklets. That ethical positions include technical information or recommendations makes them no less ethical, and their adoption no less a part of official veterinary ethics.

encourage the development of objective principles of normative veterinary ethics, a process that can involve critical examination of official standards.

Providing Forums for Discussion of Official Norms

An essential component of official veterinary ethics is the promotion of forums in which veterinarians can consider present and proposed official ethical standards. Such forums can include commentary and letters to the editor sections of professional journals, public debates, and discussions among differing groups in the profession.

Expressing Professional Values and Ethical Concerns to Nonveterinarians

Another important function of official veterinary ethics is expressing the profession's official ethical values and viewpoints to members of the public, other professions, and government. An example of such an activity was the successful effort of the AVMA to persuade the FDA to abandon its proposed policy prohibiting all extra-label use of drugs in food animals (see Chapter 21).

THE STRUCTURE OF OFFICIAL VETERINARY ETHICS

What Are the Component Organizations of Official Ethics?

Because it is the *profession* that articulates and applies standards of official ethics, only groups that can be said to be part of the organized profession can be considered components of official ethics. There can be no disagreement that the AVMA and the state and local veterinary medical associations recognized by the AVMA are part of the structure of official veterinary ethics. All these organizations are recognized by the great majority of veterinarians not as limited groups seeking to promote some kind of viewpoint or platform, but as parts of a national apparatus that in its totality speaks for the profession. Moreover, the AVMA and state and local associations all subscribe to a universal code of ethics for all American practitioners, the AVMA *Principles*.

There may, however, be uncertainty about whether to include certain independent associations of veterinarians within the official ethical apparatus. One might, for example, be inclined to include the American Association of Feline Practitioners, but then wonder whether it would be fair to exclude the American Association of Wildlife Veterinarians. (At the time of this writing, the former organization was granted representation in the AVMA House of Delegates while the latter was not.) It is, surely, a process for the profession itself to decide what groups will be considered part of its official apparatus for the purposes of articulating ethical standards. This process is an ongoing one: a group that today might not be considered part of the apparatus or on the borderline might tomorrow be recognized as part of it. For the purposes of this discussion, I want to suggest that, at the very least, any association that has representation in the AVMA House of Delegates be considered a component of the organized profession and therefore capable of taking part in official veterinary ethics. Such representation is a sign that an organization is considered a part of the organic whole of the profession.[d]

The fact that an organization can qualify as a proponent of official ethical standards does not mean that it is or should be active in the ethical area. Moreover, the fact that an organization is not part of the official apparatus does not mean that the profession should ignore its views in formulating official norms.

The American Veterinary Medical Association

The Principles of Veterinary Medical Ethics state that "(i)deally, questions of ethical behavior on the part of a veterinarian should be considered and dealt with by the local association's ethics or grievance committees" which "are familiar with local customs and circumstances, and are in a position to talk to all parties concerned" (10).

Although it is surely the case that ethical issues usually can be handled most effectively at the local level, the AVMA remains the foundation for all of official veterinary ethics. When local, state, or practice associations do act to discipline a practitioner or take a position on an ethical issue, it is the AVMA *Principles* and other official AVMA ethical pronouncements that they generally apply. (The *Principles* themselves urge veterinary associations to "adopt the AVMA *Principles* ... or a similar code" (11); because there is no other such code, it is not surprising that the *Principles* are followed.) Another reason component associations look to the national standards is that these organizations are represented in the AVMA House of Delegates and therefore play a role in the adoption of these standards. Finally, the AVMA Judicial Council is very much a general reviewing body on issues of veterinary ethics throughout the profession. The Council hears cases referred by constituent associations; it is asked to provide definitive opinions about the appropriateness of certain kinds of behavior; and it is charged with the preparation of annotations and amendments to the universally-adopted *Principles*.

The Judicial Council is the chief self-regulatory arm of the AVMA regarding official ethics. It consists of five active members elected by the House of Delegates and has "jurisdiction on all questions of veterinary medical ethics" (12). The Council can investigate complaints of an ethical nature by itself or can request the AVMA President to appoint "investigating juries" to which it can refer complaints or evidence regarding unethical conduct "which in its judgment are of a serious and substantial nature" (13). Such juries can then file complaints under the formal *Rules of Disciplinary Procedures of the AVMA* (14). These set forth the procedures by which the Judicial Council hears and adjudicates complaints. The *General Appellate*

---

[d]Article VI, Section 1 of the *AVMA Bylaws* provides criteria for representation in the House of Delegates. By 1988, the following practice associations were included: the American Animal Hospital Association; the American Associations of Avian Pathologists, Bovine Practitioners, Equine Practitioners, Food Hygiene Veterinarians, Industrial Veterinarians, Sheep and Goat Practitioners, Swine Practitioners, and Veterinary Clinicians; the American Society of Laboratory Animal Practitioners; the National Association of Federal Veterinarians; and the Society for Theriogenology. Beginning in 1988, the American Association of Feline Practitioners and the Association of Avian Veterinarians joined the list (15).

Procedures of the AVMA (16) contain rules for reconsideration of an adjudication by the Judicial Council and appeal to the AVMA Board of Governors.

The Judicial Council can make five kinds of adjudication: acquittal, censure, probation, suspension, or expulsion from the AVMA. However, the Council is not restricted to the explicit provisions of the *Principles of Veterinary Medical Ethics* or of official AVMA ethical pronouncements. It may also discipline a member who has been convicted of a "felony or a crime involving moral ineptitude"[e] or who has been "guilty of other behavior detrimental to the profession of veterinary medicine" (17).

The notion of being "detrimental" to the profession is vague and could conceivably be used in ways some might find arbitrary. Nevertheless, this provision is an important tool for the advancement of official veterinary ethics. It allows the Council to explore and define new principles much as courts do, by responding on a case-by-case basis to situations that may not be covered by existing rules.

The Judicial Council makes its views known to the profession in regular reports in the *JAVMA*. These reports provide the best evidence of what ethical issues the organized profession finds most pressing and how official norms are likely to develop. They show that for several years the major concern of official ethics has remained the proper limits of advertising, promotion, and marketing (18). For example, in its September 1986 meeting, the Council took the following actions (19): In response to a complaint by several practitioners against a colleague, it determined that it is unethical to sell "professional-type products" (i.e., those intended for use by veterinarians) without the existence of a veterinarian-client relationship. The Council issued an advisory opinion that an advertisement for a "surgical consultation-referral service" is likely to create the impression that the advertiser is a specialist and ruled that only board-certified specialists may use such a designation. The Council ruled that a veterinarian's proposed promotional involvement in an animal mortality insurance program would be unprofessional. The Council also adopted as a long-range goal the revision of the *Principles* "to simplify some of the complicated legalistic terminology and to eliminate the ambiguities." (This project was attempted in 1988. See chapter 9.) Two proposed (and subsequently enacted) amendments to the *Principles* were approved. One adds a prohibition against "advertising of discounts and discounted fees." The other replaces the old ban on displays in waiting rooms, eliminated from the *Principles* in 1986, with permission to display professional veterinary products in the waiting room. However, display of nonprofessional products would be considered "undesirable" but "permissible if such nonprofessional products are generally unavailable or are difficult to obtain in the general vicinity of the client being served."

It is impossible to relate here even a representative sampling of the activities of other bodies of the AVMA in the arena of official ethics. The following are just a few examples of such activity in 1986: development of an AVMA position statement on laboratory animal standards by the Council on Research (20); recommendations for further research and action by the Committee on the Human/Companion Animal Bond (21); a statement of concern by the Advisory Board on Specialties about general practitioners who represent themselves as specialists (22); a resolution of the

---

[e]Because this statement seems patterned after similar veterinary practice act provisions, the words "moral turpitude" are probably intended. "Ineptitude" is an inappropriate term because it denotes lack of skill rather than badness.

House of Delegates denouncing the holding of a university dean as a political hostage in Lebanon (23); representation at a White House Conference on Small Business at which the AVMA's concerns about competition from humane societies were raised (24); and a resolution of the Drug Availability Committee urging the AVMA to support a policy of increased veterinary supervision of animal drug use (25).

Finally, any overview of official veterinary ethics must mention the role of the *Journal of the American Veterinary Medical Association* not only in disseminating information about official activities in the ethical arena, but in presenting lively and provocative offerings on ethical issues.

State and Local Veterinary Medical Associations

One of the most important tasks students of official veterinary ethics must undertake is to examine the activities of the various state and local veterinary medical associations in the ethical arena. Such activities are rarely reported in national professional journals. However, my own survey of official ethics on the state and local levels indicates that there is a good deal of diversity and experimentation. Associations around the country might profit from information about what other associations are doing by way of applying ethical standards.

In preparation of this chapter, in late 1986 I asked a representative group (approximately one-half) of the state associations to describe their ethical activities and concerns. I asked whether they have their own ethical codes or standards, whether they have formal procedures governing ethical complaints, what sorts of issues are likely to be addressed in such complaints, and whether there are ethical issues of specific interest to the association.

All associations that responded in detail indicated that they have adopted the AVMA *Principles* as their ethical code. One, the Ohio VMA, includes among its official charges to its Ethics and Grievance Committee, recommending changes in the *Principles* if these are believed advisable. The Ohio VMA has also issued five detailed statements of concern about particular issues. One statement, addressing ethical issues in practice management, notes that "isolated incidents of poor marketing practices, poor interpersonal communication, less than adequate performance, higher than necessary fees, lack of professionalism and other factors continue to create client dissatisfaction." The statement recommends client surveys and analysis of state veterinary medical board complaints, and liaison to the state veterinary school and appropriate committees of the association (B. Madison, personal communication).

Most, but not all, associations have formal ethics committees. The New Jersey VMA committee had been allowed to expire but was being reorganized at the time of this writing (S.B. Weiner, personal communication). In the District of Columbia, where there are few private practitioners, a formal committee is considered unnecessary; ethical issues seldom arise, and those that do can be resolved by verbal communication to the individual practitioner from a delegation of one or more association members (D.E. Davidson, personal communication).

Associations with formal ethics committees vary in the procedure by which complaints are handled. In Ohio, which has 39 local associations, complaints registered with the state VMA are referred first to the appropriate local association, and are considered by the state group only if this process does not result in resolution. In Illinois, the state Judicial Committee, which has jurisdiction in all questions involving the interpretation of veterinary medical ethics, can appoint an investigating jury after a complaint signed by one or more members. If such a jury finds there is probable cause for action, the Chairman of the association Board of Directors may appoint a prosecutor to present charges before the Judicial Committee, which then conducts a formal hearing at which the accused may defend himself in person or by counsel (26; E.C. Larocca, personal communication). When complaints of an ethical nature are received by the Michigan VMA, the chairman of the Ethics and Grievance Committee, the executive director, or a designated representative determines whether the complaint is against a member, a nonmember veterinarian, or a nonveterinarian. Association rules provide for several possible alternatives for each category. Regarding complaints against members, the matter is first referred to the local Ethics and Grievance Committee, it being "highly recommended that a board of at least three veterinarians review each complaint. Mediation and resolution at the local level is strongly advised" (27; P.A. Prescott, personal communication). In Kansas, complaints are handled directly by the ethics committee chairman and executive director (H.K. Caley, personal communication).

If a complaint alleges malpractice or appears to raise legal issues, all associations indicated that they would refer the matter directly to the state board. However, some associations seem more likely than others to refer certain kinds of ethical complaints to their state board. The Florida VMA reports having referred only one complaint to the state board, and that involved malpractice (H.L. Gore, personal communication). The Kansas VMA refers all ethics problems that are not settled by the ethics committee or the executive director. In Illinois, ethical complaints will be referred to the board only if the accused is not a member of the association. In Wisconsin, most complaints of an ethical nature are either brought in the first instance before the state board or will be referred there by the VMA (W.J. O'Rourke, personal communication).

Among the issues that have been of greatest concern to the associations are the practice of veterinary medicine by lay persons (e.g., embryo transfer), cut-rate vaccination clinics, drastically reduced fees accompanied by hidden costs, and the practice of veterinary medicine by lay staff during the absence of the veterinarian [Georgia] (J.T. Mercer, personal communication); improper marketing of veterinary services [Illinois]; use and retention of records by a veterinarian after he joins or opens another practice [New Hampshire] (J. Zezula, personal communication); and advertising in yellow pages, newspapers, and by direct mail [Michigan].

There are several matters about which many of the associations seem to agree.

First, few associations regularly refer cases to the AVMA. This appears to indicate that the associations are indeed doing the great bulk of the actual application of official standards, and that the ethical activities of the associations deserve more sustained study than they have received thus far.

Second, while the AVMA Judicial Council tends to consider matters raised by practitioners, most complaints to state and local associations appear to be filed by clients. Moreover, most of these complaints arise from a failure in communication between veterinarian and client, or a perception that the practitioner was rude, insensitive, or had a bad "bedside manner."

Third, many ethical complaints are settled quickly. A client may simply need to talk to someone to vent his anger. A veterinarian may just need to be confronted by a committee of his peers to change his ways. When both sides are heard, the charges may not be as bad as first reported, and there may be a logical explanation or solution that can satisfy all concerned. Interestingly, several of the associations indicated that they had recently utilized formal rules and proceedings, but that these cases involved complaints by one member or members against a fellow member.

Finally, the potential for lawsuits against members who participate in ethics committee proceedings seems to have discouraged several of the associations from becoming as active as they would like to be in this area. Several were considering asking their state legislatures to enact statutes prohibiting such suits, or requesting liability insurers to provide coverage for ethics committee actions. As the District of Columbia VMA reported, "cost and [lack of] availability of association liability insurance threatens to take the teeth out of most punitive actions [and] we will generally have to rely on more persuasive measures and educational programs"(D.E. Davidson, personal communication). If such concerns are shared throughout the country, the profession may lose its control over the behavior of members, unless it can obtain adequate and affordable association liability insurance.

Practice Associations

Practice associations, whose activities are delineated by kinds of veterinary activity rather than by geographical borders, bring to the articulation of official standards especially valuable points of view. The interests of these organizations transcend regional issues but are at the same time more focused than those of the AVMA. Practice associations can articulate their own ethical rules, which can even contradict the ethical standards of other associations or the AVMA itself. For example, the American Animal Hospital Association adopted an official policy permitting the display of nonprofessional products in waiting rooms, although such behavior was prohibited at the time by the AVMA *Principles*. Practice associations can also set up their own official apparatus to assure ethical behavior. The American Association of Equine Practitioners, for example, has its own ethics committee that has disciplined members for violations of moral standards (R. J. Sheehan, personal communication).

REFERENCES

1. *Code of Ethics of the National Association of Realtors.* In Gorlin RA (ed): *Codes of Professional Responsibility.* Washington, DC: Bureau of National Affairs, 1986, pp 271-279.
2. *National Association of Social Workers Code of Ethics.* In Gorlin, RA, *op. cit.*, pp 161-167.
3. *American Library Association Statement on Professional Ethics.* In Gorlin, RA, *op. cit.*, p 187.
4. Veatch RM: *A Theory of Medical Ethics.* New York: Basic Books, 1981, p 97, emphasis added.
5. *Id.*, 110.
6. *Id.*, 100.
7. Bates v. State Bar of Arizona, 433 U.S. 350 (1977).
8. *The Veterinarian's Role in Companion Animal Welfare.* Schaumburg, IL: American Veterinary Medical Association, undated, unpaginated.
9. *The Veterinarian's Role in Food Animal Welfare.* Schaumburg, IL: American Veterinary Medical Association, undated, unpaginated.

10. "Relationships of Local, State, and National Associations on the Matter of Ethics." *1988 AVMA Directory*, p 474.
11. "Principles Applicable to All." *1988 AVMA Directory*, p 476.
12. AVMA Bylaws. Art V. Sec. 2(b)(ii). *1988 AVMA Directory*, p 464.
13. AVMA Bylaws. Art. V. Sec. 2(b)(iv). *1988 AVMA Directory*, p 464.
14. *1988 AVMA Directory*, p 455.
15. Displays and Reciprocity Emerge as Key House Issues. *J Am Vet Med Assoc* 191:625, 1987.
16. *1988 AVMA Directory*, pp 456-457.
17. AVMA Bylaws. Art. I. Sec. 8. *1988 AVMA* Directory, p 462.
18. See, e.g., Specialist Designation a Judicial Council Concern. *J Am Vet Med Assoc* 181:859, 1982; Council Proposes "Principle" Revisions. *J Am Vet Med Assoc* 184:913,1984; Judicial Council Looks at Discount Advertising. *J Am Vet Med Assoc* 189:10, 1986.
19. Discount Advertising and Waiting-Room Displays Reviewed by Judicial Council. *J Am Vet Med Assoc* 189:1408, 1986.
20. Council Comments on Laboratory Animal Standards. *J Am Vet Med Assoc* 189:14, 1986.
21. Committee Identifies Public Health Implications of Human/Animal Bond. *J Am Vet Med Assoc* 189:18, 1986.
22. Advisory Board Prepares Subspecialty Guidelines. *J Am Vet Med Assoc* 189:160, 1986.
23. Resolution Results from House of Delegates. *J Am Vet Med Assoc* 189:624, 1986.
24. White House Conferees Decry Unfair Competition. *J Am Vet Med Assoc* 189:974, 1986.
25. Committee Supports Increased Supervision of Animal Drugs. *J Am Vet Med Assoc* 189:1267, 1986.
26. Constitution and Bylaws of the Illinois State Veterinary Medical Association, sec. 8, 1986.
27. MVMA Policy Manual, p 13, 1986.

Chapter

—————— 9 ——————

Official Veterinary Ethics:
Oath and Principles

Official veterinary ethics has generated many pronouncements and standards. However, two texts, the Veterinarian's Oath and the *Principles of Veterinary Medical Ethics*, are of such paramount importance that they require separate consideration.

THE VETERINARIAN'S OATH

In 1969, the AVMA House of Delegates adopted the Veterinarian's Oath. It reads as follows:

> Being admitted to the profession of veterinary medicine,
> I solemnly swear to use my scientific knowledge and skills for the benefit of society through the protection of animal health, the relief of animal suffering, the conservation of livestock resources, the promotion of public health, and the advancement of medical knowledge.
> I will practice my profession conscientiously, with dignity, and in keeping with the principles of veterinary medical ethics.
> I accept as a lifelong obligation the continual improvement of my professional knowledge and competence.

Importance of the Oath

Although the Oath is not cited as frequently in print as, and is considerably shorter than, the *Principles of Veterinary Medical Ethics*, its importance should not be underestimated. The Veterinarian's Oath is clearly intended to be for veterinarians what the Hippocratic Oath has for centuries represented to physicians: a statement of the highest ideals and most central values of the profession, made at the time when a person graduates from being a student to becoming a member of the profession. The fact that the Oath is usually taken when the doctorate is conferred, before one has received a license to practice, is of great significance. Entry to the "practice" of veterinary medicine as this is defined by the law is controlled by government. In contrast, the Oath reflects the view of the profession that *it* has the right to admit persons to its ranks prior to, or indeed irrespective of, governmental permission to practice in the legal sense. This is not just an assertion of authority. It is a statement that, however important it might be for individual veterinarians or the profession in general, practice in the legal sense is only one possible manifestation or use of one's professional status.

Five Pillars of Professionalism: Science, Ethics, Society, Animal Health, and Self-Improvement

Despite its brevity, the Oath identifies five distinct foundations of professionalism in which all veterinarians can take pride.

The Oath begins by specifying scientific knowledge as the means through which the aims of veterinary medicine are to be attained. The Oath thus defines the veterinarian as more than a craftsman who possesses certain mechanical or technical skills. It commits each veterinarian to the study of science. The Oath also links the profession to biomedical research aimed at the advancement of veterinary knowledge and techniques.

Also identified as a foundation of professionalism is attention to ethics, in the form of conscientiousness, dignity, and adherence to the *Principles*.

Society is also given a prominent place in the Oath. Indeed, it is the benefit of society that is identified as the aim of all the activities enumerated in the second paragraph. Societal interests are also alluded to implicitly in the Oath's references to the conservation of livestock resources, public health, and medical knowledge.

Not surprisingly, the protection of animal health and the prevention of animal suffering are also included as central goals of the profession.

The Oath concludes with a pledge to engage in self-improvement, in knowledge as well as technical competence.

Criticisms of the Oath

In evaluating the Veterinarian's Oath, one must keep in mind what one can expect of a professional oath. Professor Rollin has complained that unless the aims of the Oath's second paragraph are

> elaborated and rank ordered, these values are clearly incompatible. For example, the advancement of knowledge is often at odds with the relief of animal suffering. Clearly much fleshing-out through dialogue is required to make the oath more than a pious but vacuous statement of good intentions (1).

However, it cannot be the purpose of an oath to provide a detailed elaboration or "rank ordering" of fundamental values. Fundamental values (such as kindness and honesty, or justice and happiness) by their very nature can conflict in particular cases. One might as well say that the statement of the *Declaration of Independence* of the United States of America that all people have the inalienable right to "life, liberty, and the pursuit of happiness" is vacuous – because the defense of liberty sometimes requires the sacrifice of life, or because too much liberty can lead to unhappiness. There is nothing in the Veterinarian's Oath that prevents the profession from providing further elaboration about how the Oath's five central concerns are to be ranked or applied in particular kinds of situations.

Nevertheless the Oath does raise several questions.

To whom is the Oath taken? First, it is unclear to whom one is swearing when one takes the Oath: to oneself, one's fellow veterinarians, clients, the public, or some combination of these. To whom the Oath is taken can make a significant difference. If one is swearing just to one's colleagues, one is not thereby giving clients or society the right to complain about violations of the Oath. On the other hand, if the Oath is a promise to more than just veterinarians, it would be more than a text of official veterinary ethics and would permit nonveterinarians to appeal to the Oath in ethical discussions not controlled by the profession.

Should more than conscientiousness, dignity, and adherence to the *Principles* **be included in the Oath's ethical concerns?** Conscientiousness and dignity are, clearly, appropriate virtues for a veterinarian. It is also understandable that a document of official veterinary ethics such as the Oath should mention adherence to the leading text of official ethics, the AVMA *Principles*, even though doctors might on occasion differ with the code as a matter of conscience. As we shall see, the *Principles* cannot be expected to contain the final word on ethical issues. Indeed, the code has changed over time as veterinarians have modified their ethical views. Because a professional oath proclaims the most central aspirations of the profession, one might therefore ask whether the Veterinarian's Oath ought to imply something that is clearly the desire of all veterinarians: that the *Principles* not only be followed but that they be continually improved in light of the requirements of morality.

Does the Oath give sufficient attention to animals? Veterinary medicine is a diverse profession, in which one can use one's attainments in the service of human beings as well as (or instead of) animals. Yet, the present Oath does not place caring for animals on the same level as service to people. All the enumerated aims of the Oath's second paragraph, including the protection of animal health and the relief of animal suffering, are stated as means toward the benefit of *society*, which by definition includes only people. The focus on people is reinforced by the references to conservation of livestock, public health, and medical knowledge.

I have found some hostility to the Oath among my veterinary students because of its identification of society as the ultimate beneficiary of *all* of veterinary medicine. One need not believe that animals are as important as people, or that veterinarians should favor the interests of patients over those of clients, to assert that, at the very least, caring for animals is as worthy a general goal for veterinarians as service to society. Any oath that fails to recognize this will surely fail to reflect the attitudes of many veterinarians.

A Revised Oath

The following modest revisions are suggested to stimulate discussion among veterinarians about possible modifications of the present Oath. This revised oath preserves the character and strengths of the current text while addressing the questions raised above. Its major feature is giving increased prominence to animals, animal welfare, and veterinary (as distinguished from medical) knowledge. It also makes clear, as the present text does not, that one is swearing to uphold the values of the entire Oath and not just its second paragraph.

> Being admitted to the profession of veterinary medicine, I solemnly swear to my fellow veterinarians, to my future clients, and to society:
> That I shall use my scientific knowledge and skills for the benefit of society, the protection of animal health and welfare, the relief of animal suffering, the conservation of livestock resources, the promotion of public health, and the advancement of veterinary and medical knowledge;
> That I will practice my profession conscientiously, with dignity, and in keeping with the principles of veterinary medical ethics; and
> That I accept as a lifelong obligation the continual improvement of my professional knowledge and competence and of the moral values of myself and my profession.

THE PRINCIPLES OF VETERINARY MEDICAL ETHICS

The *Principles* is a lengthy document.[a] It is therefore generally advisable to evaluate its provisions when considering the ethical issues these provisions address. However, there are several things that can be said of the code as a whole that can aid in one's approach to it.

The Nature of a Professional Code

In considering the *Principles*, one must keep in mind what a professional code is and what it is reasonable to expect of it.

Official standards result from agreement and compromise. One important difference between the standards of normative ethics (see Chapters 2 and 10) and those of an official ethical code is that the latter do derive from agreement among the members of a profession. Therefore, while normative ethics is a process of discovery of what is right and wrong, the fashioning of official ethical standards is often akin to *politics*. Typically, proponents of differing viewpoints will express their desires regarding an ethical principle, and, through a process of negotiation and compromise, a standard will be hammered out.

Because official ethical standards often reflect compromise among competing points of view, it is to be expected that they will not always embody the complete truth about a moral issue. Like a politician, a veterinarian engaged in the formulation of a proposed official ethical standard must recognize that he might sometimes have to settle for less than what he believes is morally right in order to get the best official ethical standard he can achieve. He might have to give a little on one proposed ethical standard so that he can make some headway on another.

---

[a]The *Principles* are available separately in booklet form from the AVMA, and are also printed each year in the *AVMA Directory*. Accordingly, references to the code in this chapter and throughout the text are to the titles of the sections cited as well as to page numbers in the *Directory*.

Official codes often stress obviously correct positions and accommodate competing viewpoints. Because official codes are adopted by professions for all their members, code standards must enunciate positions with which the great majority of members can be comfortable. Thus, codes such as the AVMA *Principles* are replete with statements that are obviously correct or that "split it down the middle" between opposing approaches. For example, there can be no argument with the statement that "no member shall willfully place professional knowledge, attainments or services at the disposal of any lay body ... for the purpose of encouraging unqualified groups or individuals to diagnose and prescribe for the ailments and diseases of animals" (2). And the *Principles* resolve differences about whether all veterinarians must offer emergency service with a compromise: although "every practitioner has a moral and ethical responsibility" to provide such service, this responsibility can be fulfilled by joining "with colleagues in the area to see that emergency services are provided consistent with the needs of the locality" (3).

Official codes tend to skirt controversial or divisive issues. The need for general acceptance of official ethical standards also tends to filter out of a professional code statements or references to issues that a significant portion of the profession finds divisive. Because there has been so much controversy about the propriety of limiting veterinary school enrollments in order to protect established doctors from competition, the AVMA would probably risk widespread dissatisfaction with the entire *Principles* if it attempted to address this question in the code. Likewise, there probably are too many veterinarians who are seriously troubled, or undecided, about the usefulness of the concept of animal rights (see Chapter 12) to permit the *Principles* to safely refer to this concept in the very near future. This does not mean the profession must discourage vigorous discussion of such issues among members, but only that it might not be prepared to express positions regarding these issues in its official code.

Official codes contain ambiguities and generalities. Another way official codes accommodate differing viewpoints is by building into their pronouncements enough ambiguity and generality to permit practitioners with varying viewpoints to live with the final result. This is especially important in a profession like veterinary medicine, which encompasses great diversity in values and practice styles. A good example of an abstract statement that can embrace different viewpoints is the pronouncement of the *Principles* (based on the Veterinarian's Oath) that the "principal objectives of the veterinary profession are to render service to society, to conserve our livestock resources, and to prevent and relieve the suffering of animals" (4). This statement permits disagreement about, for example, whether rendering "service to society" should include veterinarians working in hospitals operated by nonprofit humane societies, or aggressive marketing campaigns that inform consumers about available services and fees, or participation in low-cost spay and neuter clinics, or the use of animals in the testing of cosmetics. The statement also permits some veterinarians to devote their professional lives to serving society, others to alleviating animal suffering, and still others to conserving livestock resources.

Code standards change slowly. It is also more difficult for a professional association such as the AVMA to change its official ethical code than it is for a legislature to amend or repeal a statute. If adoption of a code standard has followed considerable discussion and negotiation, it can be difficult, and unfair to those who have made compromises in good faith, to reopen the entire process once again. More importantly, official ethical codes are presented both to members and the world as statements of the most fundamental values of the profession. If these codes were to change drastically from year to year, or even from decade to decade, members of the profession and the public might justifiably wonder whether the profession has very many central moral principles. This is why a code like the *Principles* can contain some standards that a good number of practitioners oppose, and why a standard that no longer reflects shared values might not be swept away until long after it has ceased to seem reasonable to the majority.

Official codes reflect attitudes and concerns of their times. Because official ethical codes are written by and for professionals, they tend to reflect what is bothering these persons. There is no better way of appreciating how a profession's values have developed and changed than to read its successive codes of ethics. Thus, in 1867, when the United States Veterinary Medical Association's first *Code of Ethics* was written, veterinarians were not yet required to be licensed. They were struggling to separate themselves in the public's mind from charlatans without legitimate scientific training. This early code therefore prohibited the advertising of "secret medicines" as well as "specific medicines, specific plans of treatment, advertising through the medium of posters, illuminated bills, newspaper puffs, etc." (5). By 1940, veterinarians had established themselves in the public's view as true professionals and were more concerned about competition from within the profession. The Code of that year devoted more than half its length to advertising. It denounced all advertising as "unethical and unprofessional." It specifically banned, among other things, calling oneself a specialist in a public directory and the "distribution of cards or circulars by mail or otherwise reminding clients that the time is at hand for rendering certain services (vaccinations, worm-parasite treatment *et al.*)" (6).

Another provision that speaks volumes about changes in the profession's attitudes was the requirement, enunciated in the 1928 *Code of Ethics*, that members of the AVMA "are expected to conduct themselves at all times as professional gentlemen" (7). This was amended in 1940 to demand "conduct characterizing the personal behavior of a gentleman" (8), language that remained in the *Principles* until 1983.

The Proposed 1988 Revision and the Federal Trade Commission Inquiry about the *Principles*

THE FTC INQUIRY

In 1986, the AVMA Judicial Council decided to undertake a major revision of the *Principles* to improve the organization of the document and to clarify certain ambiguous or problematic sections (9). This effort culminated in the preparation of a new version of the code, to which I shall refer as the "proposed 1988 revision." The document was to be voted on by the House of Delegates at the AVMA's annual convention in July, 1988. Shortly before the revision was to be considered by the House, the Judicial Committee announced that it was recommending that no action be taken on the revised *Principles*. The AVMA had received an inquiry from the Federal Trade Commission regarding the current code of ethics. The FTC requested information about a number of provisions in the code that, according to the FTC, could be in violation of federal laws prohibiting anticompetitive behavior (see Chapter 18). The Judicial Council informed the House of Delegates that any action on the new revision would be inappropriate until the AVMA had the opportunity to respond to the FTC's questions. Accordingly, the proposed 1988 revision was not considered by the House. The current 1987 revision of the code was left in force, at least until the next meeting of the House of Delegates in 1989 (10; F. L. Davis, personal communication; R. Shomer, personal communication). The House did, however, vote to include in the current code a provision dealing with impaired veterinarians. This section counsels veterinarians who are "impaired by alcohol or other drugs" to seek assistance from qualified persons or organizations, and asks colleagues of these doctors to "make every effort to encourage such individuals to obtain assistance and overcome such disability" (11). This provision was also included in the proposed 1988 revision of the code.

THE PROPOSED 1988 REVISION: ORGANIZATIONAL CHANGES

The proposed 1988 revision is worth discussing in some detail because, given its high quality, it seems likely that parts of the revision will find their way into future versions of the *Principles*.

In each of several previous years, the code has undergone minor changes, through the addition, deletion, or modification of a limited number of its provisions. The proposed 1988 revision attempted the most significant alterations of the document since the addition of the Advertising Regulations 10 years earlier. The proposed revision would have made very few changes in the substantive provisions of the code. Its major feature was a reorganization of already existing standards and an improvement in the writing and general presentation of the document.

The current code (12) contains three general "Sections:" an "Introduction," "Fundamental Concepts," and "Guidelines for Professional Conduct." It is not always clear what significance is to be attached to inclusion of a provision in one of these Sections. Each of the Sections asserts very general ideals, as well as extremely specific obligations and prohibitions (see Chapter 5). The Introduction includes a provision that is itself entitled "Principles of Veterinary Medical Ethics." This provision is composed of six "Parts." Each of these Parts enunciates very fundamental standards. The title and abstract content of this portion of the document suggests that these "Principles" are intended to be the heart of the code. However, such an interpretation is undercut by the fact that these "Principles" are placed in the Introduction of the code and not in one of its two main Sections. Moreover, there is *another* set of fundamental principles, contained in the Guidelines for Professional Conduct, and entitled "Principles Applicable to All." The fact that each of the three "Sections" contains similar kinds of provisions renders the current code somewhat rambling and disorganized. It is sometimes difficult to determine whether a given provision is supposed to set forth a very general ideal, or an obligation or prohibition violation of which could result in disciplinary action.

The proposed 1988 revision would clarify the overarching organization of the code. The proposal collected the more general provisions of the *Principles* in two sections near the beginning of the code, entitled "General Concepts" and "Guidelines for Professional Behavior." The latter would contain 10 paragraphs, many of which repeat *verbatim* the "Parts" of the current provision labelled "Principles of Veterinary Medical Ethics." The proposed 1988 revision would have made it clear that these "Guidelines" (including the current "Parts") are intended to set forth the most central and important standards of the document. Following the general "Guidelines," the 1988 revision proposed a lengthy set of "Explanatory Notes." These Notes assembled in one part of the text most of the provisions already in the code. In the proposed revision, it is clear that these specific sections are intended to explain how the more abstract "Guidelines" should be applied in particular situations. The "Notes" tend to assert concrete obligations or prohibitions, the violation of which can be expected to result in disciplinary action.

The proposed 1988 revision also suggested minor but helpful changes in the titles and wording of a number of provisions in order to clarify their meaning. Additionally, the revision pulled together related provisions that currently appear in disparate sections. For example, the current code addresses the obligations of practitioners regarding referrals, consultations, and relationships with new clients in 3 separate provisions (13). Two of these provisions even bear the same title, "Consultations." The proposed 1988 revision would have relocated all these standards in a single provision.

The organizational changes in the proposed 1988 revision would make the *Principles* a tighter, more readable, and more usable document. The proposed revision presents the entire document in a manner that shows a logical progression from the general to the particular. Specific recommendations are suggested more clearly as instantiations of, and ultimately justifiable by, general ideals. By placing the most specific provisions at the end of the document, the new revision also would make it easier for the code to adapt to changing circumstances without requiring wholesale changes in asserted fundamental principles; in most cases, one or more of the "Explanatory Notes" could be amended without suggesting dissatisfaction with the more general ideals and guidelines. The proposed 1988 revision attempted to reconcile in a most impressive fashion the need of a professional code to improve and adapt to the times, with the requirement that changes not be made precipitously or prematurely.

THE PROPOSED 1988 REVISION: SUBSTANTIVE MODIFICATIONS

Very little of substance would have been deleted by the 1988 revision. One provision that would have been removed prohibits the display of continuing education course certificates or diplomas on the grounds that such certificates "might lead the public to infer that the veterinarian to whom they are issued is a specialist in the specific subject matter" (14). This latter claim seems implausible, and the section appears to strike many veterinarians as silly and unnecessary.

As noted above, the proposed 1988 revision contained a section dealing with veterinarians who are impaired by alcohol or other drugs. The proposed revision also incorporated into the code the AVMA's definition of the "veterinarian-client-patient relationship" (15). This characterization was then used to define and prohibit the merchandising of professional products and services (see Chapter 16). The new revision would add to the code the statement that veterinarians "should consider first the welfare of the patient for the purpose of relieving suffering and disability while causing a minimum of pain or fright. Benefit to the patient should transcend personal advantage or monetary gain in decisions concerning therapy" (16). The code has long contained statements stressing the need for veterinarians to serve primarily the interests of patients rather than their own monetary gain. Proclaiming this principle in the new "Guidelines for Professional Behavior" would give it increased prominence. The reference to the prevention of pain and fright reflects the profession's growing interest in scientific studies of pain, suffering, distress, and other negative animal mental states (see Chapters 21 and 23).

WHAT IS THE FUTURE OF THE *PRINCIPLES*?

It is ironic that the FTC inquiry about the *Principles* occurred when it did. The AVMA had just decided to increase its activities in the ethical arena (17). It was about to present a brilliantly executed and forceful new revision of the *Principles* as a tool in this process. At the time of this writing, few details regarding the FTC's questions or the AVMA's probable response had been made public. Nevertheless, the following general observations seem in order. These observations apply to any attempt by government authorities to pass judgment upon the code and the official ethical apparatus of which it is a part.

First, the profession has a very strong interest in defending its official code. It is a good code. As the proposed 1988 revision shows, it is likely only to improve. If there are features of the code that violate the law, these features must, of course, be removed. If it is necessary to rephrase some of the provisions that now set forth obligations or prohibitions, as ideals – standards to which veterinarians should aspire but that cannot be used to discipline members – then such an option should be explored. Where current statements of obligations or prohibitions do comport with legal standards, the case for retaining these standards must be made forcefully and convincingly. Government employees who might not have significant experience with the realities of veterinary practice are capable of being misinformed. They can also be wrong about the law. The current *Principles* did not spring into existence overnight. The roots of the code go back over 100 years. Each successive revision has been part of a larger historical evolution. This evolution has reflected not just the changing attitudes of the profession, but veterinarians' adherence to certain immutable moral values. If the profession hastily gives up large segments of its code, it will be giving up an important part of itself.

A second reason the profession should never accede quickly to wholesale changes in the *Principles* is that the code has played an important role in encouraging dignified and professional behavior. As we shall see in subsequent chapters, the forces of commercialism within veterinary medicine are alive and well. There are those who think that a veterinarian should promote, hustle, and sell, just as a car dealership or furniture store promotes, hustles, and sells. But the forces of commercialism have not yet taken over. One reason they have not prevailed is that veterinary medicine still has a code that frowns upon placing one's own pocketbook over the interests of patients, clients, and the rest of the profession. To some veterinarians, there is much in the *Principles* that must seem an impediment, a hindrance, to the task of maximizing revenues. It is important that the profession cooperate with government officials whose aim is to assure that official veterinary ethics follows the law. Nevertheless, the profession must also assert its interest in keeping a sharp eye on those whose primary motivation is to clear an unimpeded path between themselves and the bank.

Third, government inquiries about the code could, in the long run, be a blessing. I have found that many veterinarians are not familiar with the *Principles*. The FTC's actions might generate increased interest in the code. This, in turn, could lead to greater interest in normative veterinary ethics, to which one must look for guidance in evaluating official ethical standards.

Finally, whatever happens to the *Principles*, all veterinarians must keep firmly in mind the difference between official veterinary ethics and normative veterinary ethics (see Chapters 2 and 10). If the law should prevent veterinary professional associations from prohibiting certain kinds of behavior, that does not mean it is morally right to engage in such behavior. For example, if the AVMA cannot lawfully discipline a member who advertises discounted fees (18), that does not make it morally permissible to advertise discounted fees. (Indeed, as I argue in Chapter 17, the advertising of discounted fees, as well as discounted fees themselves, are wrong.) Practitioners and ethicists engaged in exploring issues of normative veterinary ethics will always remain legally free to conclude that certain kinds of conduct are right or wrong, good or bad, just or unjust. Veterinarians will always be able to decide *individually*, as a matter of *moral principle*, that they may, may not, or must engage in certain kinds of behavior.

To be sure, normative veterinary ethics as a field of thought and inquiry can only explore; it cannot coerce or impose discipline. But recognizing that moral behavior in professional life is something each individual veterinarian must choose for himself should be nothing new or disheartening. For that is the way all of us generally operate. When there is an ethical question regarding our behavior, there rarely is someone or some organization to step in to acquit or censure us, to place us on probation, or to suspend or expel us. We all must choose for ourselves whether we shall act in accordance with the standards of morality.

In sum, even if official veterinary ethics undergoes some shrinkage in the range of activities it can address, normative veterinary ethics should prove more than able to take up the slack.

General Features of the *Principles*

It is much easier to point out the relatively few problems in a lengthy document like the *Principles* than it is to discuss its many strong points. To place in proper perspective criticisms of the code that are to follow in this and subsequent chapters, I want to state at the outset my view that the *Principles* is in general a sound code that compares very favorably with the official codes of other professions. But nothing is perfect. It is the task of the scholar to note problems and areas for improvement when he thinks he sees them.

The following are among the code's many strong points. The *Principles* recognize that a comprehensive code must not only lay down specific obligations and prohibitions, but must also identify very general values and virtues without which the promotion of ethical behavior is impossible. The document acknowledges that it cannot dictate answers for the entire field of veterinary medicine and that professional life is too complex to formulate one's moral duties into a hard and fast "set of rules" (19). Among the general values identified by the code are service to society (20), improvement in professional knowledge and skill (21), protection of the public and the profession against those deficient in moral character or professional competence (22), and the prevention and relief of animal suffering (23). The *Principles* also demand such virtues as honesty in dealing with clients and the public (24), modesty and moderation in promoting one's own name or practice (25), diligence in attending to patients (26), respect for the privacy and confidences of clients (27), and sensitivity to the needs and reputations of fellow veterinarians (28).

Many of the specific obligations or prohibitions of the code are beyond dispute. For example, the ban against commissions, rebates and kickbacks (29), and the prohibition against choosing a method of treatment based on the pecuniary gain of the practitioner (30), are intended to assure that the veterinarian works in the first instance for his patient and client. The prohibition against guarantees of cures (31) and the requirement that client confidences be respected (32) also protect clients against unscrupulous behavior. None of the healing professions has adopted a code that defines the limits of acceptable advertising as meticulously, and with as much effort at not only repeating but applying Constitutional requirements, as do the *Principles'* Advertising Regulations (33) and sections on testimonials and endorsements (34). (See Chapter 17.)

The *Principles* also contain the recommendation that the code itself be "given a thorough study with a view to clarification of certain sections and amendments to strengthen it" (35). The code thus proclaims itself as open-minded, adaptable, and receptive to sincere and helpful criticism.

Two Problems in the *Principles*

Even when the *Principles* are considered in light of what one can reasonably expect of an official code, one finds several deficiencies that detract from its effectiveness. Two very general problems I would like to discuss here are 1) the code's excessive reliance on "attitude" and the Golden Rule as keystones of professional ethics and 2) its failure to address several areas important to the profession today.

ATTITUDE AND THE GOLDEN RULE

The first substantive provision of the code is entitled "It's Attitude that Counts." The section asserts that the code is constructed broadly, as a general guide for behavior. Such an approach is justified on the grounds that veterinarians who accept the Golden Rule as a guide for general conduct and make a reasonable effort to abide by the *Principles*

> ... will have little difficulty with ethics. Those whose aggressiveness and promotional tendencies cause them to run afoul of the *Principles* would probably have the same difficulty under more specific rules (36).

The next provision of the code states that the entire code is "based on the Golden Rule" (37). These same words are repeated by yet another section of the code (38). Reference to the Golden Rule as the foundation of professional behavior occurs four times in the document.

The fundamental "attitude" referred to in the code appears to be respect for the Golden Rule, moderation in aggressiveness and promotion, or a combination of both. Unfortunately, none of these attitudes can guarantee that one will have "little difficulty" with ethics. The reason is clear. There are many difficult ethical problems for which these attitudes simply cannot provide sufficient guidance.

First, many ethical issues in veterinary practice relate to how doctors ought to treat their animal patients. The Golden Rule cannot address such issues because it makes reference only to *people*. The Golden Rule asks us to treat other people as we would want to be treated by them.[b] It does not ask us to put ourselves in the place of animals and inquire how we would want to be treated if we were they. Indeed, it is often far from clear how one would go about trying to answer such a question, and it is not always obvious that this would be a relevant or appropriate question. Likewise, attention to "aggressiveness and promotional tendencies" will often fail to address important ethical issues relating to a doctor's treatment of his animal patients. For there are many important ethical issues relating to these patients (e.g., many issues regarding the euthanasia of sick animals) that have nothing to do with competition and promotion.

Second, there are many moral problems relating to doctors' behavior toward other people that cannot be solved by an appeal to moderation in aggressiveness or promotional tendencies, or by an appeal to respect for the Golden Rule.

There can be little doubt that, as a general matter, moderation in aggressiveness and promotion is an admirable attitude. But thus stated, it is so general an attitude that it often does not provide guidance even in deciding many ethical questions that involve competition, promotion, and marketing. For example, one issue currently dividing veterinarians is whether doctors may sell nonmedical items such as pet food and toys (see Chapter 16). What sometimes separates practitioners is precisely the issue of whether such activities *are* overly promotional and aggressive. Someone who objects to them might find them overly aggressive, while a proponent of these activities will not. Thus, a judgment about whether these (and other) approaches reflect an overly aggressive and promotional attitude must be made after a conclusion is reached about their appropriateness. Appeal to an "attitude" cannot itself provide the arguments that will settle the issue, because often the point of the argument is to decide what is an appropriate attitude.

Likewise, the Golden Rule is often an admirable guide for behavior, and it can sometimes provide a specific recommendation for an ethical problem. Nevertheless, it, too, can become an overly generalized substitute for argument. It does not even reflect some of the actual positions of the *Principles* or do justice to some of the most difficult issues facing the profession. As important as it undoubtedly is, the Golden Rule cannot be, as the code suggests, the foundation of all of professional ethics.

As applied to veterinarians, the Golden Rule presumably means that each practitioner should behave toward *every* fellow veterinarian as he would want that veterinarian to behave toward him, *and* that each practitioner should treat *every* client as he himself would want to be treated if he were a client.

Regarding relations just among veterinarians, the Golden Rule often will not settle ethical issues, because veterinarians sometimes *disagree* about how they would want to be treated by other practitioners if they could change places with these doctors. A veterinarian who believes in vigorous marketing aimed at winning clients away from other doctors probably would welcome other doctors treating him in the same way. But a colleague opposed to such techniques will not want his fellow practitioners to treat him like this. One cannot decide which of these doctors is correct by appealing to the Golden Rule, because each has a different view about how he would want to

---

[b]The Golden Rule is usually phrased "Do unto others as you would have them do unto you." It derives from Matthew 7:12, "Whatsoever ye would that men should do to you, do ye even so unto them."

be treated by the other. This, and other controversies regarding how aggressively practitioners may compete against each other, will have to be resolved not by appeal to the Golden Rule – but by deciding whether certain kinds of competitive or promotional behavior are just right or wrong.

The Golden Rule also raises problems regarding the code's approach to relations between veterinarians and clients. Several sections of the *Principles* advise veterinarians never to criticize a fellow practitioner to a client, but rather to call some mistake or problem to the other doctor's attention. One is told, for example to "handle new clients, their sick animals, and the veterinarians they have consulted previously in a manner consistent with the Golden Rule. To criticize or disparage another veterinarian's service to a client is unethical" (39).

These provisions (which will be discussed in greater detail in Chapter 18) appear to apply the Golden Rule from one veterinarian to another. The problem is that if one applies the Golden Rule between veterinarian and *client*, the Rule will often require that a doctor *inform* a client about a colleague's mistakes. For it is probably the case that many clients would like to know if a previous doctor erred. (They certainly would like to know this if they ask.) If veterinarians treated clients the way they would like to be treated if they were clients, they would sometimes violate several key provisions of the code.

My point is not that the code is always incorrect in counselling at least temporary silence about a colleague's performance. Sometimes, I shall argue later, this is the best approach. Rather, as will be explained more fully in Chapter 10, the point is that there are sometimes conflicts between the interests and desires of veterinarians and those of their clients, just as there are sometimes conflicts between the interests of patients and those of clients. *Ethical deliberation very often is the process of resolving competing interests in a morally satisfactory way.* But when there are conflicts, the Golden Rule will not always provide an answer, precisely because the conflicting parties will sometimes need or want different things from each other.

The solution to these difficulties is not to discard moderation in competitiveness or respect for the Golden Rule. Rather, greater care needs to be taken in specifying which issues such attitudes can help to address. Otherwise, vague, warm-hearted talk about right "attitude" and the Golden Rule can replace careful and reasoned consideration of difficult ethical problems.

MISSING PROVISIONS

Although the *Principles* address many questions of great importance to the profession, there are conspicuous gaps in its coverage. Most of the provisions of the code that offer specific guidance are devoted to issues relevant to problems faced by private practitioners who are in economic competition with each other. Hence, the code's statement that those who restrain their "aggressiveness and promotional tendencies" will have "little difficulty with ethics."

The text offers no explicit, detailed provisions regarding the welfare of farm, laboratory, or industrial animals, even though official veterinary ethics has labored long and hard on these issues and has produced other documents that discuss them. In contrast, the American Medical Association *Principles of Medical Ethics* (40) contain lengthy sections on the obligations of physicians regarding research subjects and industrial practice.

The *Principles* also do not address the ethical obligations of practitioners regarding veterinarians, technicians, and other support personnel in their employ (*see* Chapter 22).

Despite the considerable attention official veterinary ethics has paid to the human-companion animal bond, there is missing from the *Principles* explicit reference to this concept or to many of the important ethical issues it raises – ranging from the obligations of doctors to make financial arrangements to facilitate the care of companion animals, to the ethical limits of veterinarian participation in and promotion of third-party veterinary insurance programs, to issues relating to the euthanasia of both healthy and unhealthy animals. Although many veterinarians believe that the euthanasia of companion animals poses some of the most difficult moral issues they face in practice, the word "euthanasia" does not appear in the code.

Finally, the *Principles* appear reluctant to grant something that every veterinarian believes: veterinarians have moral obligations relating *to their animal patients* as well as to people. In several of its directives, the code admonishes doctors to serve the interests of their patients. Yet, in some of its most fundamental and central sections, the text omits any reference to animals as objects of concern for official veterinary ethics. The code fails to mention animals when it states that "(p)rofessional life is too complex to classify one's duties and obligations to clients, colleagues, and fellow citizens into a set of rules" (41). (This statement appears to imply that moral obligations and ideals regarding animals are not part of a veterinarian's "professional life.") Likewise, there is no mention of animals in the declaration that the *Principles* are "standards by which an individual may determine the propriety of conduct in relationships with clients, colleagues, and with the public" (42). (This statement appears to imply that the code is not intended to contain standards by which a practitioner may determine the propriety of his conduct in relation to his patients.) Presumably, the absence of a reference to animals in these pronouncements does not reflect the view that in order to establish itself as a "real" profession, veterinary medicine must emphasize its ethical obligations to people. That the profession has such obligations is obvious. However, that veterinarians deal with, and have many moral obligations and ideals regarding animals is not an unfortunate accident. Nor is it something about which any veterinarian should feel guilty or embarrassed.

It would be easy for the *Principles* to discuss or give greater emphasis to animal welfare, employer-employee relations, the human-companion animal bond, and the status of animals as objects of direct concern to official ethical standards. Where questions (e.g., those concerning euthanasia) are especially difficult, the code need not attempt to settle them definitively, but might highlight the profession's interest in them. However, if the *Principles* are to stand as the most definitive statement of the profession's values, its focus must be expanded, so that it will speak to all areas of major concern to veterinarians.

THE LIMITATIONS OF OFFICIAL VETERINARY ETHICS

Veterinarians should be proud of their Oath and *Principles*, and the official ethical apparatus of which these texts are a part. Clearly, professional behavior has been improved, and will continue to be improved, by official veterinary ethics.

However, we are now in a position to better appreciate why official veterinary ethics can be only a part of the total ethical commitment and activity of veterinarians.

Because they must speak for the entire profession about many problems whose solution is not obvious, the Oath and *Principles* contain some provisions that do not answer questions, but rather identify important ethical concerns and channel further discussion and debate. These texts do not, and they probably cannot, determine when it is morally appropriate to euthanize a terminally ill animal, how far veterinarians should go in attempting to offer reduced fees to needy clients, to what extent veterinarians should criticize clients who have neglected their animals, to what extent sport animals may be given drugs to improve their performance, or whether paid pregnancy leave is a moral right of female doctors and employees. To answer these (and many other) questions, veterinarians must supplement the guidance of official standards with objective principles of morality – with normative veterinary ethics.

Official veterinary ethics must also comport with legal standards that restrict the effects professional associations may have upon competition and commerce. As explained above, normative veterinary ethics encounters no such restrictions. Its function is not to regulate or discipline. Its task is to question, discuss, discover, suggest, and (where possible) to exhort.

Finally, because official ethics is controlled by the profession, the process by which it approaches moral issues does not include equal input from nonveterinarians. This can sometimes lead to conclusions that do not adequately take into account the interests of patients, clients, or society. For example, I argue in Chapter 18 that where a previous doctor has been grossly negligent and has wasted a client's money and endangered the health of his animal, it will sometimes be appropriate for a practitioner to criticize the first doctor's performance to the client. Yet, the *Principles* state that it is always unethical to criticize or disparage another veterinarian's service to a client. This prohibition is motivated by the profession's legitimate desire to protect itself against litigation from clients and against bad feelings among doctors. However, in striving fervently to protect its members, any profession can sometimes lose sight of the legitimate interests of others. To the standards of official ethics there must be added a healthy dose of normative veterinary ethics, in which the interests of all must be given due regard.

REFERENCES

1. Rollin BE: Updating veterinary medical ethics. *J Am Vet Med Assoc* 173:1017, 1978.
2. "Alliance with Unqualified Persons." *1988 AVMA Directory*, p 475.
3. "Emergency Service." *1988 AVMA Directory*, p 477.
4. "Principles of Veterinary Medical Ethics," Part I. *1988 AVMA Directory*, p 474. Note that this formulation, unlike the passage from the Veterinarian's Oath from which it is derived, does not designate society as the ultimate beneficiary of the other activities.
5. USVMA Proceedings, 4th Annual Meeting, New York, Sept. 3, 1867. *USVMA Minutes Book*, pp 42-47. Quoted in Miller EB: History and Evolution of the AVMA Veterinary Medical Code of Ethics, 1867-1940. *California Veterinarian* 39:18, 1985.
6. *Code of Ethics of the American Veterinary Medical Association. J Am Vet Med Assoc* 96:92-93, 1940.

7. *AVMA Membership Directory, 1928-1929; Constitution and By-Laws.* Detroit: AVMA, 1928, p 70, reprinted in Miller, *op. cit.*, pp. 19-20.
8. *Code of Ethics of the American Veterinary Medical Association. J Am Vet Med Assoc* 96:92, 1940.
9. Discount Advertising and Waiting-Room Displays Reviewed by Judicial Council. *J Am Vet Med Assoc* 189:1408, 1986.
10. See, House of Delegates Postpones Action on Revised Principles. *AVMA Convention News.* Portland, OR: American Veterinary Medical Association, July 20, 1988, p 2.
11. Judicial Council Revises Guidelines on Displays and Discount Advertising. *J Am Vet Med Assoc* 192:14, 1988.
12. *1988 AVMA Directory*, pp 474-478.
13. "Consultations." *1988 AVMA Directory*, p 475; "Consultations." *1988 AVMA Directory*, p 476; "Professional Relationships with New Clients." *1988 AVMA Directory*, p 477.
14. "Certificates or Diplomas, Continuing Education, Display of." *1988 AVMA Directory*, p 477.
15. *Principles of Veterinary Medical Ethics*, proposed 1988 rev. "Dispensing, Marketing, and Merchandising." AVMA 1988 Annual Convention Delegates' Agenda. Schaumburg, IL: American Veterinary Medical Association, 1988, p 17t.
16. *Principles of Veterinary Medical Ethics*, proposed 1988 rev. "Guidelines for Professional Behavior," par. 2. AVMA 1988 Annual Convention Delegates' Agenda. Schaumburg, IL: American Veterinary Medical Association, 1988, p 17f.
17. Ethics and Professionalism. *J Am Vet Med Assoc* 192:1380-1381, 1988 (announcing a 5-year project by the AVMA to "mount a concerted effort to educate and stimulate improved ethical conduct and professionalism in the veterinary profession").
18. "Advertising Regulations." *1988 AVMA Directory*, p 476.
19. Section 2: Fundamental Concepts. *1988 AVMA Directory*, p 474.
20. "Principles of Veterinary Medical Ethics," Part 1; Part 6. *1988 AVMA Directory*, p 474.
21. "Principles of Veterinary Medical Ethics," Part 4. *1988 AVMA Directory*, p 474.
22. "Principles of Veterinary Medical Ethics," Part 5. *1988 AVMA Directory*, p 474.
23. "Principles of Veterinary Medical Ethics," Part 1. *1988 AVMA Directory*, p 474.
24. "Frauds." *1988 AVMA Directory*, p 474; "Advertising Regulations." *1988 AVMA Directory*, p 476.
25. E.g., "It's Attitude that Counts," *1988 AVMA Directory*, p 474; Testimonials and Endorsements." *1988 AVMA Directory*, p 475; "Advertising Regulations." *1988 AVMA Directory*, p 476; "Commercial Use of Reprints." *1988 AVMA Directory*, p 476; "Press Relations." *1988 AVMA Directory*, p 478.
26. "Principles of Veterinary Medical Ethics" Part 2. *1988 AVMA Directory*, p 474.
27. "Veterinarian-Client Relationships." *1988 AVMA Directory*, p 478.
28. "Deportment." *1988 AVMA Directory*, p 474; "Consultations." *1988 AVMA Directory*, p 475; "Consultations." *1988 AVMA Directory*, p 476; "Professional Relationships with New Clients." *1988 AVMA Directory*, p 477.
29. "Commissions, Rebates, or Kickbacks." *1988 AVMA Directory*, p 475; "Therapy, Determination of." *1988 AVMA Directory*, p 476.
30. "Therapy, Determination of." *1988 AVMA Directory*, p 476.

31. "Guarantee Cures." *1988 AVMA Directory*, p 474.
32. "Veterinarian-Client Relationships." *1988 AVMA Directory*, p 478.
33. *1988 AVMA Directory*, p 476.
34. "Testimonials and Endorsements." *1988 AVMA Directory*, p 475; "Advertising Regulations," par. 3. *1988 AVMA Directory*, p 476.
35. "Principles Applicable to All," par. 6. *1988 AVMA Directory*, p 476.
36. *1988 AVMA Directory*, p. 474. This language also occurs in the proposed 1988 revision. *Principles of Veterinary Medical Ethics*, proposed 1988 rev. "Attitude and Intent." AVMA 1988 Annual Convention Delegates' Agenda. Schaumburg, IL: American Veterinary Medical Association, 1988, p 17e.
37. "Principles of Veterinary Medical Ethics." *1988 AVMA Directory*, p 474.
38. "Fundamental Concepts." *1988 AVMA Directory*, p 474.
39. "Professional Relationships with New Clients." *1988 AVMA Directory*, p 477.
40. In Gorlin RA (ed): *Codes of Professional Responsibility*. Washington, DC: Bureau of National Affairs, 1986, pp 99-125.
41. "Fundamental Concepts." *1988 AVMA Directory*, p 474. This language is reproduced in the proposed 1988 revision. *Principles of Veterinary Medical Ethics*, proposed 1988 rev. "Attitude and Intent." AVMA 1988 Annual Convention Delegates' Agenda. Schaumburg, IL: American Veterinary Medical Association, 1988, pp 17e-17f.
42. "Principles Applicable to All." *1988 AVMA Directory*, p 476. Such a statement also occurs in the proposed 1988 revision. *Principles of Veterinary Medical Ethics*, proposed 1988 rev. "General Concepts." AVMA 1988 Annual Convention Delegates' Agenda. Schaumburg, IL: American Veterinary Medical Association, 1988, p 17f.

Chapter

─────── 10 ───────

How to Approach Problems in Normative Veterinary Ethics

Normative veterinary ethics is the branch of veterinary ethics that attempts to discover and apply correct moral norms for veterinary practice.

Normative veterinary ethics is the most important branch of veterinary ethics. When a veterinarian who is considering a moral question asks "What ought I do?" he usually wants to know what is morally right for him to do. He is not interested simply in what he or other practitioners think he ought to do, or what a government body or the organized profession might require. Understanding these things will often be relevant to a determination of what is right, or in making a decision about how one will want to act. However, there is no necessary correspondence between one's own ethical standards, or those of other veterinarians, government bodies, or the official ethical apparatus, and the requirements or ideals of morality.

Government bodies and professional organizations should also regard normative veterinary ethics as fundamental. Government bodies and the organized profession also want their ethical standards to be correct. They too must be prepared to compare their ethical judgments against objective principles of morality.

REALISTIC AIMS OF CONTEMPORARY NORMATIVE VETERINARY ETHICS

Like other branches of ethics that attempt to determine what is morally correct in an area of human endeavor, normative veterinary ethics seeks a general and systematic account of moral issues. Such an account would include a survey of the virtues that one should expect in veterinarians. It would identify the general values that the profession should inculcate in its members, and explore how these values can help to solve particular issues. Normative veterinary ethics would also attempt to formulate a set of principles that veterinarians can use in guiding their responses to particular moral questions about how they ought to act.

Normative veterinary ethics is today very far from such a comprehensive approach. The literature of normative veterinary ethics is tiny compared with that of normative medical or legal ethics. There must be more articles and books, more ethics scholars active in the veterinary schools, and more veterinarians participating in ethical discussion before normative veterinary ethics can collect enough perspectives and proposed conclusions to produce a comprehensive body of knowledge.

Because of the present rudimentary state of normative veterinary ethics, no one is in a position to offer definitive answers to all of its most important problems. Nor will this text attempt to do so. Rather, it is the purpose of the remainder of this book to survey many of the critical issues facing normative ethics today, and to provide a structure that veterinarians can use to elaborate their own thinking about these issues. Along the way I shall offer some of my own conclusions about how some of these ethical questions ought to be answered in order to stimulate discussion and debate.

THREE FUNDAMENTAL ISSUES OF NORMATIVE VETERINARY ETHICS

Normative veterinary ethics faces three fundamental issues in examining veterinary practice.

What Questions Should Be Asked?

Normative veterinary ethics must first determine when to ask questions and what sorts of questions to ask. Clearly, if there is an ethical problem that one does not see in a situation, or if one asks the wrong questions about a perceived problem, one will not do justice to the situation.

For example, I once visited animal quarters maintained by a respected laboratory animal veterinarian. The facility housed several dogs. They all appeared clean and healthy and in fact were receiving excellent veterinary care. However, the pens in which the dogs were kept contained only food, water, and bedding. I asked the veterinarian what he thought about supplying chew toys to make the animals' lives a bit more enjoyable. He responded by raising clearly relevant questions regarding whether such toys would be economically feasible and consistent with the purposes of the experiment. But the veterinarian (to his own surprise) had never thought of asking any of these questions because he had never considered the issue of supplying toys to laboratory dogs.

On the other hand, one must avoid asking too many questions, lest one invent issues where they do not exist. I always sneak into the situations I discuss with my veterinary students several problems that raise *medical* issues or in which ethical questioning should be delayed pending medical analysis. I ask, for example, what the students would do about a client who wants his animal euthanized because it is urinating all over the house. When presented with this situation in a medicine course, these students invariably focus first on possible medical causes of the problem. But when they are "doing ethics," more than a few will ask immediately whether the owner has mistreated the animal or failed in his moral duties to train it properly. This is, of course, a poor response. It illustrates the important point that asking ethical questions before one practices competent veterinary medicine is bad veterinary medicine as well as bad ethics.

Certain questions must be addressed by normative ethics simply because they are matters of controversy among veterinarians or the public. However, one's judgment about whether some questions are worth asking can depend on one's ethical views. Some veterinarians may believe that inquiring about toys for laboratory dogs is foolish because, in their view, one does not have an obligation to make such animals happy but only to prevent their experiencing unnecessary discomfort (see Chapter 11). It is clear, therefore, that among the issues normative veterinary ethics must consider is what questions are worth raising in the first place.

What Is the Best Approach to These Questions?

A second fundamental concern of normative veterinary ethics is quite obviously attempting to determine what the best approach to a situation would be.

Who Should Make the Decision?

But normative ethics has a third concern quite different from discovering the best approach – the issue of who should have the authority to make a decision regarding a problem.[a] Assuming for the purposes of argument that the dogs discussed above ought to have been given toys, it would not follow that I had any moral right to make the decision whether to give them toys. Indeed, I did not have such authority, because neither the dogs, the animal quarters, or the experiments of which the animals were a part were mine.

Although it may sometimes be obvious who has the moral right to make a decision regarding an ethical issue, this can be a matter of disagreement. For example, some veterinarians believe that they have the right to make important decisions *for* clients by assuring that the clients agree to what they have already decided ought to be done. Others (including myself) would argue that in most cases, the client and not the veterinarian has the moral right to make the decision, even if the client might make a morally incorrect decision (see, e.g., Chapter 20).

IDENTIFYING AND WEIGHING LEGITIMATE INTERESTS: A BATTLE PLAN FOR NORMATIVE VETERINARY ETHICS

As the 18th century Scottish philosopher David Hume observed (1), if everyone could have whatever he wanted or needed, and if no one ever offended the wants and needs of anyone else, justice would be a superfluous concept. In a land of milk and honey, where riches could be had for the taking, it would be a waste of time to discuss what kinds of wages would be fair to pay employees or what kinds of distribution of wealth are just. No one would bother with these questions because they would have no complaints, and no need for guidance, about such matters. If people always treated each other and all other sentient creatures with saintly perfection, and if no one ever showed disrespect for, took advantage of, thieved from, assaulted, or violated the rights of anyone else, no one would be concerned about

---

[a]One could treat the issue of who should have the authority to make a decision as part of the question of what the best approach would be. The point of separating these questions is to call attention to the fact that the matter of who ought to make a decision is frequently an important issue in its own right.

how people ought or ought not to behave. Everyone would just be happy and
would behave well, automatically.

In veterinary medicine, too, ethics is important largely because those who
participate in or are affected by veterinary practice are *not* all perfectly situated and
do *not* all have the same wants and interests. Veterinarians are concerned about how
far they may go in promoting their practices because many doctors are not doing as
well as they desire, and because many in the profession believe that certain marketing
techniques may harm the profession and ultimately the interests of clients and
patients. Likewise, euthanasia would not be an issue for normative veterinary ethics
if *everyone* felt comfortable about or behaved properly regarding the killing of
veterinary patients.

It would be a mistake to think that all ethical issues involve a difference of
interests or desires, or that those which do all require lengthy and acrimonious battle
before a resolution can be achieved. Patients, clients, and practitioners often have
the same interests. Sometimes, their differing interests can argue for the same course
of action. In such cases, it may be easy to decide what ought to be done.

Nevertheless, my experience discussing moral issues with veterinary students and
practitioners has led me to conclude that the best way of making progress in
normative veterinary ethics is to ask – at least initially – about *differences* in interests
and about potential conflicts among these interests. Such an approach moves one
quickly to the heart of the most important ethical issues facing the profession.

The following list of questions sets forth my proposed approach to normative
veterinary ethics. It is offered not just as a framework for the remainder of this
volume. It is presented as a tool that veterinary students, veterinarians, and others
can use to structure their thinking about ethical issues in veterinary medicine.

A GENERAL APPROACH TO ETHICAL PROBLEMS
IN VETERINARY MEDICINE

*In determining what questions should be asked, the best approach to these
questions, and who ought to have the authority to make a decision regarding them,
one should routinely ask the following:*

1. *What are the parties participating in, or potentially affected by, a problem or
    some aspect of veterinary practice?*

    *In answering this question, consider whether any or all of the following should
    be included as relevant parties:*

        *a. any particular animal or animals directly involved in or affected by
    the situation or issue;*
        *b. other animals that could be affected by what might be done in the
    situation under consideration;*
        *c. any particular client or clients directly involved in or affected by the
    situation or issue;*
        *d. other actual or potential clients of this or other veterinarians who
    could be affected by what might be done in the situation under
    consideration;*

    e. members of the public and society at large;

    f. the particular veterinarian or veterinarians directly involved in or affected by the situation under consideration;

    g. other veterinarians and the profession at large; and

    h. other actual or potential participants in the provision of veterinary services, including employees of the veterinarian under consideration, employees of other veterinarians, and veterinary students.

2. *What are the legitimate interests of these parties?*

3. *How should these interests be weighed, balanced, or reconciled?*

    In considering how these interests ought to be weighed relative to each other, one should ask the following questions:

    a. What are the possible alternatives that can be reasonably considered, and what are the potential advantages and disadvantages of these alternatives to the relevant parties?

    b. Does the law (including the pronouncements of the state board of veterinary medicine and other administrative bodies) attempt to choose an alternative or channel one's thinking toward or away from certain alternatives? How much weight should one give to any such legal guidance?

    c. Do standards of official veterinary ethics require that a certain approach be taken, or suggest ethical ideals useful in determining how one might act? If official norms do require some approach, how strongly should such requirements count in deciding what one ought to do?

4. *To what extent can one derive from one's response to the problem or issue, principles concerning virtues, values, and action-oriented rules for veterinarians that might contribute to a systematic approach to normative veterinary ethics?*

EXPLAINING THE APPROACH

It will be the task of the remainder of this book to demonstrate the usefulness of this suggested approach to ethical issues. However, it is important that certain features of the strategy be understood from the outset.

A Rough and Ready Battle Plan

First, the approach does not contain an exhaustive list of all questions to be asked when considering ethical issues in veterinary medicine. There are many interesting and important issues in veterinary ethics, and one could make a strong case for including questions regarding any number of them in a general strategy. One could, for example, argue that the approach should ask more specifically about factors relevant in weighing the interests of veterinary employees, veterinary students, or women practitioners. Nor does the approach specify all the possible ways of further refining and inquiring about those matters that are listed. Indeed, even the entries on my list of parties whose interests should be routinely considered are capable of considerable refinement. For example, one could further divide the category of "other animals" that could be affected into i) other animals owned by a particular client; ii) other animals owned by all one's other clients; iii) all other animals owned by clients of other practitioners; iv) all other animals located in one's geographic region; v) all nonowned wild animals; and vi) animals used in research and industry. Sometimes, as we shall see, several of these categories are among those one will want to consider in approaching an ethical problem.

Clearly, the success of any approach to ethical issues will turn on the ability of those using it to make further refinements and to ask additional questions when these are required by the issues at hand. And, indeed, it is the purpose of my suggested approach to stimulate such refinement and questions. However, I have found that too long and complex an outline of questions tends to get put on the shelf and does not get used by students and practitioners looking for a manageable way of attacking ethical problems.

The Difficulty of the Questions

Because the approach is designed to elicit important questions, and because many important questions in normative veterinary ethics raise difficult and controversial issues, the approach will sometimes stimulate many more questions than it answers. For example, balancing the interests of an animal patient against those of its human owner is not always a routine exercise. One will sometimes have to first address the ethical question of what *ought* to be recognized as a legitimate interest of the animal. This in turn will often raise the issue of whether the animal may have a moral right to be treated or not treated in a certain way, or whether utilitarian considerations ought to apply.

The task of weighing legitimate interests is complicated not only by the fact that the interests of different parties can conflict. There can be conflicts in the interests of each of the parties, the resolution of which itself can involve difficult moral issues. Thus, I argue in Chapter 16 that among the potentially conflicting interests of a veterinarian can be 1) his self-interest in increasing the profits of his practice and 2) his interest in belonging to a profession that is included among the healing arts. I shall argue that the merchandising of nonprofessional goods and services may in the short run promote the former interest for some doctors, but ultimately may injure the latter interest for the profession as a whole. However, as we shall see, one cannot resolve this conflict simply by attempting to balance against each other just these interests of practitioners. One must also weigh these potentially conflicting interests against the interest that *clients* have in obtaining products and services at a reasonable price, and the effect that furthering this interest will have upon the interests of *patients* in receiving professional services clients can afford.

Elaboration of Some Basic Concepts

The importance of several of the questions in my suggested approach has already been demonstrated. We have seen that an ethical problem may have more alternative responses than at first meet the eye (Chapter 1); how the law sometimes attempts to choose among the alternatives and how one might assign a proper weight to such a choice (Chapter 4); how administrative governmental bodies can impose their ethical judgments upon veterinarians (Chapter 7); and how official ethical standards can apply to moral issues (Chapters 8 and 9).

There remain, however, several general concepts and concerns that require further elaboration before the approach can be applied in earnest.

Chapter 11 will discuss factors relevant in determining the interests of veterinary patients, and Chapter 12 focuses on one such factor, the concept of animal rights. Chapter 13 develops principles regarding the legitimate interests of veterinary clients. Chapter 14 defines and asks some pointed questions about a concept that may have an enormous impact on veterinary practice, the human-companion animal bond. Chapter 15 discusses in general terms the legitimate interests of veterinarians and presents four models of veterinary practice that are currently struggling for the hearts and minds of doctors.

These are not the only concepts or concerns one will need in approaching issues in normative veterinary ethics. However, they will aid considerably in identifying and weighing the legitimate interests of the three most frequent participants in the arena of veterinary ethics – the patient, the client, and the veterinarian.

After establishing general principles regarding the legitimate interests of patients, clients, and doctors, the text turns to ethical issues in which the interests of these parties, and sometimes of others as well, come into play.

REFERENCE

1. Hume D: *Treatise of Human Nature.* Sec. II. In Aiken HD (ed): *Hume's Moral and Political Philosophy.* New York: Hafner Publishing Co., 1966, p 63.

Chapter

11

The Interests of Animals

There are, surely, few veterinarians who do not think that their patients have legitimate interests. Few doctors would have difficulty concluding that it is in the best interests of a cat in severe pain and near death from terminal lymphoma to put the poor animal out of its misery. Nor are judgments about what is good or bad for a patient reserved for situations in which one must contemplate ending its life. Veterinarians act in the interests of animal patients every day – by assisting them in giving birth and being born, by inoculating them against disease, by treating and repairing them when they become ill or injured, by helping them to live long and happy lives through preventive medicine and good nutrition.

The issue faced by contemporary normative veterinary ethics is not establishing that animals have interests, but how to determine what interests animals do have and how strong these interests are. About this question there is considerable disagreement, among veterinarians and the public at large.

THE ANTICRUELTY POSITION: FREEDOM FROM PAIN OR SUFFERING

According to one view, which I shall call *the anticruelty position*, the only very strong interest that nonhuman animals possess is an interest in not experiencing pain or suffering – or, if they must undergo some pain or suffering in their use by people, in not experiencing unnecessary pain or suffering.

This is probably still the predominant view regarding animals in American society today. It is found in numerous laws, and in the thinking of many in the veterinary and scientific communities. For example, the anticruelty to animals statutes of the various states do not require that people be good or kind to certain animals, but only that they *not* be *cruel* to them. (One cannot be prosecuted for failing to make one's dog happy by not playing with it or loving it as much as one might.) Moreover, according these laws, merely killing an animal or using it for food, fiber, draught, or innumerable other purposes, cannot of itself constitute cruelty. One must also have done such things in a manner causing the animals unjustifiable or unnecessary pain or discomfort.[a] Our laws also require the "humane" slaughter of food animals, which is taken to mean killing them with a minimum amount of pain or discomfort.

Likewise, the great majority of animal researchers believe that their primary moral obligation is to protect their animals from unnecessary pain (1). Most researchers also believe that there is no moral issue in using an animal in an experiment if it is anesthetized prior to the beginning of the protocol and is never permitted to regain consciousness. For in such circumstances the animal will experience no pain whatever (2).

In the food animal area, too, the anticruelty position holds sway. According to several leading livestock scientists "it is in the best interest of the American livestock producer to optimize the living conditions or environment of farm animals" (3). However, the terms "optimization" or animal "welfare" are not understood by these scientists to mean the maximization of goods or positive states, but rather "the absence of an excessive amount of stress" (4). Identification of "welfare" and "well-being" with lack of stress or negative states is also to be found in that standard reference, the *Merck Manual*. Its discussion of these concepts recommends that "from a practical stand," the veterinarian ask the following question: "Do the methods of handling, housing, and general management adopted by this owner/operator impose the least amount of distress (negative side of stress) on animals of this age, weight, stage of development, etc." (5)?

In prohibiting "unnecessary" pain or suffering, the anticruelty position presupposes the legitimacy of certain human endeavors. For what the position means by "unnecessary" pain is pain that is not required for some legitimate human use of animals. No amount of pain or discomfort is, strictly speaking, "necessary" for a food or research animal. It is not absolutely required that any animals be used for food or in research; they are so used because people decide to use them in these ways. From the point of view of the anticruelty position as it is applied in our society, pain or discomfort undergone by food or research animals would be "necessary" if it is required for the use of animals as food or in scientifically defensible experiments. For both of these kinds of animal use are considered acceptable in our society. On the other hand, if some amount of animal pain is required for a human endeavor that is thought to be *illegitimate* (e.g., organized dog fighting or experiments with utterly no scientific justification), using animals in such endeavors will be judged to inflict "unnecessary" pain and will therefore be categorized as "cruel" or "inhumane."

The anticruelty position does permit one to take into account the amount of animal pain caused by a certain kind of animal use in determining whether that use is a legitimate one and the pain is therefore "necessary." But quite often, adherents of the anticruelty position will begin with the acceptance of a certain animal use as legitimate and then require that it be conducted so as to cause no pain or no more pain than is "necessary."

The anticruelty position also permits one to view animals as having interests other than being free from pain or unnecessary pain. What characterizes the anticruelty position is that it does not view such other interests as *very strong*.

Thus, a veterinarian who subscribes to the anticruelty position can give as one of his reasons for treating a dog or cat that his care will assure the animal a better

---

[a]There are laws prohibiting the killing of other persons' animals, but these are not anticruelty laws. It should also be noted that although in many jurisdictions the crime of "cruelty" to animals once required a malicious intent to harm an animal or taking pleasure in doing so, today in the great majority of states there is no such requirement. It is sufficient that one cause an animal unnecessary or unjustifiable pain.

life. He can agree that these patients have an interest not just in being free from pain but in being positively healthy and happy. However, he will see no ethical problem in euthanizing the same animals when he is asked to do, as long as they will not suffer in the process. He may, in short, believe it would be a moral ideal, something to strive for, that clients not have their healthy animals killed. But he will view an animal's interest in living or living a healthy and happy life as so weak that it is easily outweighed by the client's desire to be rid of it. He will see his only ethical obligation to make sure that the animal will not experience any unnecessary suffering.

THE PARTIAL BREAKDOWN OF THE ANTICRUELTY POSITION

It seems fair to say that as a general position regarding the interests of *all* animals, the anticruelty position is no longer accepted by many in our society. An increasing number of people appear to be adopting the view that at least some animals are morally entitled not just to freedom from pain or unnecessary suffering, but to certain positive benefits – even if providing these benefits entails considerable expense or inconvenience for people. There are veterinarians who will not painlessly kill an animal simply because the client wants to be rid of it, but will insist at the very least that it be taken to a shelter for possible adoption. These practitioners may not believe that such animals have an unqualified right to live, but they do believe that it is wrong not to try to give some animals a second chance. Every companion animal doctor has clients who view their animal as a member of the family, and who believe that it is entitled to the best veterinary care that money can buy, even if such care is many times more expensive than a painless death. In the area of animal research as well, some animals are coming to be seen as having interests over and above being free from pain or discomfort. The federal Animal Welfare Act now requires that primates used in research be afforded "a physical environment adequate to promote [their] psychological well-being" (6). Some thinkers in the area of farm animal welfare too advocate not only the minimization of negative mental states, but also the promotion of positive well-being (7).

It would be incorrect to think that the beliefs of society or of the veterinary profession regarding the legitimate interests of animals are in total disarray. Nevertheless, it is equally true that there is not a universal consensus about the interests of all animals, on which one could comfortably rely in weighing the interests of an animal or animals. There is, surely, enough disagreement to compel those who accept the anticruelty position, as well as those who reject it, to say something in defense of their positions.

THE INADEQUACY OF THE ANTICRUELTY POSITION

My suggested decision-procedure for approaching normative veterinary ethics (see Chapter 10) is intended to facilitate discussion of moral issues and not to dictate solutions. Nevertheless, I would argue that as an exhaustive account of the interests of *all* animals, the anticruelty position is obviously incorrect.

The easiest place to find counter-examples to the anticruelty position is in the relationship between people and animals that is now termed the "human-companion animal bond." More about the nature of this bond will be discussed in Chapter 14. But for now it can be said that this relationship brings great benefit to a central aspect of the lives of human and animal alike. We may not always be able to say that an animal in such a relationship is able to "give of itself" with the "expectation" that it will receive something in response. However, we can certainly say that what such an animal gives can often make it enormously disrespectful, ungrateful, and *wrong* to treat it as having no more than an interest in avoiding pain or discomfort.

My Yorkie may not know he is doing me a favor when he greets me joyously at the door or when we play fetch with his little toys. Yet great favors and pleasures he bestows nevertheless. In light of the many benefits I have received from him over the years, I am surely obligated to attend to many of his interests. He ought to receive attention, the opportunity for exercise, and good nutrition so that he can have his happiness too. He deserves to be taken to the veterinarian regularly, not just so that he may be free of pain, but also so that he can continue to enjoy his own pleasures. None of this means that I must bankrupt myself to meet his needs, or that his interests must usually take precedence over my own. But it does mean that I must treat him as having legitimate interests that go beyond freedom from discomfort and that sometimes outweigh my desires or predilections.

What I have said about my dog is no different from what many people would say about their animals. However, once one begins to view certain animals as having legitimate interests beyond freedom from pain or discomfort, one is forced to draw some lines. There are limits to such interests. There are many times when human interests do outweigh those of animals. Moreover, it is not the case that all animals have the same legitimate interests or have them to the same degree. Once we admit that some animals sometimes have interests above and beyond freedom from pain, we must be prepared to justify our decisions about when this is the case and when it is not. To assist in this process, normative veterinary ethics must utilize principles regarding the nature and weight of animal interests.

RELEVANT FACTORS IN IDENTIFYING AND WEIGHING THE LEGITIMATE INTERESTS OF ANIMALS

The following are suggested as very general factors to be taken into account in weighing the interests of animals. Although all these factors seem intuitively relevant to weighing animal interests, many require further elaboration and research. It is, for example, easy – and surely correct – to say that an animal's capacity to experience stress is relevant to determining its interests. But how animal stress is to be defined, measured, and compared is a matter that could require many decades of solid research. The need for further work on these suggested considerations does not argue against the considerations. Rather, it points out the amount of scientific as well as ethical study that is required before a fully satisfactory approach to normative ethical issues will be possible.

Capacity to Experience Pain, Suffering, Stress, and Other Forms of Discomfort

Although some animals may sometimes have interests beyond freedom from pain or discomfort, the capacity of an animal to experience what we would call unpleasant or negative psychological states remains a crucial factor in determining the nature and weight of its interests. Although pain and other negative states can be beneficial in assuring an animal's health or safety and are undoubtedly products of natural selection, all other things being equal, it is better not to feel pain (or another negative state such as distress or discomfort) than to feel it. Moreover, intense or long-lasting pain is worse than weak or fleeting pain. Therefore, it seems intuitively clear that the interest an animal has in not suffering pain, or a certain kind of negative psychological state, is greater the more intensely and the longer it can experience that negative state. And it has a greater interest in not experiencing a severe negative state than a mild one, and in not experiencing a long negative state than a short one.

Amount and duration, however, are not the only factors. Certain negative psychological states carry extra weight. For example, when one feels a sharp pain, that is bad. But if one also feels anxiety and fear *about* the pain – if one worries about it, contemplates its potential effects, and then troubles about whether more is on the way, one will feel worse than if one just felt the pain alone. Such anxiety and fear can be so intense that they can not only continue after the pain has disappeared, but can be more unpleasant than the pain ever was.

To the extent that an animal can feel not only pain, but also stress, fear, and anxiety, its interest in avoiding a situation might be greater than the interest of an animal that might only feel pain in the same situation. Veterinarians and animal owners all know a common example of this distinction. A dog or cat may be up and about hours after surgery. If a person has a similar operation, the agony can last for weeks or months. It is possible that human pain receptors are more sensitive and that the person is really feeling more pain than the animal. However, it seems just as likely that what makes the human's condition worse is the fact that he can, and does, feel terrible in many ways about the pain – a process that itself can call attention to the pain, make it worse, and make it last longer.

Capacity to Experience Pleasure and Other Positive Mental States

If it can be in the interest of certain nonhuman animals to be spared pain or discomfort, it may also be in their interest to experience pleasure or other positive mental states. Research indicates that there are "reward circuits" in the brains of both human beings and animals (8). These pathways could have evolved as a mechanism for reinforcing behaviors that promote the survival of the individual and the species; they may also play a fundamental role in the human appreciation of beauty and the desire to learn. If animals have such reward circuits some may have the capacity to experience some of the "higher" pleasures. We may well decide upon reflection that animals, or some animals, have a much stronger interest in avoiding pain than in experiencing pleasure. Thus, animal pleasures might not weigh heavily against human needs. But if some animals do have an interest in experiencing pleasure, we also might be able to determine that they have a greater interest in experiencing a more intense pleasure than mild pleasure, and in experiencing a long positive mental state than a short one.

Intelligence

One factor that surely counts in influencing the weight of an animal's interests is its intelligence. Most people feel more uncomfortable about subjecting chimpanzees to invasive laboratory experiments than rats because the former are able to perceive and react to their surroundings in a far more complex and innovative way. Likewise, one reason there is such intense interest in protecting whales is that, although we may have little idea what is going through the minds of these creatures, we do know that they are enormously intelligent.

In many cases, intelligence may increase the weight of an animal's interests because it leads to or makes possible something else of value. Dogs, cats, and certain primates can interact and form bonds with people in part because they are intelligent. Another result or aspect of intelligence that itself may have value is self-awareness, the ability to reflect upon or understand what is happening to one. Likewise, the capacity to experience certain painful or pleasurable states seems linked to intelligence; for example, the cat that appears to take great pleasure in attempting to bat an errant insect with its paws is able to have such experiences because it is capable of sophisticated awareness and interpretation.

Although intelligence can lead to other things of value, it is itself valuable. We regard the retarded human as unlucky (but not without great worth) because we view being able to perceive and react to the world in certain ways as preferable to not having such capacities. Likewise, we view chimpanzees' extraordinary intelligence as itself a lucky and precious condition, in part because it enables these animals to take in more of the world than can a laboratory rodent or even the family dog.

Capacity to Experience or Exhibit Valuable Emotions and Character Traits

Another feature of some animals that increases their value in our eyes is their ability to experience emotions or to have traits of character that we value in our fellow humans. We admire a dog that loves its owner, and praise it for being loyal and obedient. On the other hand, a dog that is vicious, nasty, and selfish may be valued less – so much so, that an owner of such an animal will sometimes appear justified in not expending the time or resources to assist its interests as one might want him to expend upon a loving and friendly animal. It may seem unfair to favor some animals and disfavor others because of traits for which they may not be responsible. But we also favor nice and disfavor disagreeable people even though we may not be able to say that they somehow decided to be so. Just as friendliness in people is better than viciousness and belligerence, so can it be in animals, and so can it make a difference in our judgments about how strongly we ought to value their interests.

Self-Awareness

One feature of human beings that appears to give them greater value than many animals is the fact that we possess self-awareness. Not only do we experience certain things, but we are aware that it is ourselves who are experiencing them, and we are aware of ourselves as beings distinct from others. It can be worse to do something to a being that possesses such self-awareness than to one that does not. While beings that do and those that do not possess self-awareness may both be able to experience pleasure, only those with self-awareness can anticipate experiencing pleasure and can feel further pleasure at the anticipation of experiencing pleasure. Similarly, while beings that do and those that do not have self-awareness may feel pain, only the former can feel anxiety or fear at the prospect that they will feel pain, can be ashamed of fearing the experience of pain, and so on. Self-awareness is also related to autonomy, the capacity to decide on one's own that one will make decisions and long-term plans and to work to put these decisions into effect.

There is some evidence that certain animals may possess self-awareness to a limited degree. Gallup has demonstrated that chimpanzees and orangutans, but not gorillas or monkeys, are capable of looking into a mirror and recognizing that is themselves they are seeing. Gallup argues that the former animals do have a sense of self (9). Chimpanzees deceive each other, a kind of behavior that requires them to impute some thought or self-awareness to other beings (10). Dolphins may display reciprocal altruism not related to kinship (11). Elephants appear to demonstrate elaborate grieving behaviors on the death of other elephants (12). These behaviors indicate that certain animals do sometimes exhibit some degree of self-awareness and should be accorded a higher moral status than other animals.

Interaction with Human Beings

As noted above, we do think that certain animals are owed greater consideration because of their interactions with human beings. Thus, even if a pig and the family dog have comparable mental abilities, we often believe we owe something to the dog because of what it has done for us and what we have already done for it. It is not irrational and unjustifiable to single out for special treatment certain beings with whom one has interacted even though there may be others that, in the abstract, may seem as worthy. Most people believe that they have greater obligations to members of their own families than to strangers. They believe this not just because of blood lineage (some people are, of course, adopted) but because they think they owe more to those they have known, interacted with, and loved than to strangers.

The Animal's Nature

Rollin argues that animals have a biologically determined nature (he uses the Aristotelian term "*telos*") that they have an interest in satisfying and that is therefore entitled to respect (13). As Rollin points out, it seems plausible to say that it is in the interest of a dog that seems to have an innate need for vigorous activity, to be given opportunities for exercise. Likewise, as I shall suggest later, one argument against "debarking" family dogs is that it takes away from many of these animals an important part of what it seems to be a dog.

The notion that an animal's "nature" contributes to its legitimate interests is intuitively appealing, but requires considerable refinement and discussion. Do we think animals possess an interest in having parts of their "nature" respected simply because frustrating their natures causes them discomfort or prevents them from experiencing pleasures they might otherwise experience – or because there is something inherently wrong in violating their *telos*? Do some animals (predators such as wolves, for example) have natures that do not entitle them to as much respect as other animals that happen to have more benign natures? Are certain features of an animal's nature more important to it, or (not necessarily the same thing) worthy of greater respect than other features? What is the relevance of the fact that certain animals have been given inborn "natures" by humans to make them more amenable to certain human purposes?

Utilitarian Considerations

As was explained in Chapter 5, utilitarianism proclaims that the right action (or general rule for action) is one that will in the future produce no less benefit to all affected than any other action (or rule). Utilitarianism is unsatisfactory as an exhaustive normative theory because we do not believe that the only consideration in determining the morality of an action or practice is the amount of benefit or detriment that action or practice will produce in the future.

Nevertheless, comparing the resultant benefits and detriments of alternative actions is *sometimes* relevant in determining what one ought to do, and such considerations often play a role in deciding our moral obligations regarding animals. We often apply utilitarian considerations to a single animal, for example, when we conclude that we ought to euthanize a terminally ill patient because ending its life will prevent it from suffering unnecessary pain. (To be sure, one can also argue that such an animal has a right not to be kept in pain.) Utilitarian arguments are also applied from animal to animal. Thus, we sometimes justify experimentation on selected animals to develop and test veterinary drugs on the grounds that causing some pain or discomfort to these animals will produce great benefits for other animals on which these drugs will be used. Utilitarian considerations are also applied from animals to humans. The argument that animal experimentation is justified by resultant benefits to people, or that farrowing crates ought to be designed so as to maximize productivity while at the same time minimizing pain or discomfort to the animals, are utilitarian arguments.

HUMAN SUPERIORITY

I have identified several considerations that appear to be legitimate in identifying and weighing animal interests. However, it is one thing to hold that an animal may have a legitimate interest and quite another to conclude that this interest ought to be given *priority* over the interests of people or other animals in a given set of circumstances. In the area of normative veterinary ethics, recognition of this distinction is extremely important because animal interests – as indisputably present as they may be – are often less weighty than and must often give way in particular circumstances to human interests.

In applying any palatable approach to veterinary ethics, therefore, one will often find oneself appealing to the principle that the interests of a particular person or of people in general are so much more important than those of some animal or animals, that the animals' interests must give way partially or entirely.

It is beyond the scope of this text to provide a complete justification for the widely held belief that human interests are generally entitled to greater weight than animal interests. However, in recent years some philosophers and animal rights activists have claimed that there are no morally relevant differences between humans and many animals. Therefore, any discussion of normative veterinary ethics cannot ignore completely certain arguments challenging the view that human beings are superior in moral value and status to nonhuman animals.

The Argument from Animal Mental Complexity

One argument that is supposed to show that some animal interests are as important as human interests recognizes the relevance of mental sophistication to the weight of human or animal interests. But according to this argument, many animals are in fact as mentally sophisticated as most human beings, at least in respects relevant to comparing their moral value. It is concluded that human and nonhuman animals have equally weighty interests in such things as living, not being eaten or experimented on, and in not being used as a means toward any one else's ends.

One proponent of such an argument is Professor Regan. He asserts that

perception, memory, desire, belief, self-consciousness, intention, a sense of the future – these are among the leading attributes of the mental life of normal mammalian animals aged one or more. Add to this list the not unimportant categories of emotion (e.g., fear or hatred) and sentience, understood as the capacity to experience pleasure or pain, and we begin to approach a fair rendering of the mental life of these animals (14).

Regan does not reveal why he thinks all "normal" mammals have such mental complexity after they reach 1 year of age. Nor does he provide credible evidence for his contention that a laboratory hamster, for example, can be self-conscious in the same way that a human being is, has a sense of the future, or can be said to experience not just pain but such sophisticated emotions as hatred (which requires not just a negative feeling, but such a feeling directed *at* someone or something that one identifies *as* the hated object).

One should not ignore behavioral or biochemical evidence of the mental attributes of any animal. However, it is simply not the case that a hamster, cow, horse, dog, or even a chimpanzee, is capable of all the same kinds of pleasures and pains, thoughts and decisions, and autonomous life as an average adult human being. Regan's blanket generalizations are incompatible with the kind of ethical approach to animals we surely need – one that is willing to look carefully and scientifically at what animals really are and what they can do, and one that takes into account the enormous variety among animal species and individual animals of the same species.

The Argument from Deficient Humans

A second argument raised in favor of equal consideration for people and animals proceeds from the fact that there are many human beings, including young infants, the severely mentally retarded, and the profoundly senile, whom most people regard as having very strong moral rights. Included among these rights are the right not to have their lives terminated simply because they are not mentally sophisticated, and the right not to be used in biomedical research solely for the benefit of others. According to the argument from deficient humans, there are many animals that are at least as sophisticated mentally as these deficient humans. Therefore, it is concluded, if deficient people have the moral right not to be eaten or experimented on without their consent, so do these animals (15).

There are many things wrong with this argument. It is far from clear that it even makes sense to say that a human being has the same mental level as, say, a bat or hamster, because if he did he would not be a human being, but a bat or a hamster (16). Nor does the argument from deficient humans take into account crucially important differences between many deficient humans and animals that often give the former greater moral value. For example, the human infant who may at present be mentally unsophisticated is *potentially* a human adult of great mental sophistication, while the laboratory hamster will never reach this level. Moreover, many deficient human beings have become so after a long and productive life and are, we want to say, entitled to respect and care from their relatives and society in part because of what they have given to others.

However, even if we set aside the past and futures of certain deficient humans, we can still see that there are important morally relevant differences between animals and deficient humans that show there is something special about being a deficient human. These differences reinforce rather than undercut our basic moral belief that human beings are superior to animals.

The Relevance of Being a Deficient Human

One clear difference between all deficient humans as we have been speaking of them and, for example, all normal laboratory hamsters, is that the former are all deficient while the latter are not.

Because deficient humans fall short of what normal humans can experience and do, we are inclined to say the following things about some of them who are not in a temporary state of deficiency:

- They are *disabled* in virtue of their having restricted capabilities.
- They *suffer* from a disability. (We would say this even if they are not suffering because of their disability.)
- They have been *harmed* or *injured*.
- They have already been subjected to a great *evil* or *misfortune*.

None of these things would be said of the normal laboratory hamster, and several things follow from this fact.

First, in experimenting on a deficient human, one would be making him worse off than one would be making a hamster of (let us suppose) equal mental abilities on whom the same experiment would be conducted. For if we suppose that both deficient human and hamster would be treated equally (confined in the same way, caused the same amount of pain, etc.), the experiment will nevertheless bring the deficient human to a level far beneath the level of a nondeficient human than the hamster will be brought beneath the level of a normal hamster. Even before the experiment, the deficient human with the mental life of a hamster is enormously disabled, harmed, and tragic. (Remember, we are speaking here of a human being with the mental capacity of a hamster.) During and after the experiment, he may become even more so. The hamster, on the other hand, begins as a normal, nonharmed, noninjured, nontragic hamster. It can be harmed by an experiment, of course. But treating it and the deficient human equally surely can never render it worse off than the deficient human.

Put another way, in determining the extent of an injury or harm to a being, one must take into account more than the quantity or quality of unpleasant sensations it may experience. One must consider what it means that *such a being* is having these experiences.

It does not follow that we can experiment freely on hamsters or other animals or use them in any way we please. What follows is that where the total degree of harm or injury suffered by potential subjects of an experiment is a relevant consideration in determining which subjects to use, this consideration usually will argue much more strongly in favor of using an animal whose normal state might be equal at best to that of a deficient human, than for using a deficient human.

There are other reasons why the enormous degree of a deficient human's disability can weigh more strongly against using him in experiments than against using, say, a hamster. We feel a reluctance to harm someone who has suffered a great injury unless there is a very strong reason to do so. Other things being equal, it is wrong to hurt someone when he is down. Because deficient humans are already gravely disabled, subjecting them to further deprivation is like beating the fallen; it just is not fair to hurt them more. I suggest that one reason we feel less reluctant to experiment on hamsters is that they are not already deprived. Indeed, many laboratory animals have safer, more comfortable lives than they would experience in the wild.

Also, when faced with the necessity of choosing which of a number of persons must suffer some deprivation or harm (as, for example, where budget cuts make it necessary to deprive some students of low-interest loans), justice sometimes requires that those who are already deprived suffer less of the necessary burden than those for whom the new deprivation will be less of an injury. And this can be so even where none of those affected are responsible for their condition or for the need to impose a burden upon anyone. Thus, aside from our obligation to avoid inflicting harm on already disabled humans, where an experiment or some use of a living creature is appropriate (and when this is the case will admittedly sometimes be in need of discussion), justice will almost always require doing it on a normal animal first, and if at all possible, instead of, on a disabled human.

LIMITS OF HUMAN SUPERIORITY

In short, weighing animal interests will often involve recognizing the superiority of human interests. However, animal interests do count. Sometimes, these interests can prohibit a human activity entirely. Sometimes, animal interests create severe constraints on what people may morally do to animals. The strength of animal interests is reflected in the concept of animal rights, which is the subject of the next chapter.

REFERENCES

1. Loew FM: Alleviation of pain: The researcher's obligation. *Lab Anim* 9:36-38, 1981.
2. Hewitt HB: The Use of Animals in Experimental Cancer Research. In Sperlinger D (ed): *Animals in Research.* Chichester, England: John Wiley & Sons, 1981, p 170 (stating that the "painless taking of animal life" is not an immoral act; and that "I should be more upset by my having caused one animal to suffer by my neglect or ineptitude than I should be by my administering euthanasia to 50 animals at the termination of an experiment in which none had been caused suffering").
3. Friend TH and Dellmeier GR: Applied Animal Euthenics Program. Mk. II. College Station, Texas: published privately, undated, p 3.
4. *Id.,* 7.
5. Animal Welfare. In Fraser CM (ed): *The Merck Veterinary Manual.* ed 6. Rahway, NJ: Merck & Co., 1986, p 873.
6. 7 U.S.C.A. § 2143(a)(2)(B). But note that for animals in general, the Secretary of Agriculture is directed to promulgate regulations "to ensure that animal pain and distress are minimized." § 2143(a)(3)(A).
7. Fox MW: *Farm Animals: Husbandry, Behavior, and Veterinary Practice.* Baltimore: University Park Press, 1984, p 205.
8. Wise RA: Catecholamine theories of reward: A critical review. *Brain Res* 152:215-247, 1978; Prado-Alcala R, Streather A and Wise RA: Brain stimulation reward and dopamine terminal fields. II. Septal and cortical fields. *Brain Res* 301:209-219, 1984.
9. Gallup GG: Toward a Comparative Psychology of Mind. In Mellgren RL: *Animal Cognition and Behavior.* Amsterdam: North Holland Publishing Co., 1983, pp 473-510.
10. Premack D and Woodruff G: Does the chimpanzee have a theory of mind? *Behavioral and Brain Sciences* 4:515-526, 1981; Woodruff G and Premack D: Intentional communication in the chimpanzee: The development of deception. *Cognition* 7:333-362, 1979.
11. Connor RC and Norris KS: Are dolphins reciprocal altruists? *American Naturalist* 11:358-374, 1982.
12. Douglas-Hamilton I and Douglas-Hamilton O: *Among the Elephants.* New York: Viking Press, 1975.

13. Rollin BE: *Animal Rights and Human Morality*. Buffalo: Prometheus Books, 1981, pp 54-57.
14. Regan T: *The Case for Animal Rights*. Berkeley: University of California Press, 1983, p 81.
15. For an exhaustive account of several forms of this kind of argument and a defense of one of them, see Regan T: An Examination and Defense of One Argument Concerning Animal Rights. In Regan T: *All That Dwell Therein*. Berkeley: University of California Press, 1982, pp 113-147.
16. Nagel T: What Is It Like to Be a Bat? *Philosophical Review* 83:435-450, 1974.

Chapter

12

Animal Rights: Some Guideposts
for the Veterinarian

The subject of animal rights has caused considerable disquiet and discomfort among veterinarians. Some see in animal rights yet an additional challenge to the economic viability of the profession (1). For others, the concept of animal rights poses a danger to the natural order and to science and progress (2). Many veterinarians find animal rights so antithetical to the aims and values of the profession that they prefer not to speak of animal "rights" at all (3-7). One astute observer has remarked that the battle over animal rights has caught veterinarians in a "cross fire" (8) – a metaphor that might suggest to some that veterinarians are doomed, and to others that the profession must beat a quick retreat from the entire controversy.

Much of this unhappiness is justified. There is, in fact, a great deal in the animal rights movement that is morally repugnant and deeply subversive of the interests of veterinarians and many patients and clients.

As I shall argue in this chapter, a proper response to the animal rights movement is not abandonment of animal rights. Indeed, the concept of animal rights is essential in the proper identification and weighing of animal interests.

WHAT IS A RIGHT?

There is disagreement among philosophers about the nature of rights, and about who or what does or does not have certain rights, and why (9). For the purposes of this discussion, however, it can be said that there are several things that are certainly true of rights.

There Is a Difference Between Moral and Legal Rights. Some moral rights (e.g., the right of parents to receive respect from their children) are not enforced by the law. And the law can enforce as a right (e.g., the right to own slaves in the Confederacy) practices that violate moral rights. Legal rights can be a matter of political decision: if the government decrees that something is a right and backs its decision with the force of law, then it is a legal right. On the other hand, although decisions of individuals or groups of people often are relevant to their moral rights, something does not become a moral right simply because the majority, or anyone for that matter, decides that it is. Thus, when one asks whether animals "have rights," it is important to keep in mind whether one is talking about moral or legal rights, or both.

Moral Rights Mark Out Very Strong Claims. When people say that someone has a moral right to some kind of treatment, they are saying something much stronger than that it is right to treat him in this way. For example, it may be the right thing for you to give to a charity when a solicitor appears at your door. But this does not mean that the charity has a *right* to any of your money. Moral rights mark out claims that normally do not require another's permission to be respected and that cannot be overridden simply because overriding them would, on balance, produce more benefit than detriment to all affected (10). For example, because a person normally has the right to use his car as he likes, he may quite properly drive to a basketball game, and pass in good conscience a stranger who might better use the car to support his family, even though lending the car to the stranger might on balance produce more happiness for all affected. This does not mean that considerations of the general happiness or welfare or others' rights can never override a given person's right. In a snowstorm, for example, when private use of cars might endanger the lives of others and prevent cleaning of the road, one's right to use one's automobile may properly be overridden, in favor of the greater good of the greater number. However, part of the point of saying it is one's moral right to use his property as he wants is to say that one should not normally be prevented from using it as he likes, and that this ability can be overridden, if at all, only for extremely important reasons.

THE DISTINCTIVENESS OF ANIMAL RIGHTS

To say that animals have moral rights is to make a distinctive kind of assertion that is different from the claim that people have moral obligations regarding animals. Those who argue that human beings should not abuse animals because this would lead to mistreatment of our fellow human beings (11), or who assert that animals may be used in scientific experiments only if doing so will produce greater benefits for people than harm to the animals (12), are not founding their arguments on the claim that animals have rights. Thus, Peter Singer, the author of *Animal Liberation* (13), opposes the use of animals for food and in research. But he does so solely on the grounds that these practices cause more pain and harm than benefits to all those animals and human beings affected. Although his book is commonly misinterpreted as "the definitive text of the animal rights movement" (5), he is a utilitarian and does not believe there are any moral rights, either for animals or people (14).

To say that animals have moral rights is to mean that they have *some* inherent worth independent of the value we human beings place on them. It is also to say that animals sometimes have interests that must be respected, even if failing to respect these interests would result in more pleasure for people than pain for the animals.

THE INDISPUTABILITY OF ANIMAL RIGHTS

Clearly, most people already believe that some animals have some moral rights. For example, most people find organized dogfighting morally unacceptable. Most would find it so even if the aggregate of pleasure brought to those who enjoy such events outweighs the aggregate of pain suffered by the combatants. What is wrong with dogfighting is that, irrespective of the total resulting benefits and detriments, it is unfair to the animals to subject them to such treatment. Dogs count for something in their own right, and they count enough to make dogfighting a cruelty, a moral offense, to them. Like the human infant or incompetent whose moral rights can be abridged even though he may be unable to articulate a complaint, these animals have a moral claim against society (which members of society can make in their behalf) not to use them in certain ways. However, to say these things is precisely to ascribe a moral right to these animals, the right not to be used in fights for the pleasure or monetary gain of people. There is nothing radical or earth-shaking in such an ascription. It does not of itself commit one to such demands of the animal rights movement as the abolition of horse and dog racing, meat-eating, or animal experimentation.

There are numerous other moral rights that almost everyone believes animals have. Most people reject unnecessary infliction of pain on laboratory animals, or painful slaughter of livestock, or neglect and mistreatment of household pets. When people reject these things, they do not appeal merely to some utilitarian calculation of pain versus benefits. They say these things are immoral, because they are gravely unfair and a serious wrong to the animals, and are in serious violation of their most basic interests.

Because many animals do count for something in their own right, and proper treatment of animals cannot always be reduced to comparison of resultant benefits and detriments, one should not abandon the notion of animal rights when thinking about how one may morally interact with animals. People might, I suppose, try to speak only of animal "welfare," if they included in the concept of animal welfare the presence of some moral claims of animals not reducible to utilitarian calculation. But if one is willing to do this, why should one not use the term "rights," which already exists in our moral vocabulary and which appropriately captures one consideration most people want to endorse?

Surely, refusing to use the term "rights" will not cause extremists to change their views or forsake their demands. More important, there is a real danger that those who refuse to use the term "rights" may abandon the legitimate and important idea the term denotes. Suppose people decided to continue to believe in certain human rights, such as the right not to be forced to turn one's property over to others, but for some reason decided to abandon the term "rights" and to speak only about human "welfare." One could say that a component of human welfare is not being forced to turn one's property over to others. However, people surely would soon be drawn to the major thrust of the concept of human welfare, which is what is good for particular humans or humanity in general. Then, people would be drawn to the question of whether it is good for them to decide on their own how to use their property, and then to arguments about the legitimacy of someone else's deciding how people should use their own property. These may well be legitimate issues. But they are not the same issues raised by the claim that people have a right to their property. This latter claim asserts that under normal circumstances one should just be left alone to use his property as he likes, and that others generally have a duty to refrain from asking whether such use should be curtailed because one's own or others' welfare would be furthered.

Of course, there are important differences between human rights and animal rights. Many human moral rights derive from the ability of normal human adults to make deliberate decisions and life choices. Few, if any, nonhuman animals are autonomous in the same way. Nevertheless, the concept of animal rights suggests that there are some ways of treating animals that are beyond the moral pale because of basic interests the animals have. One may want to argue about the nature, extent, and foundations of inviolable areas. However, one risks aborting such necessary arguments altogether if one jettisons entirely the concept around which these issues turn, the concept of moral rights.

WHAT IS THE ANIMAL RIGHTS MOVEMENT?

Whether one classifies a certain group or thinker as a member of the animal rights movement can depend on one's point of view. For example, the International Society for Animal Rights, which opposes animal research, applies the term "regulationist" to all who would permit any use of animals in research (15, 16). On the other hand, there are those who use the words "rightist" (17) or "antivivisectionist" (18-20) to refer to anyone who questions a good deal of animal experimentation, even if he in fact endorses much animal research. There is also controversy within what most thoughtful people would call "the" animal rights movement.

Granting the impossibility of defining the animal rights movement in a way that will satisfy everyone, I want to suggest that we view as members or sympathizers of "the movement" people who subscribe to at least all the following positions: 1) The vast majority of mammals (and certainly typical companion, farm, and laboratory mammals) not only have moral rights, but have some of the same moral rights as human beings. 2) Such animals have these rights at least in part because they have many of the same mental capabilities and activities as people. 3) Just as one would be violating a person's rights if one were to eat him or use him in research without his consent, or use him merely as a means to one's own ends, so does doing these things to most mammals violate their moral rights. 4) The law should enforce such moral rights, by, among other things, allowing these animals to sue in their own behalf, just as children and other human incompetents can have lawsuits brought on their behalf by legal representatives.

I believe this definition reflects how most participants and observers conceive of the movement, and allows for important internal theoretical and practical controversies within its ranks. (For example, as I have defined it, membership in the animal rights movement does not entail approval of illegal acts, even if some members of the movement do engage in such tactics.) Among the members of the animal rights movement so defined must be counted the Animal Legal Defense Fund, the Animal Liberation Front, the Coalition to End Animal Suffering in Experiments, the International Society for Animal Rights, People for the Ethical Treatment of Animals, United Action for Animals, and philosopher Tom Regan (21).

Of course, veterinarians must not restrict their attention to the animal rights movement. Other persons and organizations sometimes level sharp criticisms at veterinarians (22), and, indeed, occasionally ally themselves with the animal rights movement. Thus, the Humane Society of the United States, the National Anti-Vivisection Society, and the American and Massachusetts Societies for the Prevention of Cruelty to Animals joined the International Society for Animal Rights in a drive to end the use of pound animals in research (23). (The latter left the coalition after moderates endorsed the use of purpose-bred and dead animals (24).) Several moderate groups also funded the lawsuit brought by the Animal Legal Defense Fund against the Provimi Corporation to stop its distribution and sale of milk-fed veal in Massachusetts (25). (The suit was dismissed by a federal court judge (26).) However, if one lumps everyone who challenges – for whatever reason and to whatever extent – currently accepted animal uses under the banner of "the animal rights movement," one distorts reality, and makes it more difficult to respond adequately to these challenges.

THREE MYTHS OF THE ANIMAL RIGHTS MOVEMENT

"One Must Choose Between Animal Rights and Animal Welfare." Some leaders of the animal rights movement insist that only the movement is entitled to advocate animal rights and that anyone who thinks animals may be used for food, clothing, in sport, or in research must talk only of animal "welfare," "humane treatment," or "animal protection" (27, 28). Quite a few veterinarians have accepted this fictitious inconsistency between animal rights and animal welfare (3, 5-7). Dr. Robert M. Miller, for example, writes that he is "opposed to the concept of animals having inherent rights ... [b]ecause, if we accept the premise that animals have such rights as the right to be "free" and to live "natural" lives, then almost every utilization mankind makes of animals must be considered immoral" (7). *However, the concept of animal rights does not entail any such particular claims about what moral rights animals might have.* Nor is there any inconsistency in advocating animal welfare, or animal protection, or humane treatment, and some animal rights.

I believe the animal rights movement dearly wants veterinarians to accept its claim to exclusive use of the concept of rights.[a] As one philosopher has observed, today "rights are the principal currency of moral, political, and legal dispute" (29). If the animal rights movement can get veterinarians to refuse to talk about rights at all – even if veterinarians would in the end want to maintain that animals have limited moral rights – they will be separated from the mainstream of ethical and political debate. The animal rights movement wants to convince society that many in the veterinary community are mired in inadequate concepts and ways of thinking. This was precisely the claim made by some (30) when the AVMA Animal Welfare Committee stated that "the AVMA believes that use of the term 'animal rights' has to do with personal philosophical values and therefore recommends that the term 'animal rights' not be used and encourages the profession to focus its attention on the welfare and humane treatment of animals" (4).

---

[a]For example, a meeting was held in 1988 between representatives of the AVMA and a group calling itself the Association of Veterinarians for Animal Rights. The report of this event in the *Journal of the American Veterinary Medical Association* indicates that the AVMA representatives, as well as the *Journal* itself, accepted the interpretation of the concept of animal rights offered by this organization's representatives. The report stated that "animal rights implies each animal has intrinsic value, apart from its utility to man. According to this viewpoint, every sentient animal has a right to live out its entire life span without any painful interference from man" (31). As we have seen, the ascription of moral rights to animals simply does not amount to, or imply, the proposition that animals have the right to live out their lives without interference (painful or otherwise) from man. The AVMA ought never to identify the advocacy of animal rights with opposition to the human use of animals.

There is also a danger that acceptance of this imaginary inconsistency between animal welfare and animal rights will lead some who would prefer to take a more moderate position into the camp of the animal rights movement. For if a veterinarian wants to maintain that some animals have rights, and if he believes that in order to advocate animal rights at all he must agree with the claims of the animal rights movement, his only choice, it would seem, is to join the movement. If the animal rights movement can (somehow) convince a veterinarian that it is wrong to use animals for human ends, that is one thing. But no one should embrace such a view merely because he believes that animals have moral rights.

"Animals Do Not Have Any Legal Rights." According to animal rights activists (32, 33), something cannot have a legal right unless it has what lawyers call "standing" to sue, which means it can sue in its own name or have someone appointed by a court to sue on its behalf, and can recover money damages or other relief directly for its own benefit. These activists note that children and other human incompetents can have such standing because lawsuits can sometimes be brought for (and thus legally by) them for their own benefit. However, civil lawsuits cannot be instituted in the same way for an animal, and cannot result in that animal's receiving money or other relief from someone who harms it. According to animal rights activists, even anticruelty to animals statutes do not give animals any legal rights. For such laws empower a public authority to bring legal action, and do not provide for the appointment of a representative or guardian to further the interests of a particular animal or animals.

The claim that animals now have no legal rights, and that legal standing is necessary for their having rights, is important to the animal rights movement. The movement will not rest on moral persuasion, but seeks to use the law to force people to behave according to many of its precepts (32). The movement knows that our society tends to enforce fundamental moral rights as legal rights. Therefore, if it can establish that legal rights imply legal standing, it can try to move people from the eminently reasonable claim that animals have some fundamental moral rights, to the conclusion that animals should be treated by the law as legal persons, with standing to sue in their own behalf.

In fact, the American legal system affords many rights the possessors of which do not have standing to enforce. For example, generally only a government authority, and not a private citizen, can sue to abate a nuisance (such as a polluting factory) that affects the public at large (34). Yet most lawyers and laymen would say that individual members of the public have a legal right not to be harmed by such a nuisance. Nor would one say that people could not have a legal right to be free from crimes if the only redress from such offenses were the criminal justice system, which in fact gives the public prosecutor, and not the victim of a crime, standing to sue, and which typically does not grant compensation to the victim.

As for animals, the eminent legal philosopher Joel Feinberg states that "there is no reason to deny that animals have general legal rights to noncruel treatment derived from statutes to protect them" (35). Feinberg explains that a being or entity can have a legal right if the law permits someone (such as a public authority) to make enforceable claims in its interest. While conceding that animal protection statutes can be weak, and poor in legal rights for animals, Feinberg recognizes that this need not be so. He notes that the British Cruelty to Animals Act confers on animals "the right to 'complete anaesthesia' before being used in 'any experiment calculated to give pain,'" and can give rise to a "criminal prosecution for violation of [a laboratory] rat's legal rights" (36).

If, therefore, one believes – as many people surely do – that animals should have some legal rights, one is not thereby committed to the demand of the animal rights movement that animals should be given legal standing to sue their owners, their veterinarians, or other people for money or other kinds of relief. The concept of legal rights for animals, like the concept of moral rights for animals, does not entail the platform of the animal rights movement.

"The Animal Rights Movement Is Good for Veterinarians." Although they see much contemporary veterinary practice as immoral, some leaders of the animal rights movement argue that veterinarians can, and should, join their cause (37, 38).

The myth that the animal rights movement will benefit veterinary medicine, unlike the first two myths I have discussed, has not yet gained much acceptance among veterinarians. However, this myth is worth addressing. If they become increasingly familiar fixtures in veterinary publications and gatherings, animal rights movement members might not appear so worrisome. More important, some are seeking to play a major role in the teaching of ethics to veterinary students.

According to the animal rights movement, it is immoral to use animals as means toward human ends. It would seem that horse racing must stop, as must commercial raising of animals for fiber, dairy products, or eggs. Using animals for draft and other work would have to end, and it would appear that people who have horses largely for the pleasure of riding or showing them also violate the precepts of the animal rights movement. Thus, gone forever would be a significant portion of today's veterinary profession, including food and fiber and laboratory animal practitioners, and the great majority of equine practitioners. Moreover, the death of these fields would probably spell doom for most veterinarians who could survive, in theory, the demands of the animal rights movement. For the profession as a whole rests on an economic base supported in significant measure by those who now require farm, sport, or laboratory animal practitioners. Without this base, it seems highly unlikely that there could exist many schools to train veterinarians or pharmaceutical and supply companies to provide them with necessary goods and services.

Similarly, given the acceptance of such a position, even companion animal practice would not long survive the animal rights movement. Many things people now do to companion animals – and that generate veterinary business – such as breeding and showing them largely for human comfort, convenience, and enjoyment, would have to stop. Indeed, it is not clear that the animal rights movement can countenance very much human keeping of companion animals. For much of what people do with these animals, including housetraining or restraining them, or using them for companionship or protection, is done at least in part for human purposes. Some in the movement believe that the number of people permitted to have companion animals should be sharply curtailed. Reduction in the number of animal owners would directly reduce the number of potential veterinary clients. Also, allowing animals to sue their owners and veterinarians would make animal ownership and veterinary services less attractive to owners and practitioners, who would face expensive and upsetting lawsuits (39). Permitting greatly increased awards against veterinarians in malpractice suits, another demand of some in the animal rights movement (40), could make veterinary care still more expensive and might reduce the market for veterinarians.

Of course, the termination of animal research conducted for the benefit of other animals would prevent the development of many new veterinary drugs, vaccines, and techniques. This would curtail the potential growth of veterinary services. Just one new kind of disease or scourge that might be controllable with animal research could wipe out most of the patients for which the veterinarians in the animal rights movement's ideal world are supposed to care. Indeed, the movement seems logically committed to the view that people should stop using on animals any drugs or techniques that have already resulted from animal research. For this, too, would be no less a utilization of benefits obtained in violation of animals' rights. This alone would decimate the population of companion animals, and veterinarians, in very short order.

That something is good or bad for business does not make it right or wrong. It is also a rare profession indeed that does everything perfectly. Doubtless many in the animal rights movement sincerely believe that their program would benefit veterinarians. However, the animal rights movement is engaging in fantasy when it proclaims its devotion to animals and veterinarians, and puts forth a program that could in fact destroy both.

WHAT MORAL RIGHTS DO ANIMALS HAVE?

One task of contemporary normative veterinary ethics is to articulate to society and government why the animal rights movement cannot be permitted to have its way. This task, I have suggested, will be made more difficult than it really is if one accepts the claims of the animal rights movement that moral rights for animals entail abolition of human use of animals, that legal rights for animals entail treating animals as legal persons, and that the animal rights movement is good for veterinarians and veterinary science.

However, normative ethics cannot rest content with confronting the animal rights movement. Moral questions regarding animal rights will remain long after the animal rights movement falls victim to its own overblown and unacceptable demands. It is far more important to investigate when animals do have moral rights, how strong these rights are, and when these rights must give way to legitimate interests of people and other animals. This task cannot be accomplished at the beginning of one's study of normative veterinary ethics, but must proceed by careful analysis of particular issues and situations. I offer the following suggestions and warnings regarding such an endeavor:

1. Not every interest translates into a moral right. A right reflects an interest that is so strong that it generally must be respected even though others' interests or the promotion of utility would suffer by respecting it. A "right" that can be overridden as a matter of course is not properly spoken of as a right at all. Thus, I would be inclined to say that a laboratory dog may have an interest in having toys for amusement and that this interest is sometimes sufficiently strong to require that such toys be provided. However, it is quite another thing to assert that such animals have the *right* to these things, because there are many considerations that can often argue against respecting the interest.

2. Moral rights can be outweighed by the interests or rights of others. The fact that one might be reluctant to respect a proposed right in all situations does not mean that one should refuse to recognize it as a right. For example, it often seems plausible to say that a veterinary patient has the right to receive nursing and medical care appropriate to its condition. However, many veterinary hospitals cannot afford to remain staffed in the evenings, and it is sometimes impossible for clients to place an animal in a facility that can provide around-the-clock care. In some cases, it seems correct to conclude that an animal's interest in receiving appropriate nursing care must be overridden by the veterinarian's interests in maintaining his practice and in the client's ability to afford veterinary care.

3. Rights can be negative or positive. Philosophers commonly distinguish between negative rights, rights not to be treated in certain ways, and positive rights, rights to certain kinds of treatment, goods, or benefits. It is sometimes possible to rephrase a negative right as a positive right, and vice versa. For example, one often can speak interchangeably of the right of animals not to be treated inhumanely and their right to humane treatment. Nevertheless, the distinction between negative and positive rights is important, and has special significance for animal and veterinary ethics. Because of the predominance of the anticruelty position, many people believe that animals have far more negative rights, rights not to be treated in certain ways, than they have rights to positive benefits. If the anticruelty position continues to lose its hold as an exhaustive account of our obligations to animals, we can expect more people to assert positive moral rights for animals, and, indeed, to verbalize some rights traditionally phrased in the negative (such as the right not to be treated inhumanely) as positive rights.

4. Rights can be general or specific. In examining particular situations, one must sometimes be prepared to identify quite specific rights. I shall argue, for example, that terminally ill patients in great and unrelievable pain have the right to a quick and painless death. On the other hand, one might say that this specific right is an example of a more general right of patients to be treated with compassion.

5. Very general statements of rights tend to raise more issues than they answer or are so obviously plausible that they do not assist in answering difficult moral questions. This does not make such statements worthless, but one must not think that they provide more guidance than they really do. For example, it seems reasonable to ascribe to animals a very general right to be treated humanely, in the sense of not being caused unnecessary or unjustifiable pain or suffering. The problem, of course, is that this statement is acceptable to almost everyone, precisely because it does not attempt to address the enormously difficult question of what does constitute sufficient justification for animal pain or suffering.

Dr. Jacob Antelyes (41) offers a plausible and important list of moral rights of veterinary patients. He urges five basic rights for all patients: 1) *respect* (the right to "dignified nursing care and medical attention, delivered with decency and sincerity"); 2) *privacy* (the right "to be housed separately in well-lit and properly ventilated quarters" and not to experience "stress created by the presence of other animals or unessential people"); 3) *purposeful death* (the right "not to suffer frivolous pain or gratuitous death for the purpose of entertainment and amusement"); 4) *unavoidable pain* (the right "to prompt relief of pain by the most effective mode possible....") and 5) *food and water* (the right "to receive food and water appropriate for its medical condition....").

One might question certain of Antelyes' characterizations of these rights. For example, it is not clear why a right not to suffer pain for frivolous purposes belongs under the general right to a purposeful death, and Antelyes provides no argument for his possible contention that any pain inflicted for the purpose of human entertainment is frivolous. But a belief in the five very general rights he identifies surely belongs in some form in the value system of every veterinarian.

Nevertheless, the rights identified by Dr. Antelyes are so clearly plausible that they do not provide much assistance in answering the most difficult questions facing contemporary normative veterinary ethics. It is doubtful whether there are many veterinarians who deprive sick animals of adequate housing, food, and water, and who tolerate harsh or inattentive treatment of patients. And if there are veterinarians who allow such things, it is not a difficult matter to show that they are acting wrongly.

The hard issues lie elsewhere. When might an animal have the right to be a veterinary patient *in the first place*? When may any such right give way to a client's economic or psychological problems in treating or keeping the animal? *How much* economic sacrifice does a patient's right to adequate and competent care require of its owner, or of a veterinarian who might have difficulty offering the owner reduced fees? *What kind* of death is sufficiently purposeful and pain sufficiently justifiable so that it does not violate an animal's rights? *To what extent* does a patient's right to respectful care place constraints on what a doctor should agree to do at the client's request? (Does it, for example, prohibit such practices as ear cropping and "debarking?")

Normative veterinary ethics must search for characterizations of animal rights that will be useful in addressing these and many other difficult issues.

REFERENCES

1. Schiller BJ: Letter. *J Am Vet Med Assoc* 183:748, 1983.
2. Jacobs FS: A perspective on animal rights and domestic animals. *J Am Vet Med Assoc* 184:1344-1345, 1984.
3. Rigdon CR: Interview. *Intervet* 21:13, 1985.
4. Guiding Principles and the Term "Animal Rights" *J Am Vet Med Assoc* 182:769, 1983.
5. Tillman PC and Brooks DL: Animal Welfare, Animal Rights, and Human Responsibilities. *California Veterinarian* 37:33, 1983.
6. Held JR: Letter. *J Am Vet Med Assoc* 182:855, 1983.
7. Miller, RM: Animal Welfare-Yes! Human Laws-Sure! Animal Rights-No! *California Veterinarian* 37:21, 1983.
8. Armistead WW: Public health responsibilities of veterinary medicine. *J Am Vet Med Assoc* 187:1110, 1985.
9. See, e.g., Lyons D (ed): *Rights.* Belmont, CA: Wadsworth Publishing Co., 1979.
10. Dworkin R: Taking Rights Seriously. In Dworkin R: *Taking Rights Seriously.* Cambridge: Harvard University Press, 1978, pp 184-205.
11. Kant I: *Lectures on Ethics.* Infield L. trans. New York: Harper & Row, 1963, p 239.
12. Seligman MEP: *Helplessness.* San Francisco: Freeman Co. 1975, p xi.
13. Singer P: *Animal Liberation.* New York: The New York Review of Books, Inc., 1975.
14. Singer P: The Parable of the Fox and the Unliberated Animals. *Ethics* 88:122, 1978.

15. Jones H: Animal Rights: A View and Comment. *Society for Animal Rights Report* October 1981:3.
16. Holzer, H: Editor's Comment. *Animal Rights Law Reporter* April 1983:15.
17. Visscher MB: Animal rights and alternative methods. *The Pharos* Fall 1979:11-19.
18. Visscher MB: The Newer Antivivisectionists. *Proceedings of the American Philosophical Society* 116:157-162, 1972.
19. Caplan A: Beastly Conduct: Ethical Issues in Animal Experimentation. In Sechzer JE (ed): *The Role of Animals in Biomedical Research. Ann NY Acad Sci* 406:159-160, 1983.
20. Miller NE: Value and Ethics of Research on Animals. *Laboratory Primate Newsletter* 22:1-10, 1984.
21. See, Harvard University Office of Government and Community Affairs: *The Animal Rights Movement in the United States: Its Composition, Funding Sources, Goals, Strategies and Potential Impact on Research.* Reprinted, Clarks Summit, PA: International Society for Animal Rights, Inc., 1982.
22. E.g., Fox MW: Letter. *J Am Vet Med Assoc* 182:1314, 1983; Fox MW: Veterinarians and Animal Rights. *California Veterinarian* 37:15, 1983.
23. National Coalition Formed to Prevent Use of Pound and Shelter Animals For Scientific Purposes. *International Society for Animal Rights Report* April 1985:1.
24. Compromises Cause ISAR to Resign from Pro Pets Coalition. *International Society for Animal Rights Report* 1986:2.
25. Praded J: The Fatted Calf. *Animals* 118:12, 1985.
26. Mazzone, J: Memorandum and Order of January 14, 1986. Animal Legal Defense Fund Boston, Inc. v. Provimi Veal Corporation. Civil Action 85-3113-MA. U.S. District Court, District of Massachusetts.
27. Holzer H: Editor's Comment. *Animal Rights Law Reporter.* April 1983:15.
28. Jones H: Animal Rights: A View and Comment. *Society for Animal Rights Report* October 1981:3.
29. Lyons D: Introduction. In Lyons D (ed): *Rights.* Belmont, CA: Wadsworth Publishing Co., 1979, p 1.
30. E.g., Wolff NR: Letter. *J Am Vet Med Assoc* 183:36, 1983.
31. AVMA Entertains Views of Animal Rights Advocates. *J Am Vet Med Assoc* 192:1030-1034, 1988.
32. Regan T: Animals and the Law. In Regan T: *All That Dwell Therein.* Berkeley: University of California Press, 1982, pp 156-157.
33. Tischler JS: Rights for Nonhuman Animals: A Guardianship Model for Dogs and Cats. *San Diego Law Review* 14:484-506, 1977.
34. Prosser W: *Handbook of the Law of Torts.* ed 4. St. Paul, MN: West Publishing Co., 1971, p 586.
35. Feinberg J: Human Duties and Animal Rights. In Feinberg J: *Rights, Justice, and the Bounds of Liberty.* Princeton: Princeton University Press, 1980, p 193.
36. *Id.,* 193-194.
37 Regan T: *The Case for Animal Rights.* Berkeley: University of California Press, 1983, p 390.
38. Tischler JS: Veterinarians: The Sleeping Beauties of the Animal Rights Movement. *California Veterinarian* 37:27-28, 1983.
39. Tannenbaum, J: Ethics and Human-Companion Interaction. *Vet Clin North Am Small Anim Pract* 15:438-439, 1985.

40. See, e.g., Benson M: East coast malpractice attorney rebuffs "quick buck" theory. *DVM* 16:30, 1985.
41. Antelyes J: Animal rights in perspective. *J Am Vet Med Assoc* 189:757-759, 1986.

Chapter

13

The Interests of Veterinary Clients

Clients also have interests that must be taken into account in determining how veterinarians ought to act. This chapter will identify some of these interests and demonstrate why they are entitled to great respect.

THE INTEREST OF ANIMAL OWNERS IN ACCESSIBLE, AFFORDABLE, AND COMPETENT VETERINARY SERVICES

Animal owners certainly have a legitimate interest in having available to them veterinary services that are accessible, affordable, and competent. Although obvious, these interests are far from trivial. As we shall see, they can play an enormous role in the determination of how veterinarians ought to act – sometimes by supporting, and sometimes by running contrary to, what veterinarians perceive to be in their best interests.

THE STATUS OF THE CLIENT AS A PURCHASER OF THE VETERINARIAN'S SERVICES

Once they become clients, animal owners have a number of important interests.

Like other kinds of people, veterinary clients possess many legitimate interests. They may have an interest in furthering their careers, in earning a decent living, in enjoying a happy life, and so on. Clients often seek veterinary services to promote some of these interests.

The most important reason a client is entitled to have certain of his interests respected by the veterinarian is not that the client has these interests, but that the client engages the veterinarian's services for the specific purpose of promoting one or more of these interests. If one had to justify why a veterinarian ought, for example, to be honest with a farmer about the condition of his animals and ought to work diligently in the client's behalf, one would not begin by pointing out that farmers are entitled to make a living. Rather, we would say that the client deserves these things from his veterinarian because he is paying for them.

There are three major reasons why paying for veterinary services entitles a client to have certain interests respected. First, the veterinarian who provides services to a client has made an agreement to serve him. An agreement to provide veterinary services is a promise, and, like other promises, it ought to be kept. Second, we believe that someone who pays for a service is in entitled to his money's worth. Third, clients place reliance on their veterinarians and arrange their lives or business affairs accordingly. It is a fundamental principle of morality that if one person relies on another to do something, and that other person agrees to let the first rely on him, the second has an obligation not to let the first person down. If I have planned my day relying on your promise that you will pick me up in your car at a certain time, and you deliberately leave me in the lurch, you have done me a wrong in permitting me to act in reliance on your promise. Likewise, the client who places his animal in the care of a veterinarian relies on him to do any of a number of things, and is likely to build part of his personal or economic affairs around this reliance.

From these three foundations of the obligations of the veterinarian to the paying client, we can derive several general interests that are possessed by paying clients and that are entitled to great weight.

Honesty

Because the client is paying for the veterinarian's services, the client has a strong interest in honesty from the doctor. Honesty from the doctor about what he will do is required for the client to be able to decide whether and under what conditions to retain the doctor's services. Honesty from the doctor about what he has done or failed to do is essential to enable the client to determine whether the doctor has fulfilled his agreements and kept his promises. As an employer of veterinary services, the client must also receive information that will enable him to determine how his animal is doing and whether he is spending his money wisely. Such information will be useless, and may even be harmful, to the client if it is not truthful.

Honesty is more than not telling a lie or telling the truth when a client specifically requests some information. Failing to inform a client about some condition or event about which he does not or could not know can also be dishonest. The following practices are all dishonest: charging a client for services not actually rendered, exaggerating the seriousness of an animal's condition in order to gain the client's business, recommending unnecessary procedures, and signing a health or inspection certificate without having examined the client's animal.

Loyalty and Protection of Confidences

Because a client hires a veterinarian to serve the *client's* interests, the client must be able to rely on the veterinarian's loyalty, his steadfast devotion to the client's interests, and his unwillingness to compromise or undermine those interests. This does not mean that a practitioner can never serve two competing clients. But it does mean that he cannot be a responsible party in determining which such client succeeds. He must, that is, either leave the competition to the clients or decline to serve one of them. For example, although an equine doctor may sometimes attend race horses of competing owners, he ought never to reveal anything about one owner's animal to another, or do anything that would put one of them at a disadvantage.

A client has more than an interest in his veterinarian's loyalty to him as opposed to other clients or members of the public. Because a client engages the services of a practitioner with the understanding that the doctor is serving his interests, the client has an interest in loyalty to him as opposed to the practitioner's own interests. This does not preclude the doctor from profiting from a professional relationship, but his profit must flow from the primary consideration of serving the client. A doctor who recommends an unnecessary procedure to increase his fee, or who refers a client to another doctor and accepts a rebate or commission from that practitioner, is committing an act of disloyalty to the client.

One way of assuring loyalty to clients is to keep confidential information that one has received in one's professional attendance upon their animals. Such "information" includes not just statements made by a client or any of his employees or agents, but also medical information gathered through diagnosis and therapy as well as one's professional conclusions regarding such information.

Reasonable Fees and Payment Arrangements

The law gives veterinarians great leeway in determining what fees to charge and how to require payment of them. Indeed, provided that a client agrees, and the fee is not so outrageous or overbearing as to be unconscionable, a veterinarian lawfully can obtain any fee arrangement from a client that he can get. However, as a purchaser of services entitled to his money's worth, a client has an interest in being charged a fee that is reasonable in the sense in which it truly reflects the amount of time, skill, materials, and training involved in the services actually provided. This does not mean that some products or services cannot be marked up so as to bear the necessary and reasonable costs of the entire practice – although there is, surely, a line between a legitimate mark-up and unfair gouging. Nevertheless, charges ought to bear some relationship to the services provided.

Clients also have a legitimate interest in obtaining payment arrangements that permit them to purchase services they can afford. The private practitioner is not a charitable institution. But he is a provider of services in an economy that is accustomed to permitting consumers to pay in installments, especially when large amounts are involved. Where a client's payment record is unreliable or incapable of verification, or where a practitioner's cash flow situation is precarious, a client's moral claim to flexibility regarding payments may rightly be overridden in favor of the doctor's legitimate needs. However, veterinarians must at least attempt to play by the rules that apply to the consumer economy generally and that make this economy possible. Just as a veterinarian would expect his car dealer or furniture store to structure their financial houses so as to permit flexible payment arrangements for him, so must he understand a client's interest in being able to make similar arrangements with a veterinarian.

THE SIGNIFICANCE OF GRATUITOUS OR REDUCED-COST VETERINARY CARE

A client's agreement to pay money to a veterinarian for professional services is an act of great moral significance that invests the client with weighty interests and rights. As a profession, veterinary medicine is not as heavily engaged in providing gratuitous services to the needy as is law or medicine. Nevertheless, as we shall see, a strong case can be made for such services, at least as a moral ideal, if not an obligation. Moreover, some veterinarians do reduce fees for certain clients with financial problems. It is therefore important to understand that legitimate client interests do not derive solely from payment for veterinary services.

The law permits veterinarians to offer less extensive services for clients who do not pay or who pay reduced fees, if such clients understand that this is what they are receiving. However, once a practitioner agrees to provide any service, the law will hold him to the same standards of competence regarding that service whether he charges his full fee, a reduced fee, or no fee at all. In general, someone who pays little or nothing has just as much right to sue his veterinarian for malpractice as a fully paying client.

Just as the law does not lower its standards for those who receive gratuitous or low-cost services, neither does morality, and for the same reasons. Such clients still rely upon an agreement by the doctor to provide veterinary services. They, too, require honest information to allow them to make appropriate medical decisions for their animals. The doctor serves them and their interests no less than he serves the paying client, and they have no less need for his loyalty. Like other animal owners they, too, have an interest, as shall now be discussed, in trustworthiness and respectful treatment from the doctor because they, too, are animal owners and can have a great deal invested in the patient they bring to the veterinary office.

THE STATUS OF THE CLIENT AS AN ANIMAL OWNER

A client's interests derive not just from the fact that he pays for or receives a veterinarian's services. Veterinary clients are not just consumers, but are animal owners who entrust a particular kind of property to the care of their veterinarians. Typically, animals for whom veterinary services are sought are of significant economic value to the client or are of great emotional importance. This fact can affect profoundly the nature and weight of the client's interests.

The economic or emotional value of the animal strengthens and colors interests that can derive from the status of the client as a purchaser of the veterinarian's services. Although all consumers need honesty from merchants, for veterinary clients, honesty can be especially important because an incorrect decision can result in economic or emotional disaster. Although all consumers have an interest in reasonable fees and payment arrangements, this interest can be enormously important when one is dealing with a living being in which the consumer can invest so much of himself. It is one thing to be denied the services of a television repairman because he insists on his entire fee up front, but quite another to lose forever a beloved companion because a veterinarian will not permit installment payments.

There are also several interests of veterinary clients that are better viewed as flowing not primarily from their status as purchasers of services, but from their status as purchasers of medical services for animals.

Trustworthiness

Although related to honesty, trustworthiness is a different concept. Trustworthiness goes beyond telling the truth. It includes carrying out a client's wishes and respecting his sensibilities. Today, when so many veterinary clients have treasured pets and economically valuable animals, trustworthiness is a central virtue that clients have an interest in seeing in their veterinarians. Indeed, trustworthiness may well be more important in veterinary medicine than it is in human medicine or in any other profession. When a person believes he has been wronged by his physician or lawyer, he is usually able to complain about it and seek redress. Animals have no such ability. Barring some physical evidence of mistreatment, or statement by the veterinarian or a member of his staff admitting wrongdoing, a client must often rely solely on the veterinarian's trustworthiness to assure that competent and caring services are provided. The client may never know that his dog was hit in order to keep it quiet, that its water bowl was kept empty because of an employee's laziness, that an autopsy was performed on his animal without his permission, or that the body of another animal was substituted for that of his animal for burial. Such things, however, are fundamental violations of the trust that clients place in their veterinarians.

Courtesy, Caring, and Respect

All consumers are entitled to be treated with at least a minimum amount civility and courtesy; they deserve this much in return for their money. But because animals can be so important to veterinary clients, clients have interests in special kinds of courteous and decent treatment. These interests can, of course, vary greatly from one kind of client to another. A dairy farmer who has a cow that must be destroyed might not want from his veterinarian the kind of emotional solace that might be expected by a client who must contemplate the euthanasia of a beloved pet. The farmer, on the other hand, may expect sincere respect for his economic needs and an appreciation of the seriousness of a decision to put down one of his animals.

It would be impossible to list all the kinds of courteous, caring, and respectful treatment in which veterinary clients have an interest. Later chapters will discuss some of them in detail. I do, however, want to list some of the kinds of behavior veterinary clients and my veterinary students tell me they find most disrespectful in veterinarians. Some of these complaints may sometimes be unjustified when one takes into consideration not just the client's interest in being treated decently, but also a veterinarian's interest in maintaining a competent and profitable practice. Nevertheless, these complaints are illustrative of what clients mean when they say – correctly – that they deserve to be treated with courtesy, care, and respect.

- Waiting two or three weeks for an appointment, and then having to sit for an hour before seeing the doctor, without receiving an apology or explanation for the delay;
- Calling the doctor at lunch break or other times when the practice is in fact staffed and being greeted with a tape recording that makes it impossible to speak with someone;
- Being urged to make important decisions quickly so that the doctor can proceed to his next appointment;
- Seeing the doctor look repeatedly at his watch during an appointment;
- Not having a private area away from the examining room to sit down with the doctor or family members so that important decisions can be made rationally and with dignity;
- Not receiving a telephone call from the doctor reporting on the status of one's animal after a major procedure;
- Not having one's telephone calls returned;
- Being told that one's valued pet is only an animal, is getting old anyway, or is not worth the amount of money required to save it;
- Being asked to state on an estimate or consent form the monetary value of one's animal;
- Being repeatedly interrupted or ignored by the doctor during an examination of one's animal;
- Receiving an impatient or rude response after expressing inability to understand the gravity or nature of the condition of one's animal;
- Having the doctor dismiss as inappropriate, or leave the room at the first sign of, one's distress or grief;
- Being served by a doctor or employee in dirty or disheveled attire.

Being Treated As an Intelligent and Autonomous Adult Entitled to Make One's Own Decisions

There is a specific kind of respect that a client has an interest in receiving from his veterinarian that derives from his status as the owner of the veterinary patient – respect in the sense of being treated as an intelligent adult who is capable of making, and is entitled to make, his own decisions concerning his animal's veterinary care.

THE ANIMAL AS THE CLIENT'S PROPERTY

Although some object to this fact, it is nevertheless a fact of our legal system and culture that animals are considered property. One can argue for a client's interest in being able to make his own decisions about his animal by appealing to a general moral right of people to own animals. But such an argument is not necessary for our purposes. A more immediate justification for permitting the client to make the decisions about his animal's veterinary care is that when client and veterinarian enter a professional relationship, they *accept* the fact that the animal is the client's property. Moreover, it is not part of the typical express or implied agreement between veterinarian and client that the veterinarian shall decide what is to be done with the client's property. Quite the contrary, both doctor and client usually understand (even if they do not state this understanding explicitly) that the doctor is working for the client, who retains the right to decide what services will be provided. In virtue of having made such an agreement, the doctor is under an obligation to keep it.

INFORMED CONSENT

Clearly, a client cannot make his own decision about what will be done with his animal unless 1) he is permitted to do so without external pressure or influence and 2) he is given all the information he would reasonably need to make a decision. These requirements are stated simply, but can place significant burdens on veterinarians. Pressure can be overt, but it can also be quite subtle. For example, the order in which a doctor states the alternatives to a client and the words he uses to state them can in themselves push the client to make a decision that in fact is more the doctor's decision than the client's. Nor is it always easy to convey to clients the information they might want. Some clients are less sophisticated than others and may require a lengthy or repeated explanation that can try the veterinarian's patience.

The law uses the phrase "informed consent" to describe the kind of decision a client must be permitted to make. Unfortunately, the legal notion of informed consent does not give sufficient guidance in characterizing the moral interest a veterinary client has in obtaining information and making his own decision. One would think, as several courts did in the early 1970s (1), that in order to make a truly informed consent, a medical client must be given all the information that a reasonable person in his circumstances would find necessary to make a decision. In recent years, however, the courts or legislatures of most states have decided that in order to make an informed consent a client must be given the information that an ordinarily competent and prudent *physician* would want to give the client – even if a reasonable client would want to know more. It might follow that if most veterinarians believe that clients should be given information in a way that steers them toward a certain kind of decision, steering them toward that decision instead of letting them make up their own minds would meet the legal requirements for obtaining an informed consent.

"Informed consent" is a useful phrase for normative veterinary ethics, provided it is not understood in its usual legal sense.

THE OWNER'S RELATIONSHIP WITH THE ANIMAL AS A SOURCE OF ENTITLEMENT TO AN INFORMED CONSENT

The veterinarian's acceptance of a client's ownership of the patient is itself an important foundation of the client's interest in making his own informed decision about his animal. However, there is often another foundation – the fact that the animal is not just any kind of property, but is something in which the owner has invested significant time, effort, money, or emotion. A farmer or horse breeder, for example, who has spent a good deal of money making an animal a part of his business operations has a very strong interest in seeing that his investment has its intended results. Such a client's commitment of time and money entitles him to decide how to handle his affairs with his animals, even if his veterinarian thinks he can help the client by pressuring him to make some other kind of decision. It is no less presumptuous, and wrong, for a veterinarian to push such a client's decisions in a certain direction than it would be for a banker to withdraw a depositor's money without authorization and use it in ways he thinks would benefit the depositor.

Regarding animals with whom clients have an emotional bond, there are different reasons arguing against intermeddling by the veterinarian.

First, veterinarians are not experts in human psychology. Nor would the few minutes they usually spend with clients enable even a psychologist to know very much about a client or his family and the precise nature of their relationship with their animal. The veterinarian may know more about the medical condition and prognosis of such an animal, and he may know a great deal about how he would feel if faced with the alternatives before the client. But although the doctor's technical knowledge should enable him to direct the client's attention to matters the client might not think of on his own, the doctor cannot presume to be able to judge for the client precisely what impact on a client's life these alternatives may have.

Second, even if veterinarians could ever know better than a client emotionally attached to an animal what is in the client's best interests, in the overwhelming majority of cases, and therefore as a general rule, the client is still entitled to make his own decision. The client has undertaken the care of the animal, he has made the personal and financial sacrifices, he has arranged his life and that of his family around and with that of his animal. Having made these commitments and decisions, he is entitled to decide, without subtle psychological pressure from a stranger who will not have to live with the decision, how his life and that of his family will proceed in the future.

An animal and human who have a significant emotional attachment and reliance upon each other have a special relationship in which others, including a veterinarian, do not participate. My Yorkie trusts me to throw him into the air in play, but will not permit strangers do so. When he barks to me and not others for his dinner or walk, he understands we have a relationship he does not have with others. Perhaps it would be inappropriate to say that he has "entrusted" me with his care (although I am not at all sure this is an inaccurate way of characterizing the matter) and that this gives me, and not the veterinarian, a special claim to make decisions concerning both of us. It is surely appropriate to say that my dog and I have established a pattern of exclusive interaction that not only makes it likely that I will want to do what is in his interests – but that entitles me to judge, for both of us, how matters of health or illness should affect the relationship.

This remarkable intermingling of the interests of animal and client brings us to the human-companion animal bond. The nature of this bond and its potential impact on normative veterinary ethics is the subject of Chapter 14.

REFERENCE

1. E.g., Canterbury v. Spence, 464 F.2d 772 (D.C. Cir. 1972).

Chapter

——— 14 ———

The Human-Companion Animal Bond

The human-companion animal bond is gaining increasing prominence in the veterinary world. "The bond" seems to be everywhere – in scholarly publications describing its value in promoting human health, in AVMA policy statements, in practice management discussions touting its value for maximizing revenues, in advertisements appealing to the bond as an incentive for animal owners to buy pet products.

The concept of "the human-companion animal bond" can serve as an important tool in ethical analysis. Unfortunately, it already is showing signs of becoming little more than a soothing, empty cliché.

WHAT IS THE HUMAN-COMPANION ANIMAL BOND?

As I understand the phrase, the "human companion animal bond" refers to a relationship between a human and an animal which has at least the following characteristics:

The relationship cannot be sporadic or accidental, but must be continuous and ongoing. We would hardly speak of a "bond," (as opposed, say, to an interaction) between two beings unless they related to each other with some degree of frequency.

The relationship must also derive not just to a benefit, but to a significant benefit of both parties, and the relationship must benefit a central aspect of the lives of each. If you and I alternate driving each other to work, our relationship is simply too trivial to describe as a "bond." If, however, we invest our life savings together in a business and work long and hard at it, that begins to look very much like a bond.

In order to be termed a "bond," a relationship must also in some sense be voluntary. Prison cellmates who are thrown together for life do not thereby necessarily establish a bond. Persons who choose to relate to each other can.

A bond must be bidirectional, with each party to the bond offering its attention to the other. I can be extremely devoted to someone, showering that person with attention and benefits. But if this attention is not returned, there is, as any unrequited lover knows, no bond.

Insofar as is possible, each party to a true bond must treat the other not simply as a means toward its own ends, but as something entitled to respect and benefit in its own right. The antebellum slave owner certainly had a strong, continuous, significant relationship with his slaves. However, this was not a bond, but bondage, because the relationship was almost entirely one-sided and was severely detrimental to one of the parties. Respect and benefit, however, are not sufficient. Churchill and Stalin had great respect for each other. They also saw themselves and their nations as entitled in their own right and for their own benefit to victory over the Nazis. But one would hardly describe their relationship as a "bond," because they hated and distrusted each other. A true bond requires at the very least something akin to admiration, trust, and genuine good feeling of each party toward the other. Often, a bond involves love.

So, as I understand the phrase, a "human-companion animal bond" means at the very least a continuous, bidirectional relationship between a human and an animal that brings a significant benefit to a central aspect of the lives of each, which is in some sense voluntary, and in which each party treats the other not just as something entitled to respect and benefit in its own right, but also as an object of admiration, trust, devotion, or love.

Admittedly, one may be using some of these terms somewhat loosely in applying them to animals. For example, a family dog does not "voluntarily" enter the relationship in quite the same way as does his family. However, there is a sense in which we would say that a dog that must be tied down to prevent its running away, and greets or interacts with its owner only when threatened with punishment or offered a treat, is not a member of a bond, precisely because it does not *want* to interact with its owner.

My definition reflects what we speakers of the English language generally mean when we talk about a "bond." It also leaves open, as I believe a useful definition of the human-companion animal bond must, questions regarding precisely what animals can be included. Some people seem inclined to restrict candidates for the animal side of the bond to dogs, cats, and caged birds. But it seems clear that other kinds of animals, such as some horses, ferrets, and members of certain other species, can also qualify. The definition also allows for the possibility of stronger and weaker bonds between humans or animals. Nevertheless, as I have suggested, there will be a point at which a human-animal relationship simply becomes too trivial, or manipulative, to be called a "bond." It will also sometimes be appropriate to speak of human-animal "companionship" that is more significant than mere human-animal interaction but that still does not constitute a bond.

THE TRIVIALIZATION OF THE BOND

There are already signs that the concept of the human-companion animal bond will not become a useful tool in ethical discussion.

First, the phrase "human-companion animal bond" appears to be turning into a synonym for "owning or interacting in some way with any kind of pet." The phrase thus seems to denote the entire gamut of human-pet interactions. For example, Dr. E. Garcia distinguishes several different attitudes towards pets, ranging from the most devoted to the almost entirely disinterested. He then asserts that "*regardless* of the type of pet owner, there is some degree of bond between most owners and their pets that seems to transcend all others....[T]he bond between the pet and the owner, whatever it may be, has always been there, even as far back as our ancient ancestors" (1). The AVMA Committee on the Human/Animal Bond also equates "the bond" with pet ownership. In a recent statement it called for research about "the human/animal bond, especially patterns of pet ownership, motives for keeping pets, functions pets serve, and the nature of the physical interaction with pets." Having identified "the bond" with pet ownership, the Committee has no problem sweeping under this concept almost all human-pet interactions, including those involving "children of all ages" and apparently even owners who "view their pets as a nuisance and are unhappy with their pets' presence in the household" (2).

There surely are important ethical aspects and implications of many different kinds of human-animal interaction. The problem with equating the human-animal bond with pet ownership, however, is that it can draw one's attention away from human-animal interactions that are legitimately described as a bond and that have distinctive ethical features.

For example, if, as studies indicate (3), people are soothed by touching a dog from time to time, or by looking at fish in an aquarium or a bird in a cage, interesting ethical issues arise. A strong argument can be made that institutions that care for the ill or elderly ought to provide such animal contacts and should engage the services of a veterinarian to keep the animals healthy. However, there are important differences between these relatively casual human-animal interactions and those legitimately termed a bond. If someone is responding solely to the *sight* of *a* bird or dog, it would be difficult to argue that an institution entrusted with his care is obligated to spend a great deal of money on veterinary care for a very sick animal he happens to be looking at, if another animal could be substituted at much less cost. On the other hand, if the same person is permitted to keep for himself and comes to love a particular animal, it might be cruel and immoral to suggest to him that because veterinary care would entail some expense, his pet must be replaced with "another just like it." Likewise, it would be unfair to such a person and his devoted pet to take the animal away from him so that it can be passed around more casually to sooth the stresses of others. On the other hand, impressing an abandoned pound animal into this kind of service seems far less objectionable, and, indeed, could be a positive benefit to such an animal by assuring its continued life and some measure of human contact.

A ONE-SIDED "BOND"?

There is a second feature of much current thinking about the human-companion animal bond that may prevent the bond from achieving its rightful role in ethical deliberation. Most people who are studying the bond appear far more interested in its human side, and in promoting the interests of its human participants, than in asking hard questions about what interests the bond might give to *animals*.

For example, Dr. Garcia remarks that appreciation of the bond "instilled in me the importance of my place in society – taking care of pets for *people*. ... [A]t no time in my practice life have I felt more an important element of society as far as contributing to *people's* happiness. ... If you look at yourself as a professional person who really does have a part in increasing the quality and happiness in *people's* lives, this should give you a warm feeling inside, and you have every reason to be proud" (4). The Delta Society, which has done as much as anyone to foster scientific study of the human-companion animal bond, states that one of its objectives is "[t]o assess the role of animal companions in society and to study the effect of the human-companion animal bond on the mental health and well-being of *people*" (5). The Society recently offered over $100,000 in grants for research on two topics: "What is the role of dogs/cats in *human* growth and development over the life-span?" and "How do human-animal (dog/cat) relationships develop? What is the meaning of those relationships for *people*" (6)? A frequently-cited paper by a founder of human-companion animal bond movement appears in a textbook of veterinary internal medicine. Yet, this paper discusses the *effects* of pet interaction on people, and proclaims the veterinarian "a member of the *human* health team" (7). There is emerging a significant body of work studying the benefits animals can bring to the mentally ill, the retarded, the physically disabled, and the incarcerated (8). But it is often difficult to find in such studies mention of what these contacts ultimately do to the animals. One does not always find a concern about their needs or interests, and an appreciation that they are beings that count for something in their own right and are not simply tools for making people healthy or happy.[a]

The conclusion of one famous report on the use of dogs in a psychiatric hospital speaks volumes about the focus of most current research into the human-animal bond. Pet-facilitated therapy, this study determined, introduces "a non-threatening loving pet to serve as a catalytic vehicle for forming adaptive and satisfying [human] social interactions" (9).

No one should dismiss the value of the human-animal bond in the promotion of human health and well-being. Nevertheless, it is inappropriate to speak of one member of a *bond* as "serving" as a "catalytic vehicle" for promoting the interests of the other. In a true human-animal bond, the animal must be seen in large measure as entitled to care and concern in its own right, not as a tool or vehicle.

Perhaps the concentration on the human side of the bond by researchers is a temporary, pragmatic approach, aimed at obtaining the respect of scientists and veterinarians before greater attention is paid to the animals. However, as monkeys begin to serve as the arms and legs of quadriplegics, or cats and dogs are shuttled in and out of nursing homes to be petted by residents, or animals are placed in jails to relax or rehabilitate hardened felons, at some point, I suggest, one must ask whether all of this is fair to the animals.

It might not be clear how much we may morally do to animals in the service of human health and happiness. However, students of the human-companion animal bond must take this question seriously. They must take more seriously the task of understanding the effects of the bond on animals. Otherwise, "the human-companion animal bond" may become just another way of describing animals merely as objects for the use and enjoyment of people. This is a view of animals that many participants in true human-animal bonds find unacceptable.

SOME HARD QUESTIONS

Being a member of a human-animal bond, as this relationship is appropriately understood, can create conflicts between animal owner and animal, as well as between both of these and others, including veterinarians and government. The following are among the hard questions raised by the bond that reflect some of these potential conflicts.

Is companion animal ownership sometimes a moral right that can be abridged, if at all, only in the most extreme kinds of circumstances?

Thus far, our society has treated ownership of companion animals not as a necessity of life, but as a luxury. This is in part why the law believes it can require

---

[a]This criticism cannot be made of the veterinarian founder of the human-animal bond movement, Dr. Leo Bustad, whose interest in human-animal interaction began with a concern for animals. Bustad's devotion to both sides of the human-animal bond has gained him a place among the great figures in the history of the profession.

that pets be licensed, or can place significant restrictions on their ownership, or under certain circumstances can prohibit their ownership entirely. On the other hand, having children is not considered a luxury, but a fundamental right most adults are thought to possess. To be sure, this right is sometimes overridden, as when the state takes a child away from its natural parents to protect it from abuse or neglect. But such intervention is, we believe, appropriate only in the most extreme kinds of circumstances, precisely because childrearing is generally considered a fundamental aspect of life.

Now if for some people pets are every bit as important in the most central aspects of their lives as children, we must at least ask whether for such people having a companion animal is a moral, and should be a legal, right. Should we make it difficult for such people to have pets, by charging them license fees they might be unable to afford, or by excluding pets from publicly supported or private housing? To what extent may we regulate how many or what kinds of pets can be possessed by participants in a human-companion animal bond? Are some common restrictions on pets and pet behavior unfair? For example, I must endure the racket caused by my neighbor's four children, because people have a right to have as many children as they want and because four children will in the nature of things make a lot of noise. Is it therefore not fair to expect my neighbor to accept without complaint the vociferous barking of my dog – because of his importance to me and the fact that such an animal will in the nature of things make some noise?

Do animals that can participate in, or have participated in, a human-animal bond sometimes have strong moral claims that can make it wrong for their owners or other people to do certain things to them, such as continuing to own or mistreat them, experimenting on, or euthanizing them?

Recently, several states abolished so-called "pound seizure" laws, which permit or require public pounds to release abandoned pets to research facilities (see Chapter 23). One of the arguments advanced by opponents of the use of pound animals in research is that because these animals once related to humans in a special way not experienced by purpose-bred animals, it is wrong to expose them to research. According to this argument, once an animal is part of a human-companion animal bond, it is unfair to treat it as a research tool; it must live, if at all, the kind of life to which it has become accustomed.

Whatever one thinks of this particular argument, it is difficult to dispute the general principle that animals that are members of a human-companion animal bond come to have *some* moral claims in virtue of their having been in such a relationship. For example, it is wrong to neglect the adult dog that one showered with affection during its puppyhood, in part because the dog was permitted, indeed encouraged, to share in the joys of human companionship and affection. It is wrong to neglect the veterinary needs of one's loyal and faithful pet, in part because it has been loyal and faithful, and thus deserves something in return.

The issue of the interests and rights of the animal party to the human-animal bond raises serious questions for veterinarians. To what extent should doctors act as advocates of the interests of patients, even if this means disagreeing with the wishes of clients? Should the profession rethink its attitude toward euthanasia, which is sometimes offered not just to clients whose animals are suffering painful terminal illness, but also to people tired of their animals or inconvenienced by their behavioral problems? In order to ask such questions, one need not be a member of the animal rights movement or assert that humans and animals are of equal value. However, it seems to me that one cannot believe in the existence of a significant human-companion animal bond without believing that the animal members of such bonds have *some* significant moral rights.

To what extent should the legal system protect the interests of animal members of human-companion animal bonds?

Some have argued that the moral claims of companion animals cannot receive adequate protection unless they are given the force of law. Therefore, it is claimed, we should test and license pet owners, prevent unworthy owners from keeping animals, and give animals legal "standing" so that their owners and veterinarians can be sued in their behalf (10). A strong argument can be made that these suggestions propose too great an intrusion by government into peoples' private lives, and would make pet ownership so expensive and aggravating to animal owners and veterinarians that they would deprive many people and animals of the advantages of the human-animal bond (11). But once one recognizes that at least some companion animals have strong interests that are not always respected, the question of whether and to what extent the law should be invoked to protect these interests is certainly a legitimate one, however we may ultimately come to answer it.

Should veterinarians pay more serious attention to behavioral problems of companion animals and their owners?

Human-companion animal bonds do not always go smoothly. Animals and their owners sometimes have behavioral problems, and not always, it seems clear, because the bond between them is too weak. Thus far, the veterinary profession has seriously neglected the field of pet behavior. Perhaps the argument can be made (as it is still made by some physicians) that psychology is not a biological, and therefore not a medical matter. However, it is hard to see who would address the behavioral problems of pets and their owners if not veterinarians. To be sure, doing so will not be easy and will itself raise difficult issues. If the human-companion animal bond can give rise to or involve behavioral problems, the cause of these problems, in either human or animal or both, will sometimes come from the human side of the bond. Therefore, veterinarians who want to address behavioral problems arising from the bond must become more knowledgeable about human as well as animal psychology. Much more effort will have to be expended by the profession and the veterinary schools to place into the hands of practitioners useful knowledge about behavioral implications of the human-companion animal bond (12).

Should veterinarians or society provide gratuitous or low-cost veterinary services to the needy, and to what extent should society subsidize the human-companion animal bond in general?

Although we do not have socialized medical care in this country, society has recognized some obligation to assist the needy in obtaining the services of physicians and hospitals. We sometimes provide public hospitals and publicly supported health insurance to the needy. We do this precisely because we believe that medical care, if not a right (and in most countries it is considered a moral and legal right), is so important and central a concern of life that society must help those with limited means to obtain it.

However, if, as research is now establishing, having a companion animal can be as important to one's physical and mental health as medical care itself, we must at least ask whether society has some obligation to help some people pay for or obtain veterinary services for their animals. Indeed, one might ask whether society sometimes ought to help those of limited means to purchase and keep companion animals in the first place.

The question of subsidized veterinary care is not one of which veterinarians need be afraid. First, it is by no means clear that government or the taxpayers can afford widespread subsidy of veterinary services. Second, just as subsidized medical care has been very good (some would say too good) to the medical profession, it might well offer veterinarians a means of substantially increasing their client base. Third, there are ways of helping the needy that do not involve taxpayer support. For example, veterinarians can volunteer some of their time, or offer financial support, to community animal clinics that serve the needy at reduced cost. If such services are limited to the truly needy, they need not cut into the regular practices of local doctors. At the very least, an appreciation of the importance of the human-companion animal bond and the concomitant need for affordable veterinary care provides an additional strong reason for veterinarians to support pet health insurance programs.

Should the veterinary profession reconsider its opposition to awards in malpractice suits for clients' emotional distress?

Veterinarians enthusiastically support "the human-companion animal bond." However, the organized profession continues to insist that courts hearing veterinary malpractice suits treat pets like other kinds of personal property, such as sofas and television sets, and deny awards for owners' pain and suffering resulting from animal loss or injury caused by veterinarian malpractice. But one cannot promote the human-companion animal bond as a vital part of clients' lives and at the same time tell pet owners that they cannot collect for their pain and suffering because animals are merely articles of personal property. Imposition of awards for client pain and suffering could make veterinary care more expensive and thus less frequent by dramatically increasing malpractice insurance premiums. However, if veterinarians are serious about their advocacy of a significant human-companion animal bond, they must begin thinking more creatively about how this bond can be recognized by the law in ways that would not threaten the affordability of veterinary services.

To what extent should veterinarians and society treat members of true human-companion animal bonds differently from participants in less significant human-animal relationships?

Insofar as the human-companion animal bond may be good for business, the veterinary profession will have a motive to sweep within the bond as many clients and animals as possible. To be sure, an animal need not be a member of a true bond to need and deserve veterinary care. However, there are good reasons for veterinarians and others to try to understand and recognize when they are dealing with a bond, properly speaking, and when with mere pet ownership or human-animal interaction. For example, an argument can be made that the stronger the bond between client and patient, the more diligent a veterinarian should be in attempting to work out economic arrangements that will permit a client to pay for the best veterinary care available. For in such a case, the doctor can be dealing with a client and an animal for whom their continuing relationship is enormously important.

Recognizing the importance of the human-companion animal bond does not always require doctors to make sacrifices. Nor does it necessarily mean making discriminations between true human-animal bonds and more casual human-animal relationships. Small, routine things often say a great deal. For example, many veterinarians place the names of patients in quotation marks when they communicate with clients or other doctors regarding these animals. What is the point of this nonsense? Will a client think that *he* is supposed to be treated by the veterinarian, unless the reminder card from the Jones Animal Hospital states that "Cindy" and "George" are due for their yearly booster shots? Does this punctuation reflect Dr. Jones' view that Cindy and George really do not have these names – that when the client summons them for a walk he calls out to "sort-of Cindy" or "kind-of George"? Are the quotation marks intended to say that these animals do not *deserve* such names, or indeed that pets are not properly named *at all*? For Muffin, Tiger, and Nipper, who do not happen to have typical human names, are no less likely than Cindy and George to be enclosed in a veterinarian's quotation marks. Whatever their intent, the quotation marks take away something that companion animals have, and are regarded by their owners as having: real names that are possessed by complete, distinctive, and important beings. This horrid punctuation demeans patients and clients because it suggests that clients are misguided in thinking that their pets have real names. The quotation marks also denigrate all veterinarians. A practitioner who believes that his companion animal patients are not important enough to bear real names is saying that his profession, which provides medical care for these patients, is not quite so important either.

A CLICHÉ OR A CHALLENGE?

The "human-companion animal bond" can be a concept that describes a real and important relationship shared by some humans and some animals, a relationship that gives strong legitimate interests to both. The concept can stimulate one to raise important questions. It can suggest considerations relevant to answering these questions. Normative veterinary ethics therefore would do well to resist those who would turn "the bond" into a soothing, hackneyed synonym for pet ownership or human-animal interaction. We must also challenge students of the bond to look carefully at both of its sides.

REFERENCES

1. Garcia E: Types of Pet Owners: Owner Attitudes and the Tie That Binds. *Veterinary Forum.* Jul 1985:16, emphasis added.
2. Committee Identifies Public Health Implications of Human/Animal Bond. *J Am Vet Med Assoc* 189:18-19, 1986. (Much of this verbiage appears to have been adopted from McCulloch M: Companion Animals, Human Health, and the Veterinarian. In Ettinger SJ (ed): *Textbook of Veterinary Internal Medicine: Diseases of the Dog and Cat.* ed 2. Philadelphia: W.B. Saunders Co., 1983, pp 228-229.)
3. Bird Ownership Is Therapeutic. *J Am Vet Med Assoc* 189:1275, 1986; Katcher AH: Physiologic and Behavioral Responses to Companion Animals. *Vet Clin North Am Small Anim Pract* 15:403-410, 1985.
4. Garcia, *op. cit.,* p 16, emphasis added.
5. *Bulletin of the Delta Society* 2(2):3, 1984, emphasis added.
6. *Id.,* 14, emphasis added.
7. McCulloch M: Companion Animals, Human Health, and the Veterinarian. In Ettinger SJ (ed): *Textbook of Veterinary Internal Medicine: Diseases of the Dog and Cat.* ed 2. Philadelphia: W.B. Saunders Co., 1983, p 234, emphasis added.
8. See, e.g., Hines LM: Community People-Pet Programs that Work. *Vet Clin North Am Small Anim Pract* 15:319-332, 1985; Ryder EL: Pets and the Elderly. *Vet Clin North Am Small Anim Pract* 15:333-343, 1985; Beck AM: The Therapeutic Use of Animals. *Vet Clin North Am Small Anim Pract* 15:365-375, 1985.

9. Corson SA, Corson EO *et al.*: Pet-facilitated psychotherapy in a hospital setting. *Curr Psychiatr Ther* 15:277-286, 1975, quoted in Schwabe CW: Veterinary Medicine and Human Health. ed 3. Baltimore: Williams & Wilkins, 1984, p 622.

10. Rollin BE: *Animal Rights and Human Morality*. Buffalo, Prometheus Books, 1981, p 168.

11. Tannenbaum J: Ethics and Human-Companion Interaction: A Plea for a Veterinary Ethics of the Human-Companion Animal Bond. *Vet Clin North Am Small Anim Pract* 15:438-439, 1985.

12. McCulloch WF: The Veterinarian's Education About the Human-Animal Bond and Animal-Facilitated Therapy. *Vet Clin North Am Small Anim Pract* 15:423-429, 1985.

Chapter

15

Weighing the Interests of Veterinarians

Thus far, we have examined general considerations that are useful in identifying and weighing the interests of veterinary patients and clients. This chapter focuses upon some of the most important legitimate interests of veterinarians.

SELF-INTEREST: MONETARY GAIN

Veterinarians bring to their professional relationships with clients an interest in making an adequate living. This is, of course, only one kind of legitimate self-interest that a veterinarian can have, but it is one shared to some extent at least by almost all practitioners.

One useful task that should be undertaken by descriptive veterinary ethics is to explore the extent to which members of the profession do value monetary gain. Current interest in practice management and marketing techniques indicates that many doctors place great value on monetary reward. On the other hand, some veterinarians may feel guilty, or may be unassertive, about their moral right to earn a living commensurate with their education, skills, and value to clients and patients.

As we shall see, it is sometimes difficult to assess how strongly a doctor's interest in monetary gain ought to count against the interests of patients, clients, employees, and others. However, one should never underestimate the dangers of undervaluing monetary reward. Veterinarians who are paid poorly may not be getting what they rightly deserve. They may also suffer a lack of self-esteem that can lead to a more general denigration of their profession and of themselves. (I have seen this in students who are convinced that their skills, and indeed they themselves, are not of great value because they can earn more driving a bus or collecting garbage than practicing veterinary medicine.) Low salaries may lead to a decline in the number and quality of veterinary school applicants. The ultimate result could be a lowering of the standards of veterinary practice, decreased public confidence in the profession, and lower revenues for all practitioners.

PROTECTION OF THE PROFESSION

As members of a profession, veterinarians have a legitimate interest in strengthening their profession as an entity and in protecting it from conditions that could impair the ability of its members to function properly. Protection of the profession can include such activities as opposing the provision of veterinary services by unqualified persons, promoting a good image of the profession in the eyes of the public, and contesting legal actions by government or private citizens that threaten the interests of veterinarians.

One reason promoting and protecting the profession is a legitimate interest of veterinarians is that it can assist in furthering their legitimate interest in earning an adequate living. But promoting a vigorous and respected profession brings other rewards. One of the benefits of being a veterinarian is enjoyment of the fellowship of interacting with one's colleagues (1). Another benefit of being a veterinarian is belonging to a profession that possesses talents not shared by members of the public generally and is respected for its values and good deeds. Just being a member of such a highly respected profession can provide rich personal satisfaction.

INTERNAL CONSTRAINTS ON SELF-INTEREST

Veterinarians are not entirely morally free to pursue their own self-interest. Some constraints on their pursuit of self-interest come, as we have seen, from the legitimate interests of patients or clients. For example, it is wrong for a veterinarian to recommend unnecessary services in order to earn more money because doing this violates a client's right to obtain at a fair cost what he and his animal really require.

Some moral constraints on a veterinarian's self-interest, however, come from within the profession itself – from the interests of its members or from its own central values.

Economic Justice

One such limitation derives from the interest that other veterinarians and veterinary employees have in making an adequate living. A veterinarian who hires employees has a moral obligation to respect their self-interest in earning an adequate living by paying them fairly for their services. As we shall see in Chapter 22, it is by no means always easy to determine what constitutes just compensation for one's employees and fellow workers. But it is clear that if a veterinarian ought to be just in his economic dealings with his clients, he must also be just with his employees, including those who are veterinarians.

Freedom to Compete

Veterinarians cannot adequately pursue their legitimate interest in monetary gain unless they are able to offer their services to the public. This means that they must be free to compete with other doctors. It is not always easy to determine how much competition is fair or is consistent with professionalism. Nevertheless, as is the case with other interests of patients, clients, and veterinarians, it is advisable to assert the interest in freedom of competition in the abstract and without too many qualifications, before considering its application in particular situations. Recognizing ahead of time the legitimacy of a general interest can place a great burden on those who would deviate from this interest.

For example, most veterinarians want to be able to compete fairly for client dollars. Nevertheless, many doctors want the veterinary schools to protect *them* from competition by reducing enrollments (2). If a veterinarian really believes in freedom of competition, he cannot seek to deprive some people of its benefits. If he believes that some people are owed special protection against competition, he must be prepared to explain why this is so. He must also show why *he* was entitled to an opportunity to become a veterinarian and to compete in the marketplace and a prospective applicant is not. He must explain why *he* should not be put at a competitive disadvantage or even kept out of practice altogether so that another deserving doctor (e.g., one with more years in practice, with specialty certification, or in dire financial straits) can prosper without competition from him.

Dedication to Animals and Clients

As the Veterinary Oath proclaims, the profession is committed to the general values of alleviating animal suffering, promoting animal health, and benefiting clients and members of the public. These are interests of the profession itself, and not just of its patients or clients. These interests can sometimes outweigh the interest of practitioners in monetary gain. This fact is recognized by the AVMA *Principles*, which require, for example, that practitioners assure the availability of emergency services (3), make a determination of therapy based primarily on the needs of the patient and client (4), and provide high quality services, regardless of the fees charged, if any (5).

FOUR MODELS OF PROFESSIONALISM

A veterinarian's interest in monetary gain, economic justice, freedom of competition, and benefiting animals and clients often must be considered in approaching particular moral issues.

Nevertheless, it is quite clear from current controversies among veterinarians about ethical issues that the problem is often not just determining the importance of certain specific interests in resolving particular issues. Rather, many veterinarians are now seeing normative veterinary ethics as a choice among competing general pictures or models of what a veterinarian ought to be. Included within each of these models is a weighting of such interests as monetary gain, animal welfare, and client satisfaction. In other words, for many practitioners, what is at stake is a definition of the veterinarian that contains an interrelated structure of valuations. From this definition there then flow conclusions about appropriate behavior and attitudes in particular kinds of circumstances.

There are many possible general models of the private veterinary practitioner. But at present there seem to be four major models that are vying for support in the profession. Not all of these models are incompatible. Indeed, there are probably few practitioners who do not combine in their moral outlook elements from more than one of these pictures. Various kinds of practice may demand certain combinations. Perhaps normative veterinary ethics will conclude that it is better for practitioners to combine elements of the models, or to adopt a picture that should be characterized as an entirely new or different model, than to accept any of these four models in their pure form.

Each of these four models is very general and permits a range of values. However, these models are found time and again in the thinking of veterinarians. In addressing issues in normative ethics it will therefore be useful to consider them and their ethical implications.

The Veterinarian as Healer

Many veterinarians see themselves primarily as healers. According to this model, the veterinarian is to animals what many people want the physician to be to people – someone interested in a patient's welfare, someone who applies the healing arts with dignity and care, someone who will work tirelessly for the patient's benefit, someone who is entitled to earn a living because he is dedicated to healing and does not engage in healing primarily in order to make money.

This model of the veterinarian is expressed eloquently in Dr. Calvin Schwabe's description of veterinary medicine as

> the gentle profession. Gentleness, compassion, and loving service to the especially dependent, helpless, and needy are qualities which most thinking individuals recognize as being basic to what we regard as humane behavior. The first veterinarians in ancient times were priests and a need for their secular ministry was never more evident than today (6).

Schwabe's characterization of veterinary medicine as a "ministry" is especially apt. It reflects the contention of this model that healing is too important, too bound up with life and death, with pain and suffering, with human as well as animal welfare, to be cheapened by such things as discount coupons in newspaper advertisements, sale of water bowls and pet toys, and aggressive self-promotion. These are seen as desecrations of the healer's calling. It is the model of the veterinarian as a healer that is at work when Dr. Robert Shomer complains that the practice of selling nonprofessional products is replacing the question "Is there a doctor in the house?" with the question "Is there a salesperson in the store?" (7).

One must be careful not to make too much of an analogy between the veterinarian as healer and the physician steadfastly committed to saving the lives or promoting the interests of human patients. Many in society, including many veterinarians, subscribe to the anticruelty position (see Chapter 11) and do not view the painless killing of even a healthy animal as a harm to it. Veterinarians participate in a good deal of killing of animals. They also sometimes suggest or acquiesce in decisions that favor the interests of clients at the expense of the interests of patients. Whether such practices are always morally correct is an issue for normative veterinary ethics. But a descriptive model of veterinary practice that is accurate must reflect what veterinarians actually think. And many veterinarians who do see themselves as healers are not always committed to the preservation of animal life, or to the promotion of patients' interests when these conflict with the desires or needs of clients.

This does not mean, of course, that the model of the veterinarian as healer excludes a doctor who refuses to kill healthy animals or who takes an aggressive stand against clients who wish to euthanize curable or troublesome animals. It is altogether possible that such attitudes will gain enough support among those veterinarians who describe themselves as healers that these attitudes will appropriately be seen as essential components of the model itself. If this occurs, we may want to split the current model of the doctor as healer into two different models, one of which opposes painless killing of healthy, curable, or troublesome animals and one which does not. Today, however, the predominance of the anticruelty position in the profession and society does not appear to justify such a division of the model of the veterinarian as healer.

The Veterinarian as Friend and Counselor

In a landmark essay in legal ethics, philosopher Charles Fried observed that a lawyer characteristically becomes so committed to serving the interests of his client that it is appropriate to characterize him as the client's friend (8). Not all professional relationships involve what can accurately be termed a friendship. Sometimes, a service is provided with little emotional attachment on the part of either practitioner or client. However, like lawyers, veterinarians do frequently come to care greatly about their clients. They listen to clients not just because they must do so in order to earn a fee, make a diagnosis, or recommend a course of treatment, but because they genuinely care about helping clients to attain their own goals.

Many veterinarians have told me that serving as a friend and counselor to clients is a central part of their definition of themselves as professionals. Being a friend can involve touching an intimate part of a client's life, as when one discusses with a client the options for a desperately ill pet. Being a friend can also involve sympathetic counselling about economic matters. The large animal practitioner who becomes involved in a personal and sympathetic way in the efforts of a farmer client to make a decent living is a paradigm of the veterinarian as friend.

James Herriot, who is rightly regarded as the profession's most eloquent chronicler of the model of the veterinarian as healer, also gives us unequaled portraits of the veterinarian as friend. Herriot tells the story of a visit to an elderly client. One of her beloved dogs has just died. She senses that she will be next. She is troubled by the fact that some people say that animals have no souls, and asks Herriot whether she will see her pets again in heaven.

> ... I patted the hand which still grasped mine. "If having a soul means being able to feel love and loyalty and gratitude, then animals are better off than a lot of humans. You've nothing to worry about there."
>
> "Oh, I hope you're right. Sometimes I lie at night thinking about it."
>
> "I know I'm right, Miss Stubbs, and don't you argue with me. They teach us vets all about animals' souls."
>
> The tension left her face and she laughed with a return of her old spirit. "I'm sorry to bore you with this and I'm not going to talk about it again. But before you go, I want you to be absolutely honest with me. I don't want reassurance from you – just the truth. I know you are very young but please tell me – what are your beliefs? Will my animals go with me?"
>
> She stared intently into my eyes. I shifted in my chair once or twice.
>
> "Miss Stubbs, I'm afraid I'm a bit foggy about all this," I said. "But I'm absolutely certain of one thing. Wherever you are going, they are going too."
>
> She still stared at me but her face was calm again. "Thank you, Mr. Herriot, I know you are being honest with me. That is what you really believe, isn't it?"
>
> "I do believe it," I said. "With all my heart I believe it." (9)

The Veterinarian as Businessperson

The most controversial model of the private practitioner that currently occupies a significant place within the profession is that of the veterinarian as a businessperson. This picture of the veterinarian is controversial for two reasons.

First, some veterinarians are so opposed to a heavy emphasis on business and management that they believe it is inherently contradictory to speak of a true doctor as a businessperson.

Second, it is probably incorrect to say that there is *a* picture within the profession of the veterinarian as a businessperson. There seem to be several such pictures, which reflect varying views about the propriety of certain business techniques. For example, Dr. Shomer includes "resorting to the tactics of merchandising and the sale of nonprofessional items"(7) within his conception of being a salesperson in a store rather than a doctor in the house. I have met some veterinarians who are so opposed to self-promotion that they reject listing their practices in the yellow pages as "being a businessman." In contrast, many veterinarians would probably object to any categorization that distinguishes being a healer or friend from being a businessperson. For them, management and promotion is no more than a means of achieving a veterinarian's traditional interests of helping animals and clients, and earning a living.

For the purposes of ethical discussion in which people of all points of view can partake, it does little good to maintain that there can be *no* appropriate characterization of a veterinarian as businessperson that is different from other models. Nor will dispassionate ethical analysis be assisted by building into one's characterization whatever one finds objectionable (or acceptable) in business practices. It is difficult at this stage in the development and acceptance of practice management techniques to find a succinct or generally acceptable characterization of the veterinarian as businessperson. But it is an indisputable fact that some veterinarians do define themselves as businesspeople and that this general perception of themselves colors their views about ethical behavior.

Persuasive proof of the emergence of a distinct model of the veterinarian as businessperson can be found in a recent editorial in *Veterinary Economics*. The editorial opposed the recently enacted provision of the *Principles of Veterinary Medical Ethics* permitting practitioners to sell nonprofessional items if such products are generally unavailable or are difficult to obtain in the client's general vicinity. The editorial discussed two successful doctors for whom merchandising of nonmedical products has proved very profitable. It characterized them as "young, talented, and innovative entrepreneurs." They "didn't feel obligated to carry on the customs of a dominant mentor like James Herriot. ... [They] changed traditional customs and blueprints to fit their career goals, rather than altering the end to fit the means" (10).

The editorial suggests brilliantly what differentiates the model of the veterinarian as businessperson from more traditional conceptions. The use of some practice management techniques (e.g., computerized billing or cost control) would not of themselves qualify one for inclusion in this model. These things can just be means of garnering income that is ancillary in a practitioner's mind to something else. It is the term "entrepreneur" that best summarizes the veterinarian as businessperson. An entrepreneur is by definition someone who sees himself *as a businessperson* and not as someone who must run a business in order to support his professional activities. He regards running a successful business and making money from it as at least as important as the goods or services the business provides. He views himself as entitled to engage in ordinary commercial practices that other entrepreneurs or tradespeople use, such as advertising and retailing. This does not mean that he recognizes no ethical limits upon what he may do. But neither will he necessarily treat traditional values or approaches as providing boundaries within which his interest in monetary gain must operate.

Some veterinarians who like to think of themselves as entrepreneurs may object to this characterization. They may find it too cold. They may want to insist that they, too, can be, and indeed often are, as warm-hearted and devoted to animals and clients as a James Herriot.[a]   Such objections do not, I believe, vitiate my characterization of the model. Rather, these objections reflect the inability of many veterinarians to accept the model in its entirety. This is not surprising. For, as I shall argue later, there are aspects of the model of the veterinarian as businessperson that are not morally admirable.

The Veterinarian as Economic Manager or Consultant

There is a new model of veterinary private practice that might be even more foreign to traditional attitudes than that of the veterinarian as businessperson. A picture of the veterinarian as a general economic manager and consultant is now being urged as a way of assuring the continued existence and profitability of farm and food animal practice.

This model views the veterinarian as first and foremost a provider of herd management advice. Such advice typically is not in the form of answers to particular questions or medical problems. Rather, as Dr. David Galligan puts it, such practitioners "offer a full-service program," the purpose of which is to "determine which combinations of services will offer the greatest return with the minimum risk on the dollar for the farmer" (11).

Several things follow from the primary aim of providing a general profitable management system for animal herds. First, the veterinarian is no longer seen as someone whose primary function must be to examine animals, diagnose conditions, or dispense medications. Part of the veterinarian's "program" may involve hands-on veterinary care. However, he might willingly leave most of this to clients, and may concentrate instead on providing advice about what animals to buy, supervising the purchase of feeds, designing methods of housing and husbandry, and advising clients about when to sell and how much to charge for their products. As Dr. Galligan observes, he might "make more economic impact for the farmer pushing a pencil rather than pushing a syringe" (11).

Another aspect of the model of the veterinarian as economic manager is its disavowal of health as a necessary goal of the veterinarian. As Drs. Barbara Straw and Robert Friendship note, "the concept of 'health' has traditionally conjured up images of a pathogen-free, or 'healthy' animal or herd; and customarily efforts have been directed toward control or elimination of the pathogenic agent to attain this state of 'health.' More recently, the veterinary professional has begun to appreciate that perfect health may not be synonymous with maximum productivity or maximum profitability" (12). "For years," states Dr. Galligan, "we have recommended wiping out all disease in a herd, but now we're finding that this might not be cost effective. It might be more profitable for farmers and consumers to live with low levels of disease in herds" (11).

---

[a]On the other hand, James Herriot is a favorite target of those who reject more traditional pictures of veterinary practice. No defense of the models of the veterinarian as businessperson or as economic manager seems to be complete without an unkind reference to the "myth" or supposed "death" of James Herriot (13), or to "the traditional approach . . . epitomized by the now renowned James Herriot" (14). Opponents of more traditional models of practice rightly perceive Herriot's great popularity – among veterinarians as well as the public – as an obstacle to their views. However, they do not add to their persuasiveness by making light of a figure who has done so much to elevate the popular regard for all veterinarians. If some of the arguments of this text are correct, Herriot will remain a great moral beacon for the profession for some time to come.

The model of the veterinarian as economic manager does not represent a complete break from the past. Veterinarians have long advised clients about herd management. They have provided guidance about matters not strictly speaking of a medical nature. They have recognized that economics sometimes dictates not treating certain animals or providing less extensive or expensive treatment than is available.

Nevertheless, the model of veterinarian as manager involves a momentous shift in attitude. Some farm animal practitioners tell me that when they have a situation in which it is cost-effective not to treat certain members of a herd, they tell the client that the *veterinary* approach would be to treat. They then either leave it to the client to decide whether he wants to go the veterinary route (or the best veterinary route), or they will advise the client to favor productivity with the understanding that this may not be the veterinary approach. Likewise, when these practitioners provide advice about feed, housing, or production that does not have medical consequences, they characterize what they are doing as providing a general program of management advice one of whose components is veterinary service.

In contrast, the model of the veterinarian as manager includes within the role of the practitioner *as a veterinarian* advising clients about purely economic, nonmedical matters and counselling toleration or promotion of certain kinds or levels of disease.

I suspect that veterinarians who are accustomed to the model of the veterinarian as manager may not appreciate how surprising the model is to the typical layman. Veterinarians, laymen are likely to say, are supposed to be *doctors*, they are supposed to promote health and alleviate disease. It would be a mistake to dismiss this response to the model of the veterinarian as manager as reflecting an ignorance of the economic needs of farmers or practitioners. Laymen can understand such things. They can also understand that because animals are not people we may often allow a farm animal practitioner to do in the name of economics what would never be tolerated from a physician.

What the layman is expressing in his puzzlement about the model of veterinarian as manager is a question about the appropriateness of calling such a person a "doctor" – as opposed, say to a "herd profitability manager" or "herd productivity and disease expert."[b] For the dictionary does define the term "doctor" (in the medical and not just the degree-possessing sense) as someone "skilled or specializing in *healing* arts" (15). Puzzlement about the model is not necessarily a condemnation, but it is a reflection of how new and different a picture of the veterinarian this model presents.

REFERENCES

1. Herrick JB: The bond of being a veterinarian. *J Am Vet Med Assoc* 191:26-28, 1987.
2. Enrollment under the knife. *Veterinary Economics* Mar 1986:28-39.
3. "Emergency Service." *1988 AVMA Directory*, p 477.
4. "Therapy, Determination of." *1988 AVMA Directory*, p 476.
5. "Fees for Service." *1988 AVMA Directory*, p 475.
6. Schwabe CW: *Veterinary Medicine and Human Health.* ed 3. Baltimore: Williams & Wilkins, 1984, p 634.

[b]Interestingly, the title of a regular series of articles in the *Compendium on Continuing Education for the Practicing Veterinarian* was changed from "The Swine Health Advisor" to "Swine Production Management" (16).

7. Shomer, RR: Letter. Is there a doctor in the house – or a salesperson in the store? *J Am Vet Med Assoc* 190:245, 1987.
8. Fried C: Lawyer as friend: the moral foundations of the lawyer-client relation. *Yale Law Journal* 85:1060-1089, 1976; 86:573-587, 1987.
9. Herriot J: *All Creatures Great and Small.* New York: Bantam Books, 1973, p 308. Copyright (c) by James Herriot. Quoted with permission from St. Martin's Press, Inc., Harold Ober Associates, Inc., David Higham Associates Ltd., and James Herriot.
10. Sollars M: Memo from the Editor. *Veterinary Economics* Feb 1987:1.
11. Quoted in Enrollment Under the Knife. *Veterinary Economics* Mar 1986:32.
12. Straw B and Friendship R: Expanding the role of the veterinarian on swine farms. *Compendium on Continuing Education for the Practicing Veterinarian* 8:F69, 1986.
13. Sollars MD: Rest in peace famed James Herriot. *Veterinary Economics* March 1986:2.
14. Stein TE: Marketing health management to food animal enterprises. *Compendium on Continuing Education for the Practicing Veterinarian* 7:S330, 1986.
15. *Webster's Third New International Dictionary.* Springfield, MA: G & C. Merriam Company, 1961, p 666, emphasis supplied.
16. *Compendium on Continuing Education for the Practicing Veterinarian* 9(2):101, 1987.

Chapter

——————— 16 ———————

The Sale of Nonprofessional
Goods and Services:
Toward the Choice of a Model
of Veterinary Practice

There are many moral issues that are forcing veterinarians to choose among competing models of practice. No issue has created more controversy within the profession, or is more crucial to its self-definition, than the question of how far veterinarians may go in order to increase practice revenues. Different commercial activities raise different ethical concerns. This chapter focuses upon the selling of nonprofessional goods and services. Chapter 17 will discuss marketing techniques in veterinary practice.

THE MERCHANDISING OF PRODUCTS

What Is Merchandising?

Merchandising in the veterinary context can be defined as the selling of a product or service not involved in or necessitated by the direct medical care of a patient (1). Merchandising in this sense is distinct from "dispensing," which refers to the sale or supply of products (e.g., drugs or pesticides) to clients for medical reasons by the doctor, or by his facility under his direct orders.

Merchandising can include the sale of nonprofessional products such as ordinary commercial pet food, toys, bedding, and clothing. Merchandising can also encompass selling an ordinarily professional product for other than direct and legitimate medical reasons. This can occur where a doctor has been given oral information by a client insufficient to justify dispensing a product for medical reasons, where a client insists on purchasing a product for his own reasons, or where a doctor simply wants to make some money. Merchandising also includes selling professional products to people who have no professional relationship with the practitioner.[a]

As I use the term, "merchandising" is distinct from marketing, which can be defined as the promotion of services or goods to the public. It is possible to market one's practice without engaging in merchandising, by promoting purely professional services. And one can merchandise professional or nonprofessional products without marketing, by selling them with a minimum of promotion within the confines of one's office.

It is important to understand the distinction between merchandising and marketing. I have found that many veterinarians erroneously interpret arguments against the former as criticisms of the latter. As I shall argue, although merchandising by most veterinarians is morally objectionable, many forms of marketing are acceptable (see Chapter 17).

When Is a Product a "Medical" or "Professional" One?

Virtually anything a veterinarian might sell could, under certain circumstances, have a direct and legitimate medical purpose and therefore not be a "merchandised" product. For example, a fabric halter might be indicated medically for a dog injured by a metal collar. Nevertheless, few people would be inclined to say that halters, scratching posts, beds, sweaters, conditioning shampoos, or any of a myriad of other things that could conceivably be of medical importance are *generically* medical products.

However, it might not always be clear whether a product ought to be characterized as medical/professional. Moreover, insofar as merchandising is perceived to be profitable, there might be a tendency to categorize ambiguous products as generically medical/professional in nature – and thereby sweep them within the veterinarian's traditional role as a dispenser rather than merchandiser (2). Such a tendency is already apparent with regard to pet food. One discussion counsels veterinarians who sell commercial, nonprescription pet food to call a waiting room display of these products the "nutrition center." The doctor is told that many pet owners "would like the confidence in selecting a pet's diet that comes with your recommendation." He is urged to add to the product display brochures about

---

[a]The AVMA *Principles* define "merchandising" as "providing products for lay use, only on the supposition that the veterinarian has had knowledge of the particular case or general conditions which apply to the particular farm or kennel. ... Merchandising is buying and selling of professional veterinary products without due consideration for the patient receiving such products" (3). This is not a good definition. Most veterinarians speak of the "merchandising" of nonprofessional products and services; indeed, this seems to be the predominant usage of the term (1). The proposed 1988 revision of the *Principles* offered (4) a new definition of merchandising, as the "buying and selling of professional veterinary products without a veterinarian-client-patient relationship." The latter relationship is defined as including, among other things, a) a doctor's having "sufficient knowledge of the animal(s) ... to initiate at least a general or preliminary diagnosis" and b) his being "readily available for follow up in case of adverse reactions or failure of the regimen or therapy." This definition also errs in limiting "merchandising" to the sale of professional products and services.

feeding pets during the different stages of their lives; this will help educate clients as to what foods, vitamins, and minerals are necessary.... Then, when clients come into your exam room, you can ask what the dog or cat is being fed and remind clients about the nutrition information and foods (5).

This example shows that although it is generally useful to distinguish between the merchandising of medical/professional and of non-medical/professional products, in considering the morality of merchandising, one should not become fixated on the question of how to define what is a medical or professional product. This is a difficult question that is not entirely ethical in nature: it relates to, among other things, the issue of whether the healing professions ought to be as concerned with preventing disease as curing it, and therefore ought for medical reasons to consider such things as nutritious food to be medical products.

The major ethical issue regarding merchandising now confronting the profession is not whether veterinarians may morally recommend a number of things that are good for patient health or well-being. The issue is whether veterinarians may morally sell items that *generally* can be sold by nonveterinarians – because these items are not directed toward a specific medical condition, do not generally cause medical problems if misused, or do not require continuing medical supervision for their use.[b] In order to facilitate discussion, I shall refer to all such items as "nonprofessional" or "nonmedical." There still might be some dispute about whether certain things should be categorized as nonprofessional items in this sense. But certainly ordinary commercial, nonprescription food, as well as such products as water bowls, clothing, grooming accessories (brushes, combs, perfumes, etc.), bedding, and toys should be included in such a definition of "nonprofessional" products.

The Argument Against the Merchandising of Professional Products

It is not difficult to appreciate why merchandising medical products is wrong. By definition, such products require dispensing by a veterinarian in order to protect the patient, and often the client and other persons as well. A veterinarian who merchandises medical products can cause patients to become ill and clients to suffer economic, physical, or psychological damage. He also endangers his own interests. Because it involves the sale of a medical product without a legitimate medical justification, merchandising medical products is negligent veterinary practice. It can subject a doctor to legal action by a client or one's state veterinary board.

The AVMA *Principles* unequivocally condemn the merchandising of medical products (6). There appears to be little opposition to this view, at least in principle.

---

[b]The "sale" and "selling" of nonmedical products are not restricted to instances in which a client takes possession of the products at the veterinarian's facility. A doctor who recommends nonprofessional items that are purchased elsewhere, in return for his receiving a commission or other kind of monetary benefit from the manufacturer or sales outlet, would be engaged in the sale, and merchandising, of these products. So would a veterinarian who receives payment from the manufacturer for taking orders for nonprofessional products that are delivered by the manufacturer directly to clients. It should also be noted that the receipt of a commission, rebate, or kickback, even for the sale of a nonprofessional product, violates the *Principles* (7) and is morally wrong (see Chapter 19).

However, there are things veterinarians do that normally can be medically appropriate but can cross over the line between legitimate dispensing and merchandising. One such practice is diagnosing and prescribing over the telephone. If a doctor knows the animal and client, this can be perfectly appropriate medical practice, but without adequate first-hand information, it can constitute merchandising. Among other practices that under certain circumstances can constitute merchandising are the following: selling clients professional items by mail order upon their written or telephone requests; selling a client enough medication to be used over an extended period of time on his animal; supplying additional amounts of a medication without examining the animal to determine whether the drug is still indicated; and permitting one's receptionist to sell professional items (such as prescription diets) originally dispensed for medical reasons without obtaining current knowledge about the animal's condition.

The merchandising of professional products need not be motivated by greed, although, of course, it can be. A doctor who merchandises a medical product might believe sincerely that he is acting in the interests of patients and clients. What characterizes the merchandising of professional items is the absence of adequate familiarity with the patient. Therefore, it will sometimes be more appropriate to describe the merchandiser of a medical item as negligent rather than unscrupulous. But whether negligent or mercenary, the merchandising of professional products is objectionable from a moral standpoint.

The Argument Against the Merchandising of Nonprofessional Products

There are few controversies in the profession more intensely fought than that regarding the propriety of merchandising nonprofessional products. The literature is fairly bursting with denunciations and defenses of the practice.

I have suggested that problems in normative veterinary ethics should be addressed, at least initially, by considering how various alternative approaches to these problems would affect the legitimate interests of all concerned. Such an analysis, I submit, argues *very strongly* against the merchandising of nonprofessional products, at least by the great majority of veterinarians.

THE INTERESTS OF DOCTORS: IS IT PROFITABLE?

The argument raised most often in favor of the merchandising of nonprofessional products is increased profits for the veterinarian. There is no shortage of reports about practitioners who have made a great deal of money by such merchandising (8).

However, the question for the profession is not whether certain veterinarians have increased their revenues through merchandising, but rather whether, for the profession as a whole and in the long run, merchandising will prove profitable.

As the late Dr. Robert Knowles observed (1), it is far from clear that merchandising will increase the incomes of most practitioners. Selling nonprofessional products has a relatively small profit margin. Ordering, storing, displaying, and selling such products requires time and space that might be devoted to professional services. Moreover, most businesses engaged in moving large quantities of pet products (such as supermarkets, animal feed and supply stores, and grooming establishments) are far better merchandisers than veterinarians. Once such establishments perceive that veterinarians are making inroads into their profits, they can quickly undercut veterinarians' prices. They can use their advertising and marketing expertise to make even the most ambitious veterinary "nutrition center" or pet product display an unprofitable nightmare.

The most dangerous potential result of the merchandising of nonprofessional products, however, is the erosion of the model of the veterinarian as a healer, and of the image of veterinary patients as beings entitled to first-class medical care. These views of the veterinarian and his patient did not spring into existence overnight. It has taken the profession generations to improve its scientific base and the techniques, drugs, and services it can offer to animal owners. The profession has also labored hard to inculcate in the public an appreciation of the value and importance of pets as well as other animals. It did so long before the popularity of the concept of the "human-companion animal bond" or even before the advent of modern veterinary drugs and techniques. It did so by discouraging crass commercialism and by insisting that veterinarians strive as far as possible to approach their animal patients with much the same dignity and professionalism people expect from their physicians.

Veterinarians can now take advantage of this fortunate confluence of advancing veterinary science, traditional professionalism, and an enhanced appreciation of animals to improve revenues. People who care greatly about their animals and who consider veterinary medicine to be a calling as worthy and scientifically advanced as medicine will pay for competent and caring veterinary services.

But it would be a grave mistake for veterinarians to take high regard for their profession for granted. Many people still do not look upon veterinarians as "real" doctors. As every veterinarian knows, for every animal owner who seeks high-quality veterinary services, there are many who do not. There is still much more work to be done to convince animal owners and society at large of the value of veterinarians and their animal patients.

The routine merchandising of nonprofessional products threatens to reverse this continuing elevation of the veterinarian and the potential for profitability this elevation promises.

What would we think of a pediatrician who might sell bassinets, baby bottles, and tricycles, or of an internist who peddled exercise equipment or granola? Aside from immediate revulsion, we would suspect that they do not consider themselves, or their medical areas of expertise, to be good or valuable enough to enable them to earn a decent living. We would also think that they are more interested in their own monetary gain than in helping their patients. We would say that they are showing their patients great disrespect.

Such reactions are not attributable simply to the historical fact that physicians happen to have been able to survive without merchandising nonmedical products. These reactions stem from our fundamental belief that the physician's power over matters of life and death, and health and illness, is so important that medical care must be approached in a dignified manner and with as few trappings of commercialism as possible. We afford the physician an elevated status because of the importance we attribute to *ourselves*, his patients, and the momentous reasons for which we seek his assistance.

A veterinarian who merchandises nonprofessional products is telling his clients and the world *not* to be offended by commercialism in the veterinary context. He is sending the message that *animal* health and disease, pain and suffering, life and death, are not important enough to be separated from ordinary commercial activities. He is in fact promoting precisely the view that has prevented veterinarians from achieving the respect long afforded physicians and dentists – the view that the *veterinarian's* patients are "only animals."

Ironically, the veterinarian-merchandiser is also mounting a direct assault against what is potentially the profession's most powerful marketing tool, the human-companion animal bond itself. For if the bond means anything at all, it implies that many animals ought to be given love, respect, and dignified medical care, in virtue of their great worth and importance.

There is hard evidence that dignified veterinary practice can be profitable. Practitioners who treat animals that are increasingly coming to be seen as beings of great worth and value are doing better. Between 1983 and 1985 mean gross practice incomes rose 14% for mixed animal practices, 21% for equine predominant practices, 27% for small animal predominant practices, and 29% for small animal exclusive practices (9). These figures show that people, especially those with companion animals, are willing to pay for first-class veterinary care.

THE INTERESTS OF PRACTITIONERS: BEYOND THE PROFIT QUESTION

The potential for increased revenues, however, does not constitute the only, or indeed the most important, reason for concluding that the merchandising of nonprofessional products is not in the interests of the profession as a whole. As Dr. Robert Shomer notes in a recent critique of merchandising (10), veterinarians receive many nonmonetary benefits from placing greater emphasis on professional services than on material award. They can rest assured that they are indeed serving the interests of their patients, clients, and society. They also benefit from perceiving themselves, and by being perceived, as more than shopkeepers but as true professionals who, by virtue of special training, skill, and service deserve a *special* kind of respect and admiration afforded only to the few. If veterinarians sometimes must choose between their heritage of professionalism and acting like ordinary storekeepers in order to make some extra dollars, it still remains very much in their interests to choose professionalism. As Dr. Robert M. Miller warns, "when veterinary medicine loses its image as a decent, caring, dignified profession, we will have lost everything. When we achieve the supermarket or used-car-lot image of a huckster, all of the gains of the 20th century will be wasted" (11).

THE INTERESTS OF CLIENTS AND PATIENTS

There are also many reasons why the merchandising of nonprofessional products is not in the interests of most clients and their animals.

First, such products will usually cost clients more at veterinary facilities than at retail stores, especially large chain operations that buy in great bulk and can pass their savings along to consumers. On items purchased infrequently, the difference might be trivial. But on pet food, a client could pay substantially more over an animal's life by buying from a veterinarian. This money could be used for other worthy purposes, including veterinary care. Supporters of merchandising frequently claim that clients are getting their extra money's worth in the expertise of the veterinarian and in the convenience of being able to buy pet items when they are at their veterinarian. These are spurious arguments. Many nonprofessional items require no veterinarian recommendation or advice. Regarding others (such as pet foods), the veterinarian can still recommend without actually selling; this approach would enable clients to benefit both from lower prices and professional recommendations. In fact, convenience argues for the selling of nonprofessional items in supermarkets or department stores, which most people frequent far more often than their veterinarian.

Aside from increased costs to clients, there are potentially darker sides of veterinary merchandising. Some clients will undoubtedly buy such things as pet toys or snacks because they feel guilty they have made their animal endure an examination or treatment. Veterinarians should not take advantage of such fictional anthropomorphizing by clients.[c] Some merchandisers will surely fall prey to the temptation of appealing to the model of the veterinarian as healer – a model that rejects commercialism – to sell nonmedical items. This may be accomplished by playing upon the belief of most clients that *veterinarians* do not recommend things for their own monetary gain but to benefit patients and clients. Even if a veterinarian does not consciously appeal to the image of a healer for monetary gain, the client may still be influenced into buying something simply because the *doctor* recommends it. (Of course, merchandising will eventually kill the goose that can lay these golden eggs. For once clients come to see veterinarians as shopkeepers rather than doctors, they will not be so impressed by product recommendations.) Finally, because the primary motive for merchandising nonmedical items is profit, there is a distinct danger that a merchandiser will push a particular product or brand not because it is the best one for his patients, but because it yields a higher profit for himself.

Some veterinarians will insist with sincerity that *they* can merchandise without manipulating clients. However, once one begins to accept maximization of profit as a legitimate aim of one's practice, one is subjected to enormous pressure to push clients to do things they would not otherwise consider. For that is sometimes the only way to persuade customers to part with as much money as they can be motivated to spend. For example, among the techniques recommended by one recent discussion are the following:

> Use wood shelving wherever possible to promote a look of warmth and permanency.

> Line up at least two consecutive rows of each item if possible; grocery stores use this technique to attract the eye of hurried customers (12).

Another proponent of waiting room displays reports that

> (i)n a recent survey conducted by the Point of Purchase Institute regarding the purchase of pet accessories, nearly 80% of those questioned stated that they did not

---

[c]One advocate of merchandising reports the following "classic scenario:" a "Mrs. Doty" purchases for her dog Oakley "a red collar and matching leash for $12.50, increasing the [veterinarian's] sale from $32 [for medical services] to $44.50, nearly a 40% increase." According to this author, "Mrs. Doty is extremely pleased because she has purchased a quality pet product that her veterinarian has recommended, and Oakley is happy because he looks like a million bucks. What's so unprofessional about this" (13)?

plan on making that purchase ... five minutes before they did. What does this tell you? Pet accessories are primarily an impulse sale. Did you ever wonder why your local supermarket crams all those candy bars, safety razors, nylons, and magazines at the checkout stand? You guessed it. Idle minds make for impulse spending (14).

These discussions belie the claim that merchandising only gives clients what they want. To the aggressive merchandiser, the client is no longer a person whose own desires are paramount and to be served, but someone who is to be manipulated.

Additionally, the inevitable temptation that will be faced by many merchandisers to manipulate clients raises an extremely frightening question: if veterinarians get a taste for increasing revenues by inducing clients to buy unnecessary nonprofessional items, will they eventually seek to push unnecessary professional services?

ARGUMENTS OF THE MERCHANDISERS

Because there is significant support among veterinarians for merchandising nonmedical products, it is useful to consider briefly some of arguments commonly offered in its favor.

"Merchandising does not compromise my skills." One argument advanced in support of merchandising is that it is possible to sell nonmedical items and still provide highly skilled veterinary services (15). As I argued earlier, this is a dubious proposition regarding some doctors, who will have to expend time and money that could otherwise be spent practicing or improving technical skills. However, even if merchandising did not affect a practitioner's technical proficiency, this would not defeat the argument I have made against it. The most important issue raised by merchandising is not one of skill, but whether veterinarians want to be perceived as doctors or storekeepers. Auto mechanics and plumbers can be extremely skilled and still merchandise. However, these tradespeople do not occupy the same position of admiration and respect accorded to medical professionals. Perhaps some technically skilled veterinarian-merchandisers will be able to make a good living. But ultimately they will not occupy the elevated status of healers, and will not benefit from the many advantages that this status can bring.

"I can't be a physician, and should not feel guilty or inferior about it." Some supporters of merchandising accept the fact that their position is incompatible with the high level of professionalism we expect of physicians, but maintain that it is foolish for veterinarians to think they can ever be like physicians. Veterinarians, it is said, should accept the fact that they are veterinarians. They should realize that their rung on the professional ladder is not incompatible with merchandising. Those practitioners who resist merchandising are diagnosed as frustrated physicians who are attempting to hide their feelings of inferiority by espousing unattainable professional ideals. As one supporter of merchandising puts it, "if these insecure, ultraprofessional veterinarians want to look, act, feel, and smell like a physician, why didn't they go to medical school" (16)?

The notion that veterinarians cannot be perceived as occupying as elevated a status as physicians is simply inaccurate. Many people already regard veterinarians at least as highly as physicians (11). To be sure, veterinary patients are animals, and animals will never be regarded as the equals of human beings. Therefore, veterinarians can never expect to be viewed exactly as are physicians. But it hardly follows that veterinarians should not behave in many important respects as do physicians.

The detractors of "ultraprofessionalism" are themselves making a fundamental conceptual mistake. *They* are the ones who begin with a picture of the physician as the purest and most exalted practitioner of the healing arts. They then measure veterinarians against this model. They believe that other veterinarians who want to behave in certain ways as do physicians must also be measuring themselves against physicians. And because the merchandisers understand that there cannot be a complete fit between this pure physician model and veterinary practice, they attribute some misunderstanding or psychological infirmity to veterinarians who strive to apply some of the ideals of human medicine to veterinary medicine.

In fact, there is no need to measure veterinarians against some idealized picture of physicians. What is obligatory or ideal in veterinary practice will flow from features of veterinary practice itself. Sometimes these features will demand of veterinarians kinds of behavior one would expect of physicians; sometimes they will not. If veterinarians should behave similarly to physicians in certain respects and under certain circumstances, it does not follow that they are to this extent approaching *closer* to becoming physicians. It means that veterinarians share certain moral obligations and ideals with another healing profession. That veterinarians might want to appeal to medicine, dentistry, law, or other learned professions to illuminate issues in veterinary ethics does not mean that they are really striving to be members of any of these professions.

"My clients don't mind my selling nonprofessional products." Another argument made by supporters of merchandising is that their clients do not find the practice offensive and do not have a lowered image of them as professionals because they merchandise. Studies have not yet been done regarding how the merchandising of nonprofessional products affects the public's image of veterinarians. There are, surely, many clients who will stay away from practices that merchandise. Other clients might dislike merchandising, but will remain with a practice out of convenience or because they like a particular doctor. That a merchandiser can maintain or even increase his client base does not prove that clients in general accept merchandising, but only that there are some clients who do not mind it and some who do not mind it enough to go elsewhere.

Let us grant for the purposes of argument that some veterinary clients do not find the merchandising of nonprofessional products offensive or unprofessional. If this is so, it would only show that in the minds of these people, veterinary medicine is still not regarded as belonging on the same level of professionalism as medicine or dentistry. This should surprise no one. Every practitioner has seen clients who do not regard their animals, or veterinarians, with great admiration or respect. Other clients might be accustomed to a view of veterinarians that distinguishes them from "real" doctors, and therefore might forgive in them a kind of commercialism they would not tolerate in physicians or dentists.

The issue for the profession is whether it wants to foster an image of veterinary practice that so elevates the practitioner, the patient, and the client, that selling nonprofessional products will be considered offensive by clients and the public.

"Merchandising nonmedical pet products is necessary in today's market." The argument raised most frequently in support of merchandising is that it is forced upon practitioners by current market conditions, especially the influx of many new doctors into the profession. Indeed, it is now common to hear that unless they sell nonprofessional products, practitioners will be committing economic suicide (16).

If the profession as a whole really had to choose between merchandising and extinction, one would have to tolerate merchandising, however offensive it might be. It would be wrong to insist on a prohibition that would force the profession to close down. That would cause great harm not just to doctors but to clients and animals, who would be without veterinary services.

There might be some doctors who must choose between merchandising and economic suicide, but I have yet to find a small animal practitioner who can make the case convincingly. A practitioner's economic "suicide" would mean more than that his present practice cannot survive, but that he cannot practice veterinary medicine *anywhere*. Moreover, to show that a particular practice faces the choice between merchandising and suicide, not only must it be shown that the practice will literally fold without the sale of nonmedical products. It must be the case that nothing else can be done to cut costs or increase revenues to keep the practice afloat. If a practice requires the sale of commercial pet food or dog leashes to survive, it is surely already in very bad shape.

In fact, almost all veterinarians who claim that they "must" merchandise nonprofessional products mean either that they cannot maintain present income levels without merchandising, or that they cannot make as much money as they would like without merchandising.

There are two appropriate responses to these claims.

First, as shall be discussed in Chapter 17, most veterinarians have at their disposal an enormous range of potential professional services that can be used to maintain or increase revenues. Moreover, these professional options can be promoted by a wide range of professionally dignified marketing techniques.

Second, it might simply be the case that the ethical standards of the profession place limitations on what some practitioners can earn. In this regard, veterinary medicine is no different from any of the other professions, each of which prohibits certain activities that could arguably earn its members more money. (Lawyers, for example, are not permitted to encourage their clients to commit crimes so that they can then earn a fee for defending these clients in court.) Some veterinarians appear to believe that *their* profession is treated especially badly by the marketplace, and for that reason is entitled to engage in merchandising to raise incomes to higher levels. But in fact there are many valuable and hard-working professionals (including public school teachers, college professors, nurses, social workers, government attorneys, and public hospital physicians) who probably will never be able to earn what most veterinarians can. Our economic system does give veterinarians who want significant economic reward the opportunity to try to attain it. However, life is not always fair, and there is no guarantee that a veterinarian's income will reflect his value to his patients and clients, or to society.

A POSSIBLE EXCEPTION: FARM AND FOOD ANIMAL PRACTITIONERS

The argument against merchandising nonmedical products turns in large measure on the worth and importance of the veterinary patient. Among those kinds of animals that most people would regard as sufficiently important to merit dignified care are dogs, cats, caged birds and other family pets, as well as many pleasure, show, and race horses.

However, some veterinary patients are not regarded, and are never likely to be regarded, with great love, admiration, or respect. A draft horse or dairy cow might be an object of affection for some owners, but it is more often viewed as an economic asset. Cattle, chickens, pigs, sheep, and goats produce – or indeed can themselves *become* – products in the marketplace. A veterinarian who treats such animals need be no less skilled or dignified than a small animal practitioner. But it seems paradoxical to ask veterinarians whose very professional activity is aimed at putting products into the stream of commerce, to refrain from "engaging in commercialism" connected with the merchandising of nonmedical products.

Additional arguments can be made in favor of the merchandising of nonprofessional items by farm and food animal practitioners. Much of this practice is economically depressed, and additional sources of revenue might well be imperative. Moreover, although some farm animal practitioners decry this fact, many farmers do not want their veterinarian to be the sole dispenser of medical goods or services. Some clients purchase medical items from nonveterinarians and medicate their animals themselves; others want to be able to administer medications left by the doctor. Farm animal practitioners might rightly wonder whether it makes sense for them to restrict themselves to dispensing medical products if their clients do not even regard them as the sole source of medical items.

These arguments do, I believe, provide some support for the view that farm and food animal veterinarians may merchandise nonmedical products. However, there are also counter-arguments.

First, even if it does not appear inherently offensive for farm animal practitioners to merchandise, the profession as a whole might still have a strong interest in discouraging such merchandising. For merchandising by farm animal doctors could make it difficult for other veterinarians, who constitute the great majority of the profession, to convince the public that merchandising in their kinds of practices is inappropriate.

Second, to be successful, merchandising in farm animal practice might have to involve the kinds of activities recommended by the model of the veterinarian as economic manager (see Chapter 15). There probably is not a great deal of money to be made selling occasional farm implements or food supplements; successful merchandising to farm clients might require large-scale sales of feed and equipment necessary for sizable herd management programs. However, such activities might in the long run injure the interests of many veterinarians, clients, and farm animals. Veterinarian merchandising of nonmedical items might make it even more difficult for doctors to convince clients that veterinarians should administer medicines – and thus could reduce revenues that practitioners would otherwise gain from providing professional services. Additionally, it is undeniable that many food and farm animal practitioners are simply not trained to provide the kinds of services required of a large-scale economic manager (17). Other doctors might find the model of the veterinarian as economic manager aesthetically displeasing or morally unsatisfactory (*see* Chapter 21). Widespread adoption of the model could drive into extinction many of these traditional, hands-on, medicine-oriented practitioners. This could harm not only these doctors, but also clients who want or can afford the kinds of services they have been providing.

As the AVMA *Report on the United States Market for Food Animal Veterinary Medical Services* acknowledges, much investigation is required before the profession can determine "what services are needed by producers and how veterinarians can economically deliver those services" (18). Time will tell whether the economic survival of food and farm animal practice requires significant merchandising of nonmedical goods and services, and whether practitioners who engage in such merchandising can do so with a level of professionalism that is consistent with the interests of the profession as a whole.

THE AVMA REPEAL OF THE PROHIBITION OF MERCHANDISING

In 1986, the AVMA House of Delegates voted to eliminate a 32-year-old provision of the *Principles of Veterinary Medical Ethics* which considered it "unprofessional for veterinarians to display leashes, collars, meats, foods, and other nonprofessional products in their offices, hospitals and waiting rooms" (19). The vote on repeal of this provision was close and followed heated debate. AVMA President Dr. A. F. Hopkins (who stated he himself had "no intentions of displaying leashes, collars, dog food dishes, and the like") predicted that the prohibition could well be reinstated in the future (20).

In 1987, the AVMA House of Delegates defeated a proposal to reinstate the old prohibition. Instead, it added the following statement to the *Principles*:

> It is permissible to display professional veterinary products in the waiting room. The display of nonprofessional products is undesirable, but is permissible if such nonprofessional products are generally unavailable or are difficult to obtain in the general vicinity of the client being served (21).

As supporters of merchandising were quick to note, this language can be interpreted as intended to reinstate the old prohibition against selling nonprofessional products (22). For it is rarely the case that nonprofessional products such as pet food and supplies are unavailable or are difficult to obtain in a client's community. Moreover, the new standard can place practitioners in difficult situations. It seems to require doctors to differentiate between clients who live in areas in which nonmedical products are available and those in which such items are not available or are "difficult" to find. How are veterinarians to make such determinations? Should they ask clients what kinds of stores operate in their communities? How wide a "vicinity" must a doctor inquire about? Are practitioners likely to make objective judgments regarding the availability of nonprofessional products if they want to sell such items? Moreover, how can one maintain a waiting room display if one is supposed to tell some clients that certain displayed items cannot be sold to them?

Clearly, the new code standard reflects the fact that many veterinarians cannot bring themselves to accept the routine merchandising of nonprofessional products as ethical. If some of the arguments of this text are correct, such misgivings are not likely to disappear. The increasing value that veterinary clients are placing on their companion animals is creating a *force*, a momentum, that *will* draw doctors who want to satisfy many of these clients away from commercialism and toward an image of the veterinarian as a dignified and caring healer.

GROOMING

The term "merchandising" is generally used to refer to the sale of merchandise, i.e., products. However, veterinarians can also offer services that are not medical/professional in nature. One nonprofessional service frequently urged as a source of increased revenues is grooming.

Ancillary and Cosmetic Grooming

There are two very different kinds of grooming that can be provided by a veterinarian. The first, which I shall call "ancillary grooming," is not performed because the client has the independent purpose of grooming his animal, but because the animal is already at the facility for a medical reason and ought to be groomed during this time. Typically, ancillary grooming is performed because it is necessary for the health or comfort of the animal, as when an inpatient is bathed after it has come in contact with its own excrement, or a horse receives a routine brushing and a cleaning of its hooves. Ancillary grooming also includes the situation in which an animal (such as a show dog) normally receives nonmedical, purely cosmetic grooming at regular intervals and is groomed in a veterinary facility because it is present there – for medical reasons – at one or more of these times. Ancillary grooming can also include grooming a patient prior to discharge from the hospital so that the client can have his animal in the same condition in which it was admitted.

Ancillary grooming is quite different from the services provided by a professional grooming establishment, to which owners bring their animals specifically for the purpose of being groomed. I shall call such a service provided in the veterinary office or hospital "cosmetic grooming." Clients might bring their animals to a veterinarian solely for cosmetic grooming, or it can be provided to them in addition to some medical service such as a general physical exam. The latter would be an instance of cosmetic and not ancillary grooming because the animal could be groomed even if it were not present at the facility for a medical reason.

Those who recommend grooming as a source of practice revenues typically have cosmetic grooming in mind. Moreover, they do not envision the groomer as someone who happens to be physically present at the veterinary office as a convenience to clients. Rather, it is the veterinary facility that is supposed to offer the service to the public and to collect the fees for it. The groomer is to be retained as a regular employee or an independent contractor, with the doctor taking a percentage of the grooming receipts (23).

The Argument against Cosmetic Grooming

There need be nothing wrong with ancillary grooming. It can be no different from giving a human hospital patient a shave or bath during his stay, for his health or comfort. Moreover, it seems perfectly appropriate for a veterinarian to charge for ancillary grooming and to take a reasonable mark-up for supplies and labor, just as he would for supplies and labor expended in providing professional services.

The typical arguments made for cosmetic grooming are the same ones that are raised for merchandising nonprofessional products: revenues, client convenience, patient welfare, and still more revenues. According to one proponent,

> (t)he groomer can detect skin, ear, dental, and other problems that can be referred to a staff veterinarian. Vaccination programs that have been lagging can be brought up-to-date. Sales of home grooming supplies and equipment can be stimulated. Proper nutrition can be counselled. Sales of ... coat conditioners ... can be stimulated (24).

These words undoubtedly are motivated by a sincere desire to help patients and clients. But the picture that emerges unavoidably from such a passage – and I, submit, will ultimately be perceived by the public – is different. The veterinary office will no longer be seen as a place where sincere, dedicated people seek to serve the patient and client. It will rather be like a group of vultures, who swoop about patients, twice a month if possible, picking over their skin, teeth, and whatever, seeking relentlessly to find another way to take another bite out of clients' wallets.

Can anyone seriously doubt that using grooming to get clients and their dollars into the office will lead to the purchase of unnecessary nonprofessional and professional items? Can anyone think that clients for whom the veterinary office becomes a place of successive requests for money will be *more* eager to visit the veterinarian, or will be *more* trusting of his recommendations?

But even if we suppose that some doctors who offer in-office cosmetic grooming will never manipulate clients for their own monetary gain, these practitioners, too, will be assisting in the demise of the image of the veterinarian as a dignified provider of medical care. Poodle cuts, shampooing, colognes, and fancy ribbons do not belong in the same place in which momentous issues of life and death are confronted by a healer. These things, together with the sale of nonmedical products, will inevitably transform the veterinary hospital into a one-stop animal supply store and service station.

None of this means that grooming is unimportant or that professional groomers should not play a role in promoting animal health. A professional groomer who discovers or suspects a medical condition can suggest that the owner see his veterinarian, and can recommend a doctor if asked to do so. Likewise, if an animal needs grooming for its health or comfort, the doctor can suggest that it be taken to a groomer. However, a beauty parlor does not belong in a medical office.

SEPARATE GROOMING FACILITIES

Some veterinarians do not have a groomer within their veterinary office but nevertheless profit directly from a grooming business. The doctor might own all or part of a grooming establishment, which might be adjacent to the veterinary office. Or he might lease space located in another place to a groomer in return for some percentage of the groomer's gross revenues. A veterinarian can also lease space to a groomer for a fixed rent. Such a doctor will have a stake in the groomer's business in the sense that the groomer's success will assure the doctor his rent.

The unprofessional appearance of a beauty parlor in the veterinary office can sometimes be avoided by separate veterinary and grooming establishments. (However, there are adjacent veterinary and grooming facilities with identical storefront designs that make their connection obvious.) Nevertheless, separate facilities can still pose some of the same problems as in-office cosmetic grooming. Indeed, these problems can be even more insidious. For when a client visits a veterinarian with an in-office groomer, he will at least suspect that there is a financial connection between the two. Even where facilities are separate, the trip to the groomer can be used as a pretext for urging appointments with the veterinarian. And the doctor or his staff can still make it a practice to comment on the appearance of patients, and thereby use the sanctity and authority of the medical office to get the client's animal into the beauty parlor.

It is perfectly appropriate for doctors to recommend grooming for legitimate health reasons. But it is no more professional for a veterinarian to recommend grooming for purely cosmetic reasons than it would be for a physician to comment on a patient's hairdo and urge a trip to a human beautician or barber. If a veterinarian's separate grooming and medical facilities conduct themselves separately and professionally, it might be possible for a doctor to avoid manipulating clients by trying to sell them one kind of service each time they are utilizing the other.

BOARDING

In-facility boarding offers far less potential for manipulation of clients, and can constitute far less a departure from the image of the veterinarian as a medical person, than does cosmetic grooming or the sale of nonprofessional products. The decision to board an animal is not as likely to be made on impulse or to be influenced by subtle commercialistic appeals. Moreover, although some boarding establishments do have a veterinarian on call, for many clients, leaving their animal at a veterinary facility has special advantages. It can assure prompt medical attention if something goes wrong. Special diets or prescribed medications can be administered. Some clients feel more comfortable leaving an animal in a facility whose essential professional service includes the prevention of illness. If an animal is boarded with its regular veterinarian, its records will be available should medical care be required. Unlike a veterinarian who operates a grooming parlor, the doctor who boards animals can give his clients not just a service they may want, but one that is directly related to his special professional training and expertise.

Some people might be inclined to think that it is as offensive for a veterinary hospital to board healthy animals as it would be for a human hospital to set aside several floors as a hotel for tourists. But there are important differences between hotel guests and boarded animals. The latter need assistance and supervision in order to remain healthy and indeed to survive. Many are in a real sense bereft of their families and companions, and in such unaccustomed surroundings, they can be in special need of kind and considerate caretakers. It is more accurate to compare the boarding of a pet in a veterinary facility to the temporary stay of a person who is not ill but nevertheless in need of supervision, in a custodial care facility. We do not consider it offensive or unprofessional for such facilities to be owned and operated by physicians, precisely because good medical care should be available to people who must stay in them.

THE OFFICIAL POSITION ON BOARDING

The AVMA *Principles* state that

> A boarding kennel may be owned by a veterinarian but should not be operated under the veterinarian's name, and the telephone number should be separate from that used by the veterinarian in the conduct of the practice. Persons answering the boarding kennel telephone should not answer by giving the name of the veterinarian or hospital (25).

It is not clear whether the prohibition against operating a boarding kennel "under the veterinarian's name" is meant to require that such kennels be physically separate from the veterinary facility, in an adjoining building or wing with an entirely separate entrance, for example. Nor is it clear whether the code provision prohibits any use of a veterinarian's name in the sign or letterhead of his boarding kennel or forbids only the inclusion of the doctor's name in that of the boarding facility.

This section of the code appears intended to assist practitioners who operate boarding kennels to maintain a professional image, and this purpose is made explicit in the section dealing with boarding kennels in the proposed 1988 revision of the *Principles* (26). However, the code (in its current and proposed versions) does not appear to prohibit a doctor from indicating his connection with his boarding kennel, or the fact that boarding is available at his hospital, together with the telephone number, address, name, or directory listings of his *veterinary facility*. The code does not explain why a professional image would be undercut if a boarding kennel includes in its name its connection with its veterinarian-owner, but would not be undercut if a doctor's veterinary facility includes the name of the boarding kennel in that of his hospital.

Certain ways of associating a doctor's name with a boarding facility will detract from a professional image. Inclusion of the veterinarian's name in that of his kennel, *or* the name of his kennel in that of his hospital (as in "Dr. Jones' Boarding Kennel," or "The Jones Animal Hospital and Boarding Kennel"), will lead some people to doubt whether a doctor's paramount priority is really veterinary medicine. Similar doubts might also be fostered by certain telephone responses, such as a routine question by a receptionist to all callers asking whether they are phoning for veterinary services or boarding. I would also argue that a professional image is undercut by advertisements (including those in the yellow pages) that make excessively prominent mention of the fact that a doctor owns a kennel or offers boarding in his hospital.

However, there are dignified and professional ways of informing the public of the connection between a practitioner and his boarding facility that do not imply that veterinary medicine is not the doctor's paramount concern. For example, the letterhead and client invoices of the hospital might include a statement (perhaps in smaller print than the rest) to the effect that boarding is provided. Likewise, the letterhead and invoices of the kennel could state unobtrusively that the facility is owned and operated by Dr. Jones, who provides continuing veterinary supervision.

The *Principles* allow a veterinarian to operate a boarding facility in his hospital or elsewhere. If clients do not know of the connection between a doctor and his kennel, prohibiting him from making *any* mention of his name or that of his hospital together with that of the kennel will deprive some clients of information they might want. If clients do know of the connection, such a prohibition is pointless. Nor is such a prohibition necessary for the preservation of the image of veterinarians as first and foremost, medical professionals.

REFERENCES

1. Knowles RP: Merchandising in Veterinary Medicine. *Trends* 2(3):49-50, 1986.
2. See, e.g. Clark R: *The Best of Ross Clark on Practice Management.* Lenexia, KS: Veterinary Medicine Publishing Co., 1985, p 75 (listing "fly repellents, pet colognes, spot removers, medicated shampoos, vitamins, coat conditioners, and chew bones," and stating that "most of these products are health-related and not only help improve our income but help provide a one-stop service for the client as well").
3. "Dispensing Versus Merchandising." *1988 AVMA Directory*, p 475.
4. *Principles of Veterinary Medical Ethics*, proposed 1988 rev. "Dispensing, Marketing, and Merchandising." AVMA 1988 Annual Convention Delegates' Agenda. Schaumburg, IL: American Veterinary Medical Association, 1988, p 17t.
5. Lofflin J: Use Marketing Leverage to Lift Your Bottom Line. *Veterinary Economics* Oct 1986:89-94.
6. "Dispensing Versus Merchandising." *1988 AVMA Directory*, p 475.
7. "Commissions, Rebates, or Kickbacks." *1988 AVMA Directory*, p 475.
8. E.g., Walterscheid E: Retail Displays Pump New Life Into Practice Income. *Veterinary Economics* Feb 1987:36-48; Shouse D: Making the Move to Merchandise. *Veterinary Economics* Jul 1988:46-56.
9. Wise JK: 1985 US veterinary practice income, expenses, and financial ratios. *J Am Vet Med Assoc* 190:1594-1598, 1987.
10. Shomer, RR: Letter. Is there a doctor in the house – or a salesperson in the store? *J Am Vet Med Assoc* 190:245, 1987.
11. Miller RM: Don't Tarnish the Image. *Veterinary Economics* Mar 1986:88.
12. Walterscheid E: Retail Displays Pump New Life Into Practice Income. *Veterinary Economics* Feb 1987:46.
13. Levy JC: Merchandising in Veterinary Medicine: Another View. *Trends* 2(5):52, 1986.
14. *Id.*
15. Dunn TJ: Alternatives to Economic Suicide. *Veterinary Economics* Mar 1987:124.
16. Dunn TJ: Alternatives to Economic Suicide. *Veterinary Economics* Mar 1987:124; Gragg C: Those Who Merchandise Will Survive. *Veterinary Economics* Feb 1987:43.
17. Wise JK: US market for food animal veterinary medical services. *J Am Vet Med Assoc* 190:1532-1533, 1987.
18. *Id.*, 1532.
19. *Principles of Veterinary Medical Ethics.* 1985 rev. "Displays in Waiting Rooms." *1986 AVMA Directory*, p 454.
20. AVMA Says OK to Product Displays and Merchandising. *Veterinary Economics* Sept 1986:11.
21. Displays and Reciprocity Emerge as Key House Issues. *J Am Vet Med Assoc* 191:625, 1987; *Principles of Veterinary Medical Ethics.* 1987 rev. "Displays in Waiting Rooms." *1988 AVMA Directory*, p 476.

22. Sollars M: Editorial. *Veterinary Economics* Feb 1987:1.
23. Clark R: Practice Management Q&A. *Veterinary Economics* Sept 1986:42.
24. Clark R: *The Best of Ross Clark on Practice Management.* Lenexia, KS: Veterinary Medicine Publishing Co., 1985, pp 85-86.
25. "Boarding Kennels." *1988 AVMA Directory*, p 476. The proposed 1988 revision of the *Principles* would clarify some of the ambiguities in this section. For example, the proposed provision states that a boarding facility "should be separated from the veterinarian's practice either physically or by appropriate identification." "Distinguishing Commercial Enterprises from Veterinary Practices." AVMA 1988 Annual Convention Delegates' Agenda. Schaumburg, IL: American Veterinary Medical Association, 1988, p 17p.
26. *Principles of Veterinary Medical Ethics*, proposed 1988 rev. "Distinguishing Commercial Enterprises from Veterinary Practices." AVMA 1988 Annual Convention Delegates' Agenda. Schaumburg, IL: American Veterinary Medical Association, 1988, p 17p.

Chapter

——— 17 ———

Promotion and Marketing

WHAT IS PROMOTION AND MARKETING?

In this text I shall use the terms "promotion" and "marketing" interchangeably, to refer to the activity of urging people to purchase one's services or products. Some people might object to this definition. They might, for example, want to reserve "marketing" for selling techniques, such as advertising, directed at large numbers of people (i.e., at "the market"). Others might be offended by any application of the word "marketing" to veterinarians, on the grounds that the term has connotations of commercialism and manipulation. I am as opposed to unprofessional commercialism in veterinary practice as anyone. However, it is more important to determine what kinds of sales techniques are morally acceptable than to spend a great deal of time passing judgment on terminology – especially because the word "marketing" has already gained acceptance within the profession.

Many different kinds of marketing can be employed by veterinarians. Some, which can be called "internal," take place within the practitioner's office or during direct contact between veterinarian and client. Other marketing techniques can be termed "external" in the sense that they are directed toward clients or other members of the public when these persons are not in the doctor's facility. Marketing by veterinarians can be aimed at a wide range of audiences, including potential new clients, current clients, former clients, the public at large, and other veterinarians. The goals of marketing can be specific (e.g., to remind clients to bring their dogs in for a heartworm test) or extremely general (e.g., to educate the public about the benefits of good veterinary care.) Marketing can be undertaken by individual doctors for their own practices, and by veterinary associations for their members or for veterinarians in general. Veterinarians can also participate in promotional campaigns of nonveterinarians, such as pet food companies.

There are many different ways of promoting one's practice, ranging from overt appeals for business in advertisements, to more subtle statements in one's letterhead, newsletter, or announcements of new staff. Indeed, virtually any contact between a practice and the public (including the manner in which the receptionist handles clients and how employees speak about the practice to others) can afford opportunities for promotion (1). As the profession becomes more interested in marketing, creative and hitherto undreamed-of promotional techniques can be expected to surface. Some of these might prove to be morally objectionable. This discussion will not attempt to address the ethical implications of all current and potential marketing techniques, but

160

will focus on several that have recently aroused interest or controversy in the profession.

CAN MARKETING BE PROFESSIONAL?

One of the general themes of this text is that veterinarians will benefit themselves, their clients, and their patients by not viewing monetary gain as the overriding aim of their professional lives. Monetary reward is important. But a veterinarian should, I have urged, try to earn a decent living *through* practicing in a dignified and professional manner, and should not view practice as primarily the road toward an income.

There is no doubt that almost any marketing technique can be used for commercialistic and unprofessional ends. Moreover, as we shall see, some techniques are so undignified, dishonest, or predatory that they must be considered inherently unethical. It is also clearly the case that many veterinarians are becoming increasingly interested in marketing because they want to maintain or increase practice income.

However, it does not follow from any of these things that all marketing is necessarily unprofessional. Certain promotional techniques can be used out of a sincere desire to convince clients to take advantage of veterinary services because these services are medically beneficial.

THREE GUIDEPOSTS FOR PROFESSIONAL MARKETING

Each proposed marketing technique must be considered in its own right with due attention to how it might affect the legitimate interests of patients, clients, practitioners, and others. Nevertheless, I want to suggest three general requirements that any marketing technique must meet if it is to be professional.

Dignity and Tastefulness

First, a marketing technique must exhibit the dignity and tastefulness that is expected of a member of a medical profession. Such things as singing radio commercials, flashing or neon practice signs, and client drawings for free puppies clearly do not accord with the conservative behavior people expect of a professional who deals with matters of health and illness. It might not always be easy to decide whether a certain kind of marketing approach meets the requirement of dignity and tastefulness. Indeed, attempting to make such decisions might sometimes involve defining the boundaries of what we mean by the terms "dignity" and "taste." But few veterinarians dispute that marketing must be dignified and tasteful, even if they might sometimes disagree about what this means in practice.

Honesty and Respect for the Client

As the discussion of the merchandising of nonprofessional products emphasized, one objectionable feature of the commercialization of veterinary practice is its tendency to manipulate clients. Treating clients as autonomous decision-makers requires honesty toward them and respect for their ability to decide for themselves (see Chapter 13). This requirement is especially important in the case of veterinary marketing. Many clients have a soft spot in their hearts for their animals and understand that veterinarians know a great deal more about animal health than they do. They are therefore likely to believe whatever a veterinarian says. An advertisement claiming that Dr. X is a specialist, when in fact he is not board-certified, can induce clients to make a choice they might not otherwise make. A newsletter that ominously threatens the demise of clients' cats if they are not brought in immediately for leukemia vaccinations puts undue (and dishonest) pressure on clients. Our society is accustomed to marketing techniques that shade the truth and exaggerate the importance of goods and services. If veterinary marketing is to remain professional, it must avoid such tendencies.

Fairness to Fellow Practitioners

Promotion can affect not only clients but other veterinarians as well. An advertisement or telephone directory announcement stating that Dr. Y has "the most modern facilities anywhere" is doubtless directed at potential clients. But it appeals to clients by making an explicit or implicit claim about *other doctors*. If such a statement is false or misleading, it can treat the public unfairly by depriving it of important correct information. It can also be unfair to other veterinarians by making statements about them that they are unable to contest.

Marketing can place pressure on doctors even when it is not intended consciously to draw clients away from other veterinarians. For example, some practices distribute their own client leaflets on medical topics. With the advent of computerized "desk-top publishing," such offerings can look professionally printed. A doctor who produces such brochures might have no intention of belittling other veterinarians. Nevertheless, clients who visit neighboring facilities might wonder whether these doctors are as up-to-date as the veterinarian with the fancy leaflets.

No veterinarian can claim a lucrative client base as a moral or legal right. However, if veterinary marketing turns doctors against each other, forces them to expend resources that would otherwise be devoted to the improvement of skills and facilities, and makes flashy promotion more appealing to the public than good medicine, many good veterinarians, clients, and animals will suffer. Determining the proper balance between a doctor's right to promote himself and the interest all veterinarians have in practicing a profession in which promotion must always remain secondary to medicine, is one of the most challenging tasks faced by normative veterinary ethics.

INTERNAL PROMOTIONAL TECHNIQUES

Good Medicine

Good, thorough medicine may well be the most profitable – and is certainly the most dignified – marketing tool available to veterinarians. There is an enormous range of professional services that veterinarians can recommend because they constitute good medicine. Dr. Robert Knowles offers the following examples of procedures that can be suggested to caring pet owners: laboratory examination before each surgery; electrocardiography on all aged surgical patients; pre- and postoperative radiographs on all orthopedic patients; chest radiographs on all aged surgical patients; tracheal wash and cytology on all chronic coughers; rabies vaccinations and FeLV tests and vaccine for cats; vigorous promotion of heartworm prevention; and annual physical examinations (2). Dentistry is another service that is being recognized as a significant source of additional practice revenue (3).

The following thoughts of Dr. Knowles are more valuable than any extended dissertation on good medicine as a marketing tool:

> Be pleasant, friendly, genuinely interested in your client, your patient, and their problems. Offer high-quality veterinary medicine, encourage your clients to accept the care that their pets should have. Don't do so timidly, but boldly and with confidence that this is what is needed and confidence that your client WILL accept that care you offer. You will far outstrip the merchandiser and have a meaningful measure of pride in the doing (4).

Display of Professional Products

Many veterinarians display professional products such as prescription diets and certain flea preparations. Although it is true that physicians do not display professional products, most physicians do not sell drugs or other medical items. In this regard, veterinarians are more like pharmacists, many of whom do place part of their stock of drugs in public view.

Displaying professional products (including some veterinary drugs) need not be undignified or unprofessional. A tasteful display can inform clients about items the doctor can recommend should the need arise. It can also educate clients about the fact that today's veterinarian has at his disposal a scientifically sophisticated armamentarium of drugs and medical products.

It is negligent and unethical for a veterinarian to relinquish to a client the decision of whether a medical product will be recommended. The *doctor* must suggest medical goods and services, and he must do so only when he believes they are medically indicated. Therefore, a display of professional items should *never* be used to encourage or induce clients to purchase specific displayed products. Clients certainly may be permitted to ask whether a displayed item would help their animal, and they may ask general questions about a displayed item. But if a doctor is going to recommend a displayed item, he must do so only for medical reasons, irrespective of whether it is displayed and whether the display has caught the client's attention.

Informational Brochures and Leaflets

Some veterinarians provide clients with brochures that contain information about certain diseases, conditions, and treatments. These publications range from professionally printed booklets with color illustrations to one-page photocopied handouts. They are sometimes devoted solely to medical matters, but might also contain information about the practice and its services. They can be produced by or for individual doctors, or by veterinary associations. There are also booklets printed by nonveterinary enterprises (such as pet food companies) that contain advertisements for these companies' products.

Informational brochures, like displays of professional items, can enhance clients' image of their veterinarian and of the profession as a whole. This, in turn, can assist doctors in convincing clients to accept their recommendations for medically indicated services or products. Brochures can also help clients to make their own informed and voluntary decisions by providing them with explanations of medical problems and suggested treatments. Thus, client brochures have an enormous potential in benefiting the interests of patients, clients, and veterinarians.

There are, however, potential dangers. As is the case with the display of professional items, brochures should never be used to urge clients to ask for something only a veterinarian should recommend. Dr. Mary Beth Leininger notes (5) that many clients are especially impressed by printed documents; they tend to believe that if something is in writing, it must be so. Doctors must therefore be careful not to use written material that is untruthful or that tries to influence clients other than by an appeal to rational argument. Entitling a client handout "Do You Want *Your* Dog to Survive This Year's Heartworm Epidemic?" would be an example of an unacceptable appeal to client fear and insecurity.

One ethical issue raised by client brochures concerns publications produced by commercial enterprises that contain advertisements for or references to these companies' products. (Some of these publications feature discount coupons, which clients can take directly to their local supermarket or pet supply store.) Such publications might enable a doctor who does not have a large promotional budget to provide informational pamphlets to clients. The problems, of course, come from the impression that such publications will undoubtedly give some clients. Some may think that the doctor endorses this particular brand when in fact he might not. Moreover, whether or not a doctor endorses the brand that supplies his booklets, he becomes part of a third party's promotional campaign for a commercial product. He leaves his role as a healer and becomes an advertiser.

The AVMA *Principles* correctly observe that "participation by veterinarians in coupon redemption schemes may be regarded as endorsement of or testimonial for a commercial product and is unprofessional" (6). Providing booklets with advertisements and coupons for commercial products is no less susceptible of being interpreted as an endorsement. Doctors who want to distribute informational material should find that the client brochures prepared by the AVMA, or their own photocopied handouts, do the job quite well and are appreciated by clients.

EXTERNAL MARKETING TECHNIQUES

Practice Names

Often, the first contact a potential client has with a practice is seeing or hearing its name. The AVMA has attempted to avoid confusion and prevent abuse of practice designations through its "Guidelines for Naming of Veterinary Facilities" (7). The Guidelines define such terms as "Animal Medical Center," "Hospital," "Clinic," "Office," and "Mobile Facility." For example, an animal medical center is "a facility in which consultative, clinical, and hospital services are rendered and in which a large staff of basic and applied veterinary scientists perform significant research and conduct advanced professional educational programs." A hospital is "a facility in which the practice conducted includes the confinement as well as the treatment of patients."

The AVMA definitions seem useful in preventing misleading practice designations. However, there are probably so many possible ways of abusing practice names that a complete set of guidelines would be unfeasible. Among the kinds of designations not mentioned by the AVMA that might sometimes mislead the public are the following: those that couple the name of the region of the country or state with a term like "animal medical center;" use of the name of a neighboring college or university in the practice designation when it has no connection with the educational institution; and practice designations that imply the facility provides better care than others.

Signs

The 1940 AVMA *Code of Ethics* stated that "display signs of reasonable size and dimensions on veterinary hospitals are not regarded as objectionable, provided that they do not announce special services, such as bathing, plucking, clipping, x-ray work, etc., which characterize the ways of the charlatan" (8). The current code does not include a section on signs, but the matter of signs does seem worthy of some consideration. Many practices are located in commercial districts in which businesses normally vie for attention by confronting the public with large, and sometimes extremely ugly and distracting signs. A veterinarian might feel compelled to erect a conspicuous sign or billboard so that his facility does not get lost in the morass.

Even when it is located in a commercial district, a veterinary hospital, clinic, or office is still a *medical* facility. Practice signs must therefore be of a reasonable size. They should avoid style or content that is demeaning to a medical professional, such as garish colors, flashing or neon lights, juvenile animal caricatures, commercialistic slogans, and insipid spelling or diction (e.g., "We care 4 pets"). Signs should also avoid making statements that are themselves unethical, for example, that the hospital provides better veterinary care than others in the area.

Newsletters

Perhaps the most exciting recent development in veterinary marketing is the advent of practice newsletters (9). Newsletters afford doctors the opportunity to reach clients in a dignified manner with information that will assist them in making informed decisions about veterinary care. Newsletters can avoid the appearance of commercialism so often associated with advertisements in the print or broadcast media, for, unlike the latter, newsletters need not be presented alongside of usual commercial appeals for consumer products. Moreover, newsletters that are targeted to current clients are less likely to be seen by other doctors as an attempt to steal away *their* clients.

Because the distribution of newsletters is still an emerging area of veterinary marketing, it is premature to attempt to set forth specific ethical guidelines concerning them. However, one might keep in mind the three general requirements of all marketing: dignity and tastefulness; honesty and respect for clients; and fairness to other doctors. Dignity includes treating medical matters with seriousness (though not necessarily without some humor); informing clients about available services, office hours, and clinicians without making blatant appeals for business; and not bombarding clients with so many newsletters that they will believe they are being hustled rather than informed. Honesty and respect for clients includes not attempting to influence them with sensationalistic language that frightens them or with scientific prose they cannot understand. Fairness to other doctors means, in part, that a newsletter should attempt to inform clients about medical issues and the opportunities their doctor provides for addressing them – and should not be a disguised attempt to compare one's own virtues with alleged shortcomings of other practitioners.

As is the case with client brochures, newsletters should avoid giving the impression that the doctor is endorsing nonmedical products. Likewise, newsletters should not be produced by commercial firms in return for inclusion of advertisements for their products, nor should commercial advertising be accepted in order to defray publication costs. (Including an announcement of a nonprofit organization, such as a humane society animal adoption service, need not be undignified or improper.)

Because much of a newsletter's impact depends on its appearance, design components such as titles and artwork should be dignified and tasteful. The entire production should reflect the doctor's sincere desire to provide truthful and useful information.

Reminders and Sympathy Cards

If newsletters are an appropriate means of informing and reminding clients of a doctor's services, so are direct mailings to clients reminding them that their animals are due for tests, vaccinations, scheduled visits, and routine physical exams. Nor does it seem particularly undignified to send a reasonable number of additional reminders to follow up an initial mailing.

Some practitioners send sympathy cards to clients after the death of an animal. Although such mailings might in fact improve clients' image of their veterinarian, *sympathy cards should not be considered a marketing tool* and should never be sent with the intention of promoting the practice. The death of a beloved animal is simply too sensitive and intimate a matter to be used as an opportunity for promotion. Indeed, to avoid the possibility of misinterpretation, it is important that sympathy cards not even give the appearance of having a promotional aim. Thus, while the signature or the name of the doctor would be appropriate for such a message, such things as the hospital's office hours or a list of its services are not.

Discounts and Giveaways

Some veterinarians offer discounts on services to attract new clients and to motivate current clients to bring in their animals. Clients can be given a volume discount, i.e., they can be charged a certain percent less than the normal fee for each animal if they bring in more than one during a visit. Or, a doctor can offer a discount off his regular fee; this can be done, for example, for new clients only, or for all clients who bring in a specified species of animal, or for clients who bring in their animals during a specified time period. A variant of discounting is offering a "free" service or product with the payment of the usual fee for some service. Offering discounts or giveaways is usually a means of getting someone into one's practice. Discounts are therefore typically offered in public advertisements, although they can be presented in client newsletters or in redemption coupons distributed in such places as pet stores and grooming parlors.

As I have argued, it is in the interest of veterinarians, clients, and their animals that veterinary patients be viewed as important beings entitled to first-class, dignified medical care. Such a perception is undercut by discounts. We would be revolted by a pediatrician who offered a discount for each additional child brought to the office. ("One baby, $30, two for $55, three for $80.") We would say that such a marketing technique cheapens the patient. Veterinary discounts analogize veterinary patients not to human medical or dental patients but to such commodities as tires, cans of motor oil, and lawnmowers, for which volume or seasonal discounts are commonplace. By cheapening the patient, discounts also cheapen the image of the veterinarian.

It is difficult to believe that there are many clients who would pay, say, $15 for an examination for one cat but would bring in a second only if its exam cost $2 or $3 less. Moreover, there are more dignified ways of allowing clients to pay less than one's usual fee and thereby to encourage them to obtain care for their animals. One can reduce one's fee, not as a discount, but as a special accommodation to a client in need. Certain basic services such as heartworm tests or vaccinations may be offered for a lower fee than is charged for extensive examinations. Like medical health maintenance organizations, one can offer prepayment plans encompassing a range of services that, if paid for individually, would cost clients more. Some doctors, for example, offer prepaid puppy and kitten packages that include several examinations and vaccinations (10). Participation in a pet insurance program can also translate into reduced cost per visit for clients.

Veterinarians should not assume that the public will accept discounts and giveaways. One doctor mailed coupons offering a free flea collar or canister of flea powder to clients who would bring in their cats for routine vaccinations and a fecal test. The coupons were sent to 10,000 households. There was one response. Interestingly, the doctor interpreted the results as an indication of "the reluctant feline client" (11).

In 1987, a provision was added to the *Principles of Veterinary Medical Ethics* prohibiting the advertising of discounts and discounted fees (12). In 1988, the Judicial Council decided to approve a limited exception to this rule: the advertising of services for senior citizens in so-called "Silver" or "Golden" telephone directories would be permitted, provided such advertisements do not make any reference to a discounted price. (A statement reflecting this decision was placed into the proposed 1988 revision of the *Principles*.) The Judicial Council maintained that permitting such advertisements would represent a commitment to "social responsibility" and would bring the profession public relations benefits (13).

It is not clear why a provision that is inconsistent with the prohibition against the advertising of discounts is necessary to enable veterinarians to assist senior citizens who might be in need of special consideration. (For whatever it is or is not called, a service that is advertised in so-called "Silver" or "Golden" pages is still a discounted service, and everybody knows this.) It would be preferable to place in the *Principles* the statement that veterinarians are always encouraged to make accommodations for clients with special needs, including certain senior citizens (14). Such a statement would show a more generalized sensitivity to social responsibility. Nor would such a statement carry the implication (which, I would argue, is highly objectionable), that all people who are over a certain age need, or deserve, economic assistance from their veterinarian.

Advertising

The AVMA *Principles* define "advertising" as "newspaper, magazine, and periodical announcements; professional cards, professional announcement cards; office and other signs; letterheads; telephone and other directory listings; and any other form of communication designed to inform the general public about the availability, nature, or prices of products or services or to attract clients" (15). This definition is extremely broad and includes several marketing tools (such as simple telephone listings, letterheads, and business cards) most people would usually not include within that term. There is, however, an important point to such a definition. It draws attention to the fact that veterinarians who market their practices to the public can be doing much the same thing whether or not we would, strictly speaking, call their promotions "advertisements." The broad definition also enables the *Principles* to set forth guidelines applicable to a wide range of marketing techniques.

THE LEGAL SITUATION

In 1977, the United States Supreme Court struck down as violative of the First Amendment to the Constitution, a total ban on advertising of prices imposed upon attorneys by a state bar association that all lawyers in the state were required to join

(16). This decision is frequently misinterpreted as standing for the proposition that veterinarians and other professionals have a legal right to use "established marketing and advertising techniques" (17).

In fact, although the Supreme Court did hold that restrictions on certain kinds of professional advertising violate the Constitutional protection of freedom of speech, the Court did not give professionals a blank check to use any advertising technique acceptable in the commercial world. The Court held that false and misleading advertising by professionals could be banned either by state boards of registration or professional associations. It left open the possibility of restricting in-person solicitation and advertising claims about the quality of services. The Court speculated that it might be proper for government and professional associations to regulate the time, place, and manner of professional advertising. The Court also warned that "the special problems of advertising on the electric broadcast media will warrant special consideration" (18). The Court made it clear that government and professional associations have a legitimate, though limited, role in the enforcement of ethical standards regarding advertising by professionals.

In recent years, the Supreme Court has increasingly emphasized false, deceptive, and misleading advertising as legitimate targets of state and professional association regulation. In one decision, the Court stated that commercial speech that "is *not* false or deceptive and does not concern unlawful activities ... may be restricted only in the service of a *substantial* governmental interest, and only through means that directly advance that interest" (19). One example of potentially truthful advertising the Court still considers open to regulation is in-person solicitation by lawyers (20). However, the Court has cast doubt on whether it would allow government authorities or professional associations to regulate advertising by professionals that is undignified or tasteless if such advertising is in fact truthful (21).

THE AVMA RESPONSE

The AVMA response to the 1977 Supreme Court decision was to place in the *Principles* its "Advertising Regulations" (22). The section is in my view among the best in the code. It attempts to articulate important, and sometimes quite specific, legally enforceable moral standards. Among the practices prohibited by the Advertising Regulations are the following: guarantees of cures or results; testimonials for commercial nonveterinary products; paid advertisements or solicitations designed so as to hide their promotional character; statements of quality of services not susceptible to verification by the public; words stating or implying that a doctor who is not board-certified is a specialist; false and misleading claims; and statements about the price of services that do not include disclosure of relevant factors that would affect advertised fees.

ADVERTISING IN THE PRINT AND BROADCAST MEDIA

I have found that some practitioners and clients feel comfortable about modest advertisements in newspapers or magazines but object to veterinary advertising on radio or television. Perhaps because broadcast advertising is usually expensive, it has not yet become a major issue among veterinarians. There has, however, been no shortage of undignified newspaper advertisements. A typical tasteless veterinary advertisement might include multiple coupons for various services. The coupons might offer discounts (e.g., $1.00 off a cat spay) that an unsuspecting client might not know are minuscule. The coupons might also contain tiny expiration dates, so that the public knows they must be redeemed before it is too late, just like supermarket coupons for laundry detergent. There might be an offer of a package deal for a series of related services - with a large "X" drawn through the usual price total, and a new, much lower amount emblazoned in enormous type. The advertisement might be further decorated with a cartoon of one or more animals reminding the reader about the great savings to be had.

The Advertising Regulations of the *Principles* do address some of the offensive features of such advertisements. However, the Regulations are restricted to prohibiting unacceptable substantive claims and offers and do not address what is often the most important problem with advertisements: their disregard for style and taste. One task that normative veterinary ethics can usefully undertake is an exploration of appropriate standards of taste for advertisements in the print and broadcast media. Such an exploration is not prohibited by the fact that federal law might prevent *enforcement* of such standards by state veterinary boards or professional associations. Professionals can still try to be dignified in their communications with the public, even if they can no longer be compelled to be so.

YELLOW PAGES ADVERTISEMENTS

Advertisements in yellow pages telephone directories can present many of the same kinds of ethical problems as do other promotional techniques. There are yellow pages advertisements that, for example, claim a doctor specializes in an area not yet recognized as a specialty by the profession (e.g., "Specialist in Behavioral Disorders"); that use impressive but undefined terms ("A Full-Service Veterinary Hospital"); that falsely imply a facility is the only one of its kind in the area ("Podunk's Full-Service Animal Hospital"); that falsely imply a hospital has features not possessed by others in the area ("A Hospital with Surgical Facilities on the Premises"); that violate the *Principles* by not only using the doctor's name for a boarding facility, but giving each equal prominence ("Dr. Jones' Veterinary Hospital and Kennel"); or that make or imply a claim of higher quality service not susceptible to verification by the public ("High Quality Facilities to Serve You Better"). Some advertisements also now appear in red - an adaptation of the flashing or neon sign to the print medium.

Yellow pages advertisements can be truthful and dignified. They can state, for example, the name of the facility, its staff members, hours of operation, location, and emergency services.

However, there appears to be an inherent drive within the medium toward exaggeration and tastelessness. Unlike other forms of advertising, the yellow pages impose severe pressures upon doctors to advertise. Doctors know that the yellow pages are usually consulted by people who are looking for a veterinarian. If a doctor is not listed, he will have no chance of obtaining the patronage of such people. Many doctors rightly wonder whether a basic listing of name, location, and telephone number is sufficient, for to most people, one veterinarian's name will mean no more than another. Most people probably are attracted to a listing that contains more information. Many undoubtedly will be attracted to the largest advertisement for a practice in their locality.

Thus, a distinct burden is placed on veterinarians to place a full-blown advertisement (as opposed to a simple listing of name, address, and telephone number) in the yellow pages. And the larger or flashier the advertisements of competing doctors, the more pressure there will be to place an advertisement at least as conspicuous as those of one's competitors. To distinguish himself from others, a doctor may feel compelled to do what ordinary commercial advertisers do to attract attention to their messages – puff and puff again until the truth is stretched beyond recognition.

To their credit, many veterinarians have managed to resist the tide of exaggerated and undignified listings. But for some, the yellow pages war is like a mini-nuclear arms race. Once they have begun placing large and flashy advertisements, it can become impossible to stop, as they feel compelled to outdo each other for their own survival. (I invite anyone skeptical about this characterization to compare the last several years of veterinarian yellow pages listings for his area. One will probably find a steady increase in the number of full-blown advertisements, their size, use of color, and the number of exaggerated and misleading claims.) Who loses as a result? The public, which is subjected to misleading claims. And honest doctors, who can lose clients and suffer the consequences of a diminished image of the profession.

It is not clear precisely how far state boards and professional associations may lawfully go in compelling adherence to standards governing yellow pages advertisements. Certainly, the courts would not uphold the requirement of the 1940 AVMA *Code of Ethics* that all veterinarian telephone directory listings have "identical visual prominence" (23). However, there is no legal impediment to the enforcement of current administrative and official prohibitions against false or misleading advertisements (24). Application of these prohibitions to the yellow pages might bring the added bonus of eliminating much of the tastelessness, because deceptiveness and tastelessness often seem to be found together.

SOLICITATION

Solicitation is advertising directed toward specific persons. Solicitation can be done through the mail. It can also be done by means of an oral or in-person communication with prospective clients by a veterinarian or someone hired by him to promote his practice.

The official codes of several of the professions view solicitation as inherently coercive, and therefore generally prohibit it outright. For example, the 1983 American Bar Association *Model Rules of Professional Conduct* state (25) that "a lawyer may not solicit professional employment from a prospective client with whom the lawyer has no family or prior professional relationship by mail, in person, or otherwise, when a motive for the lawyer's doing so is the lawyer's pecuniary gain." As the ABA *Rules* explain, a person who is solicited

> often feels overwhelmed by the situation giving rise to the need for legal services, and may have an impaired capacity for reason, judgment and protective self-interest. Furthermore, the lawyer seeking the retainer is faced with a conflict stemming from the lawyer's own interest, which may color the advice and representation offered the vulnerable prospect.

These arguments seem no less relevant to solicitation by veterinarians, especially when the practitioner making a solicitation knows that the potential client has an animal in need of treatment. Moreover, direct solicitation will sometimes involve trying to win over people who are satisfied with their current veterinarian. It is unclear how the peace of mind of such people, and the good names of other doctors, will survive a solicitor's message that clients will be happy with *his* services.

The AVMA *Principles* (26) take a relatively permissive attitude toward solicitation. Written solicitation is deemed to be "permissible provided it does not exert undue influence, pressure for immediate response, intimidation, or overreaching." Oral or in-person solicitation is "undesirable," i.e., it is not prohibited but is nevertheless disfavored, because it cannot be examined by a regulatory body as can a written solicitation.

Practitioners who are disposed to engage in solicitation are not likely to admit that *their* solicitations exert undue influence or pressure. Indeed, the position of the *Principles* that written solicitation is permissible unless it exerts undue influence or pressure or is false and misleading, appears to set up a *presumption* that such solicitation is acceptable, unless proven otherwise. As the ABA code recognizes, solicitation tends by its nature to exert undue influence. If solicitation must be permitted under certain circumstances, it would be far better to presume that any kind of solicitation exerts undue influence, unless the solicitor can prove otherwise.

One kind of situation in which the solicitation of a client by a veterinarian can be morally permissible is that in which a practitioner happens *unintentionally* upon an animal that requires *immediate* medical care. Here, the animal's need for treatment would appear to outweigh the potential dangers of manipulation inherent in solicitation. However, even in such a situation, the interests of the animal owner would argue strongly in favor of the doctor encouraging the owner to seek continuing or follow-up care from his own regular veterinarian.

THE VETERINARIAN AS A PROMOTER FOR OTHERS

Free Supplies and Waiting Room Advertisements

It is not uncommon for veterinarians to permit for-profit businesses to use the veterinary office to market their products or services, even if doing so provides no direct economic benefit to the practice. This can be done by displaying free supplies (such as puppy food or grooming supplies), or by permitting businesses to place advertisements or brochures in the waiting room.

A doctor who permits such third-party marketing might be motivated by a sincere desire to assist his clients. However, turning one's office into a billboard for businesses raises the same ethical problems as does distributing brochures containing advertisements for nonmedical products. It gives the impression that the doctor is endorsing products generally and without the need to tailor a recommendation to the particular patient. It also makes the veterinary office an arm of the promotional activities of a nonveterinary business.

Nothing prevents a doctor from, on occasion, recommending a puppy food, pet photographer, grooming parlor, or pet-sitting service to clients who ask his advice about such matters. Moreover, if a doctor believes that a certain product can be recommended on legitimate medical grounds for a particular patient, there seems nothing wrong in his giving the client a free sample of that product provided by the manufacturer. But imagine what one's reaction would be if one encountered in a pediatrician's office a display of free baby foods or brochures for a baby photographer. A veterinarian who permits similar third-party marketing in his practice need not, surely, be committing a heinous moral offense. However, he is undermining the image of the veterinary office as a *medical* facility as opposed to a general all-purpose animal advice and service center. As I have argued, this latter image is not in the long-term interests of patients, clients, or veterinarians.

Third-party Coupon Redemption Programs

A perennial issue relating to the ethics of marketing concerns third-party promotional campaigns, in which veterinarians participate not only with the purpose of marketing their own practices, but with the effect of promoting the business of someone else. Although the *Principles* unequivocally condemn participation in third-party coupon redemption programs (27), time and again, veterinarians have become mired in such schemes. Repeatedly, the result has been widespread aggravation and discord.

In a typical third-party promotion, a nonveterinary business will supply to animal owners a coupon or certificate entitling them to free or discounted services from a participating doctor. In order to obtain these coupons, owners must, of course, purchase the company's products. Coupon redemption schemes need not entail that the participating veterinarian be reimbursed by the company; the expected benefit to the doctor can be solely the entrance of a client into his facility.

As was noted in the discussion of informational brochures, coupon redemption programs are unprofessional because they tend to imply doctors' endorsement of commercial products, and because they turn veterinarians into an arm of a commercial enterprise interested in selling its own, nonmedical products for profit.

But these are not the only evils of coupon redemption schemes.

They can lead the public to make unnecessary and invidious comparisons among doctors. Those who choose not to participate must explain to clients why, and risk being perceived as greedy or unhelpful. Sometimes, certain doctors may not be permitted to participate. This occurred when the American Animal Hospital Association and 9 Lives® cat food announced a program entitling consumers to services at AAHA hospitals. The promotion led many non-AAHA doctors to complain that the public would think they were not as competent as AAHA members (28).

Coupon redemption schemes can also give the impression that the entire profession endorses a company's products. This happened in 1987, when the Friskies Pet Care Division of the Carnation Company announced a program in which purchase of its Friskies® brand foods would entitle consumers to a "free checkup" from a member of the AVMA. Many *veterinarians* thought there was endorsement of the campaign by the AVMA. The AVMA and the Company explained that there was no such endorsement, and Carnation agreed to send all AVMA members a letter stating that the AVMA was not a cosponsor of the program (29).

It is unrealistic for the profession to blame pet supply companies that want to use the good name of the veterinarian to promote their own products. These businesses undoubtedly do wish to promote good pet care. But they are not charitable institutions. They cannot be expected to market veterinary practices without some return for themselves. If anyone is to blame for misunderstandings or misinterpretations, it is the profession itself, for allowing its image to be associated with third-party promotional programs. There is only one appropriate response when companies attempt to garner explicit or implicit support for their promotions from veterinary associations – a clear and resounding *No!*

Testimonials and Endorsements

Veterinarians can also participate in promotional campaigns of businesses by giving testimonials for or endorsements of their products or services. There are three potential problems with such endorsements. First, they render veterinarians part of the promotional activities of commercial enterprises. This process can sometimes involve undignified, commercialistic behavior by someone who ought to be viewed as a healer or a friend (see Chapter 15). Such behavior can make it difficult for the profession to present itself as interested first and foremost in helping patients and clients. Second, some people might tend automatically to believe an endorsement by a veterinarian, especially if the doctor is well-known. Third, when a doctor is compensated for an endorsement or has some personal connection with the company using it, his words can be motivated more by self-interest than a desire to state the truth; the public will therefore want to know of the connection in order to evaluate the endorsement's credibility.

Two provisions of the *Principles* deal with testimonials and endorsements. Endorsements of nonveterinary (i.e., nonprofessional or nonmedical) goods or services are treated in the code's Advertising Regulations. These regulations prohibit any testimonial by a veterinarian for a nonveterinary product or service "to the extent that the testimonial or endorsement represents implicitly or explicitly that the endorser's knowledge as a veterinarian gives him or her expertise with respect to any feature of or characteristic of the nonveterinary product or service..." (30). A limited exception is made for endorsements on behalf of certain kinds of nonprofit organizations. Endorsements of nonveterinary items that appeal to the status or special expertise of the veterinarian are not prohibited on the grounds that they are inherently unprofessional. Rather, such endorsements are listed as one of 14 kinds of statements that are deemed by the code to constitute false, deceptive, or misleading advertising.

A separate section of the *Principles* (31) is devoted to testimonials for and endorsements of veterinary goods or services. Such endorsements (including claims that the endorser uses the product or has expertise regarding it) must be truthful and capable of substantiation. The veterinarian-endorser must also have the expertise he is represented to possess, and his endorsement must be backed by his actual use of the product and his own exercise of his expertise in evaluating it. Additionally, "where there exists a connection between the endorser and the seller of the advertised product which might materially affect the weight or credibility of the endorsement, such connection must be fully disclosed."

Given the recent trend of Supreme Court rulings emphasizing false, deceptive, and misleading advertising as appropriate targets of regulation by the professions, the code's attempt to regulate endorsements by demanding that they be true and capable of substantiation seems reasonable. Nevertheless, the code's treatment of endorsements of nonveterinary goods and services is significantly better, both from legal and moral standpoints, than its approach to endorsements of veterinary products. Testimonials for nonveterinary products by veterinarians are virtually eliminated. For it would be a rare advertisement indeed that will not utilize a veterinarian's endorsement of a nonveterinary product without attempting to state or imply that a *veterinarian* must have special expertise regarding the product. The code astutely places such endorsements in the legally approved category of the "false, deceptive, or misleading," by recognizing that there is nothing in a veterinarian's training or knowledge that could give him special expertise regarding a *nonveterinary* product or service.

The problem with the code's approach to the endorsement of veterinary products is that it appears to leave it entirely to an endorser and company to decide whether there is a significant danger that their connection might affect the endorsement's credibility. However, an endorser and advertiser will not easily find that there is such a danger if they believe (as many surely will) that disclosure of their connection will detract from the endorsement's effectiveness. One would have thought that *any* financial or personal connection between an endorser and advertiser is material to evaluating an endorsement's credibility and should therefore be disclosed. Ironically, this problem would have been corrected by the proposed 1988 revision of the *Principles* (see Chapter 9). The proposed new section on testimonials and endorsements for veterinary products (32) would add to present provisions a requirement that disclosure of the connection between the veterinarian-endorser and advertiser must always be made when the veterinarian has been solicited for the purpose of giving the endorsement, or when he is compensated either monetarily or with product. Additionally, the proposed new section would interpret "adequate substantiation" to imply the publication of a report regarding the endorsed item "in a journal wherein articles are subjected to peer review or in a publication recognized by reputation as a source of reliable scientific information." This requirement would apply the same standards of substantiation to veterinary products that the veterinary community itself demands regarding scientific claims about veterinary procedures. Such a requirement would provide a reasonable way of protecting the profession and the public against false, deceptive, or misleading claims about veterinary products. For if an advertiser is appealing to a veterinarian's expertise to sell an essentially medical product or service, that advertiser is, in effect, himself stating or implying that the veterinarian-endorser's statements meet the standards of credibility that veterinarians would apply to claims of a medical-scientific nature.

REFERENCES

1. Pace PE and Culbertson J: *Successful Public Relations for the Professions.* Edwardsville, KS: Professional Publishing Co., 1982, p 2-1.
2. Knowles RP: Merchandising in Veterinary Medicine. *Trends* 2(3):49-50, 1986.
3. Beale S: Add Dentistry To Your List of Services. *Veterinary Economics* Feb 1987: 64-73.
4. Knowles RP: Merchandising in Veterinary Medicine. *Trends* 2(3):50, 1986.
5. Quoted in Newsletters – Keep You in Touch With Your Clients. *J Am Vet Med Assoc* 190:957, 1987.
6. "Redemption Coupons." *1988 AVMA Directory*, p 477.
7. *1988 AVMA Directory*, p 485.
8. *Code of Ethics of the American Veterinary Medical Association.* "Advertising by Display Signs." *J Am Vet Med Assoc* 96:93, 1940.
9. See, e.g., Newsletters – Keep You in Touch With Your Clients. *J Am Vet Med Assoc* 190:955-958, 1987.
10. McBride J: Keep Your Clients Coming Back. *Veterinary Economics* Jul 86:44.
11. Lofflin J: Practice Growth Comes from Feline Favor. *Veterinary Economics* Mar 1986:68.
12. "Advertising Regulations." *1988 AVMA Directory*, p 476.
13. Judicial Council Revises Guidelines on Displays and Discount Advertising. *J Am Vet Med Assoc* 192:14, 1988.
14. See, e.g., *American Bar Association Model Rules of Professional Conduct*, Rule 6.1 (stating that each lawyer "should render public interest legal service" and may discharge this service by "providing professional services at no fee or a reduced fee for persons of limited means or to public service or charitable groups or organizations . . . and by financial support for organizations that provide legal service to persons of limited means"). In Morgan TD and Rotunda RD (eds): *Selected Standards on Professional Responsibility.* Mineola, NY: Foundation Press, 1985, p 150. This rule sets forth an ideal (see Chapter 5) that is not to be enforced through disciplinary proceedings.
15. "Advertising Regulations." *1988 AVMA Directory*, p 476.
16. Bates v. State Bar of Arizona, 433 U.S. 350 (1977).
17. McCurnin DM and Thompson A: Professional advertising. *J Am Vet Med Assoc* 188:1387, 1986.
18. Bates v. State Bar of Arizona, 433 U.S. at 384.
19. Zauderer v. Office of Disciplinary Counsel of the Supreme Court of Ohio, 105 S.Ct. 2265, 2275 (1985), emphasis supplied.

20. *Id.*, at 2277.
21. *Id.*, at 2280 (asserting that "although the State undoubtedly has a substantial interest in ensuring that its attorneys behave with dignity and decorum in the courtroom, we are unsure that the State's desire that attorneys maintain their dignity in their communications with the public is an interest substantial enough to justify the abridgement of the First Amendment rights").
22. *1988 AVMA Directory*, p 476.
23. *Code of Ethics of the American Veterinary Medical Association.* "Directory Advertisements." *J Am Vet Med Assoc* 96:93, 1940.
24. See, Legal Advertising as Perceived by the BEVM. *California Board of Examiners in Veterinary Medicine Newsletter.* Spring 1988:1 (announcing that California practitioners will be given 2 years to correct "illegal advertising in the yellow pages or any other advertising medium," including fraudulent or misleading price advertising or the use of "misleading phrases such as 'as low as,' 'and up,' 'lowest prices,' or any other inexact comparative expressions").
25. Ethical Rule 7.3. Direct Contact with Prospective Clients. *ABA Model Rules of Professional Conduct.* In Morgan TD and Rotunda RD (eds): *Selected Standards on Professional Responsibility.* Mineola, NY: Foundation Press, 1985, pp 156-157.
26. "Advertising Regulations." *1988 AVMA Directory*, p 476.
27. "Redemption Coupons." *1988 AVMA Directory*, p 477.
28. See, e.g., Shomer R: Letter. Objects to examination-coupon program. *J Am Vet Med Assoc* 182:852, 1983; Friedman J, Smith L, Farber A, and Menez G: Letter. Alleged discriminatory advertising. *J Am Vet Med Assoc* 182:1300, 1983.
29. No AVMA Sponsorship of Carnation's Free Checkup Program for Pets. *J Am Vet Med Assoc* 190:1087, 1987.
30. "Advertising Regulations." *1988 AVMA Directory*, p 476.
31. "Testimonials and Endorsements." *1988 AVMA Directory*, p 475.
32. *Principles of Veterinary Medical Ethics*, proposed 1988 rev. "Testimonials and Endorsements Relating to Veterinary Products, Services, and Equipment." AVMA 1988 Annual Convention Delegates' Agenda. Schaumburg, IL: American Veterinary Medical Association, 1988, pp 17j-17k.

18

Competition and Collegiality: The Strains of the Marketplace

One fact with significant implications for normative veterinary ethics is that many practitioners are uneasy about their ability to continue to earn a satisfactory living. Although mean gross practice incomes have increased substantially in recent years (1), veterinarians are in general not nearly as well-compensated as members of some other professions. In 1985, the mean pretax income of United States veterinarians in private practice was $48,056. Their median income was $37,730 (2). A 1985 AVMA Manpower Study predicted that the real incomes of private practitioners will have declined by 25% between 1980 and 2000 (3).

Doctors' concerns about their ability to earn an adequate income have contributed not just to a general interest in finding new ways of attracting revenue, such as merchandising and marketing, but also to questions about how practitioners can coexist with their colleagues in the marketplace. Issues regarding competition and relations among veterinarians can be expected to grow in number and intensity as perceived economic pressures on the profession increase.

LEGAL ASPECTS OF COMPETITION

The general issue of competition among veterinarians is fraught with legal dangers. A number of federal and state laws protect certain competitive practices and prohibit or restrict others. Some veterinarians have not been beyond suggesting solutions to ethical issues that could expose them to very serious legal troubles.

The Sherman Antitrust and Federal Trade Commission Acts

The most important laws affecting competition among veterinarians are the federal Sherman Antitrust Act and the Federal Trade Commission (FTC) Act.

The Sherman Act prohibits "(e)very contract, combination in the form of trust or otherwise, or conspiracy, in restraint of trade or commerce among the several States, or with foreign nations" (4). The Act also states that "(e)very person who shall monopolize, or attempt to monopolize or combine or conspire with any other person or persons, to monopolize any part of the trade or commerce among the several states, or with foreign nations shall be deemed guilty of a felony" (5). In addition to providing criminal penalties for violators, the statute permits private persons (such as veterinarians or veterinary clients) who are damaged by anticompetitive practices to sue violators (such as other veterinarians or veterinary associations), and to recover triple damages, court costs, and attorneys' fees. Consumers can also institute class action suits against violators.

The Federal Trade Commission Act provides that "(u)nfair methods of competition in or affecting commerce, and unfair or deceptive acts or practices in or affecting commerce, are declared unlawful" (6). This statute is enforced by the Federal Trade Commission. Although the FTC Act is technically not part of the antitrust laws, any conduct violating these laws will also constitute a violation of the FTC Act.

The FTC keeps a sharp eye on professional associations as well as state licensing boards. In its desire to promote freedom of competition, the Commission has not always exhibited sensitivity to the special problems the learned professions face regarding misleading and deceptive practices by members. Sometimes it issues legal interpretations that are at least open to debate. For example, the FTC recently commented on proposed changes in the regulations of the Virginia Board of Veterinary Medicine. The Commission applauded the withdrawal of certain restrictions upon truthful advertising, but criticized proposed regulations prohibiting claims of superiority and the use of solicitors to attract business (7). But, in fact, the United States Supreme Court has specifically recognized that claims of superiority and in-person solicitation by professionals pose special dangers and may therefore be prohibited by state licensing boards (8). It remains to be seen whether the FTC's inquiries about the *Principles of Veterinary Medical Ethics* (see Chapter 9) will reflect adherence by the Commission to its legal mandate, or overreaching into areas that a profession such as veterinary medicine should be permitted to regulate.

Antitrust and unfair trade law is complex and technical, and it is impossible to summarize it here. Basically, the purpose of this body of law is to prevent *unreasonable* restraints upon competition. The law does not provide an exhaustive list of illegal activities; among the anticompetitive practices it clearly forbids are organized boycotts against a selected enterprise in order to drive it out of the marketplace, and price-fixing.

Current debates about competition in the profession reveal a troublesome lack of concern about potential violations of antitrust law. For example, many who are urging the AVMA to put pressure on the veterinary schools to reduce enrollments in order to protect existing practitioners from competition seem oblivious to the fact that such campaigns might well violate antitrust and unfair competition laws. I have heard some veterinarians recommend that their local associations determine "acceptable" fees for spays and neuters to prevent "unfair" competition from certain doctors. Some doctors have not been beyond expressing the view that practitioners should refuse to accept referrals from mobile clinics "to run the s.o.b.'s out of town."

Serious attention to legal requirements is especially important in the area of competition because certain ways of making points are permissible. Antitrust law does not prohibit attempts to influence federal, state, or local government even when the basic objective of such attempts is anticompetitive, provided that government is not being used as a "cover" or "sham" to achieve protection from the antitrust laws (9). Thus, although concerted attempts to run mobile vans out of town to reduce competition would be unlawful, veterinarians may express to their state boards sincere and good-faith reservations about the ability of particular facilities to provide adequate care to certain kinds of patients.

State Antitrust and Unfair Trade Practices Acts

Many states have statutes that are modeled on federal antitrust laws. These state laws also prohibit businesses and professional people from engaging in anticompetitive and unfair trade practices, such as price-fixing. These statutes usually are enforced by the state attorney general. Because many states also prohibit anticompetitive behavior in their veterinary practice acts (see Chapter 7), it would not be difficult for a state veterinary board to refer a complaint of this nature directly to the attorney general for a full-scale investigation or prosecution.

State Civil Causes of Action

Veterinarians should also be cognizant of state laws that permit them to be sued (or to sue) for actions relating to competition. In many states, business and professional people may be sued for wrongful interference with a competitor's right to seek and retain customers. Among such civil causes of action are the following:

1. injurious falsehood: "the publication of matter derogatory to the plaintiff's title to his property, or its quality, or to his business in general, or even to some element of his personal affairs, of a kind calculated to prevent others from dealing with him, or otherwise to interfere with his relations with others to his disadvantage" (10);
2. interference with contractual relations: the intentional and improper interference with the performance of a commercial contract between another and a third person by the intentional inducement or causing of the third person not to perform the contract (11); and
3. intentional interference with prospective advantage: the deliberate attempt by wrongful means to prevent the plaintiff from carrying on his trade, including such tactics as harassment of the plaintiff's customers or employees; obstruction of the means of access to his place of business; threats of groundless suits; and inducing employees to commit sabotage or to undermine the plaintiff's business (12).

A veterinarian who makes false statements so harmful to the reputation of a competitor as to deter clients or colleagues from associating or dealing with him might also find himself sued for defamation of character (13).

SOME CURRENT CONTROVERSIES REGARDING COMPETITION

Competition from Humane Societies

One of the most bitter controversies regarding competition for veterinary clients concerns the operation of veterinary facilities by nonprofit humane societies. Because such organizations are tax-exempt, some are able to charge clients much less than private practitioners for the same services. A number of veterinarians have responded to this situation by asking the courts to close down humane society veterinary hospitals, and at least one such suit has been successful (14). In 1983, the AVMA, the American Animal Hospital Association, the American Humane Association, and the Humane Society of the United States joined in proposing model legislation "limiting the full-service humane hospital or government veterinary hospital to service only those who cannot afford private veterinary care" (15). The AVMA has adopted two policy statements relating to veterinary services provided by humane organizations, the 1982 Memorandum of Understanding for Humane Organizations and Veterinarians (16) and the 1983 Guidelines for Veterinary Associations and Veterinarians Working with Humane Organizations (17). The former document encourages private doctors and veterinary associations to "provide veterinary service to animal shelters at a mutually agreeable fee."

The argument usually raised in favor of full-service, low-cost humane society hospitals is that they benefit both clients and animals by making veterinary care less expensive. In the short range, this could be so. But over time, there is a distinct danger that some private practices that cannot compete with humane societies will disappear. This will harm the interests of clients and animals. A reduction in the number of doctors would not only make it more difficult for clients to obtain veterinary services; it would reduce the diversity of practices and approaches that a thriving community of competing veterinarians can offer the public.

The full-service, low-cost humane society hospital is also profoundly unfair to private doctors with whom it competes, even if these doctors can maintain satisfactory revenues. Competition among veterinarians is unavoidable. The problem comes from the fact that the government, by exempting such facilities from taxation, subsidizes their operation in a manner in which it does not subsidize the ordinary practitioner. This arguably might be acceptable if only the needy were being served by humane society hospitals – helping the needy is a traditional governmental function. But by permitting tax-exempt organizations to offer the *same* services to the *same* clients at a lower cost, the government is, in effect, stepping into the market and giving selected participants a competitive advantage without there being any compelling governmental need to do so.

The debate about humane society veterinary facilities is likely to continue for some time. The following suggestions are offered for consideration by the profession and government:

1. Humane societies should be permitted to operate full-service hospitals without imposition of taxes upon these facilities if they do not use their tax-exempt status to undercut fees charged by private practitioners, and if they charge fees that are within the normal range of those generally charged in their communities. Although humane societies ought not to be given a competitive advantage because of their tax-exempt status, neither would it be fair to make it more difficult for them to compete with private doctors just because they are operated by nonprofit organizations.

2. An argument (though not, in my view, a very strong one) can be made for permitting humane society facilities to provide at reduced cost to all members of the public a limited number of veterinary services essentially related to the mission of these societies. Because these organizations are viewed as serving a public function in protecting people from animal disease and predation, it can be maintained that they ought to be permitted to offer low-cost rabies vaccinations. Because they are involved in efforts to control animal populations and place unwanted animals, it can be argued that they may offer the public low-cost sterilizations, certainly of animals that they themselves place for adoption, as well as euthanasia of unwanted animals that would otherwise become a public nuisance. An argument can also be made that, given their traditional concerns with animal suffering and their function of ministering to injured animals on public ways, humane organizations should be allowed to maintain emergency facilities that can serve all emergency injury cases.

3. Because assisting the needy is widely recognized as a legitimate function of government, a strong case can be made for permitting humane societies to offer full services at reduced cost only to such persons. However, the problem of defining "need" in the veterinary area requires considerable thought before one can be comfortable about government subsidization of humane society veterinary services. When a human medical patient requires an operation costing many times his annual income, it is not difficult to conclude that he might need financial assistance or a publicly subsidized facility. In the veterinary area, however, where fees are usually much lower, it is often the case that a client can literally afford a procedure – but comes to the conclusion that he does not *want* to pay for it, or that paying for it would be an undue burden. Such clients might well say that they "need" help, and their pleas can seem especially poignant if they give us the choice of subsidizing them or having their animals killed. It seems grotesquely unfair to clients whose love for their animals enables *them* to dig deep into their resources, to subsidize other people who might place a relatively low value on their animals. Those who urge that humane society facilities should serve the needy must be prepared to engage in the difficult and unpleasant task of determining whether some clients believe they are in "need" not because of financial hardship, but because they do not have as much regard for their animals as they ought to have.

4. Ideally, humane societies providing lower-cost services should use local practitioners to staff their veterinary facilities. Local practitioners might be more likely than salaried humane society staff to care about whether the facility is indeed providing an essential public service or assistance to the needy, rather than unfair competition against established private practices.

5. Under no circumstances may veterinarians serving in humane facilities provide inferior medical care or deviate from their usual ethical obligations to patients and clients.

Vaccination and Testing Clinics

Whenever there is a legitimate medical objection to some activity, it is proper for the profession to raise it, even if it might appear to some that the objection is being made for economic reasons. Approaches that are bad medically cannot be good morally.

This is the problem with vaccination clinics in which veterinarians immunize or test large numbers of pets without being able to conduct a physical examination, take a history, or advise clients regarding follow-up immunization and health care. The *Principles* distinguish between mass clinics designed to protect the public, such as rabies vaccination programs, and those designed to protect the animal patient's health. The code recognizes that the former function can usually be accomplished without the opportunity for examining the animal. However, "when the primary objective is to protect the animal's health, clinical examination of the patient including proper history taking, is an essential and necessary part of a professionally acceptable immunization procedure" (18).

Supporters of animal health-oriented mass clinics might respond that it is better that animals be vaccinated or tested, even if this means that some will suffer because they cannot be examined properly. But veterinarians, who are committed to animal health and competent care, should not settle for such a choice. When brought an animal for the purpose of protecting its health, they should impress upon the client what must be done to fulfill this purpose. Veterinarian participation in clinics without adequate medical attention can only perpetuate acceptance by some of the legitimacy of a choice between poor care and no care.

Spay and Neuter Clinics

Some veterinarians offer clients greatly reduced fees through spay and neuter clinics, in which large numbers of animals are processed through a limited surgical service. (Often these clinics are operated by humane societies, whose tax-exempt status contributes to the lower fees.) Some practitioners believe that these clinics, like mass vaccination programs, can lead to medical problems because of their limited focus. Dr. Richard Fink, for example, has had patients that must undergo subsequent surgeries because procedures (such as removal of papillomas) were not conducted during limited sterilization clinics (19).

The approach of the *Principles* to spay and neuter clinics is obscure. The relevant section states that doctors should always "exercise individual judgment in deciding whether to undertake the care of any particular patient, regardless of whether the patient is referred by a humane organization, a spay and neuter clinic, or others" (20). This section does not appear to deal with the propriety of participating in a spay and neuter clinic itself (as opposed to taking a referral from such a clinic), a matter that ought to be addressed if such programs are in fact harming some patients. Because doctors must always exercise "individual judgment," it is unclear what the section is supposed to mean. Presumably, it is not meant to condone turning away an animal in need of follow-up or referral care in order to voice one's opposition to a low-cost sterilization clinic or humane society hospital.

Mobile Veterinary Facilities

The AVMA "Guidelines for Naming of Veterinary Facilities" define a "mobile facility" as a "practice conducted from a vehicle with special medical or surgical facilities or from a vehicle suitable only for making house or farm calls" (21). A mobile facility is thus to be distinguished from the situation in which a veterinarian who maintains a fixed-premise facility visits a home or farm in a motor vehicle containing a limited supply of medicines or implements to be used in or on the client's premises.

Today's mobile veterinary facility is usually a motor trailer or large van. Some provide only vaccinations and testing. In others, animals are also examined and treated. Some doctors with mobile facilities practice only in such facilities. Some mobile facilities are part of practices that include a fixed-premise office, clinic, or hospital in which animals are regularly seen or to which they are referred when they cannot be adequately diagnosed or treated in the mobile unit.

In certain locations and under certain kinds of conditions, mobile facilities can play an enormously beneficial role in providing veterinary care. To those in the inner city without means of transporting an animal to the doctor, to many elderly, to residents of nursing homes and public housing projects, and to inhabitants of rural areas that cannot support a fixed-premise veterinary office, a mobile van might be the only source of veterinary services. Some of these people might also have difficulty affording standard veterinary fees and would not frequent a standard fixed-premise facility with higher fees, even if it were available to them.

The reason there has been considerable opposition in the profession to mobile facilities is that many of them seek clients who can come to, and can afford the fees of, fixed-premise practices. Such mobile facilities are perceived as just another variant of the common street peddler, whose low overhead enables him to undercut the prices ordinary establishments must charge, who might not contribute his fair share of taxes, and who cannot offer the variety or quality of services available in more standard kinds of businesses.

"UNFAIR" COMPETITION

To some doctors, the mere fact that mobile facilities do not have the same overhead costs of fixed-premise hospitals gives the former an unfair competitive advantage. Some practitioners also believe it is unfair that a mobile facility can simply show up at a shopping center or parking lot and lure away from them, through lower fees or the convenience of the facility itself, clients whom they have served for years.

The quickest answer to such complaints is that these complaints contradict certain basic features of our economic system. Our system does not regard as unfair – indeed, it rewards – those who can find less expensive ways of serving the public's needs. The fact that a mobile facility is cheaper to operate than a fixed facility does not *of itself* make the former unfair, any more than a fixed-premise hospital that can cut costs by hiring fewer but more productive employees is being unfair to its fixed-premise competitors.

VIOLATION OF ZONING ORDINANCES; FAILURE TO PAY APPROPRIATE TAXES AND FEES

A much stronger charge of unfairness can be brought against any mobile facility that might operate in violation of local zoning ordinances. Zoning rules represent a community's collective judgment concerning esthetic values and the proper manner of reconciling the interests of various segments of the population. Some communities ban street vendors altogether. Some permit them only in certain locations and at certain times and only after receiving a permit. Still other communities require that all street operations be conducted by businesses with a permanent location in the area.

A mobile practice that knowingly violates zoning rules is showing contempt for a community by attempting to profit from it while rejecting rules it has set down for all businesses. There is little doubt that if a fixed-premise veterinary facility attempted to violate zoning rules either by placing a building in an inappropriate area or by operating its own mobile facility in violation of zoning standards, city officials would be able to find and stop it. If fixed practices must abide by zoning rules, so must mobile ones. If mobile practitioners find a community's zoning rules overly restrictive, they can, like anyone else, ask for a variance or challenge the rules as is prescribed by law.

A mobile facility would also be unfair to fixed practices and to the community if it failed to pay all required taxes and permit fees. Just as the owner of a fixed facility must pay property taxes and other kinds of fees to support community services that protect and support his practice, it would be wrong for a mobile facility to benefit from such services without paying all mandated taxes and fees.

POOR QUALITY SERVICE

The argument against certain mobile facilities most likely to impress the public and government is that they provide inadequate veterinary care. This charge can certainly be made against patient health-oriented mass veterinary clinics offered through mobile facilities. As noted above, such operations are deemed medically inappropriate by the AVMA. All practitioners, as well as the state veterinary boards, have an interest in preventing mobile facilities from accepting patients they are not equipped or qualified to handle.

Nevertheless, doctors who object to mobile facilities that do provide high quality care and obey the law might find that the public will interpret their criticisms to be motivated by naked self-interest. It is much safer (both from a legal and public relations standpoint) to try to beat the mobile facilities at their own game of competition. Fixed practices can explain to clients why their fees sometimes must be higher than those of mobile vans; they can include examinations within vaccination fees; they can conduct their own lower-cost vaccination clinics (with the possibility of appropriate examinations); they can sponsor or participate in community clinics for the needy; and they can explain to clients the advantages of bringing animals on a regular basis to a full-service fixed facility.

MORAL OBLIGATIONS OF MOBILE FACILITIES

Mobile facilities have some very important moral obligations that flow from their nature as limited and movable operations.

First, these facilities must never attempt to undertake diagnoses or perform procedures that can only be accomplished, or can be accomplished better, in a larger fixed-premise hospital. All veterinarians are morally obligated to make treatment choices based primarily on the needs of patient and client and not their own pecuniary interests. It would be profoundly immoral for a mobile facility to fail to inform clients of alternative approaches because these options cannot be done at such a facility.

Second, any veterinary facility must be able to be found on a continuing basis by clients and regulatory authorities. Otherwise, patients in need of follow-up care will be left in the lurch, and it will be impossible for state boards and other appropriate government bodies to determine whether good quality care is being provided.

The Veterinary School Enrollment Debate

The issue of whether veterinary schools ought to reduce enrollments to lessen the burdens of competition on all practitioners is too complex and controversial to be settled by a brief discussion. The following observations are offered to assist veterinarians in framing their approach to the debate:

1. Veterinarians should be wary of actions that would violate federal or state antitrust statutes. Ours is a culture that believes strongly in both education and competition. As hesitant as it is to allow restraints upon competition, the law will be even less likely to tolerate restriction of competition by means of reduced educational opportunities.

2. Most veterinary schools are funded by state government. Thus, their mission is to serve the people of their states, and to a lesser extent the people of other states whose governments contract with them for the education of students from these states. Because veterinarians constitute a very small portion of the population, it is not veterinarians' interests, but those of the public at large that must be of greatest concern to state governments in determinations of how to fund their veterinary schools. Therefore, those who urge enrollment reductions will have to show the states that current enrollments threaten the interests of their citizens. Such a threat could materialize some day in some states – if a surplus of veterinarians leads a significant number of doctors to leave practice or causes a diminution in the quality of those who enter or remain in practice. But today, the argument that the *public's* interest demands drastically reduced enrollments across the nation is unconvincing. Many clients must wait weeks for an appointment, and are likely to welcome fee reductions that some veterinarians find so abhorrent. Additionally, many in state and federal government appear to believe that *more* veterinarians are needed, for meat inspection, in animal and human disease control, to protect the welfare of laboratory animals and wildlife, and to assist in biomedical research.

Most veterinarians were able to attend school because of the generosity of the taxpayers of their states. The public constructed the facilities, paid the faculty, and then further subsidized the tuition. Doctors therefore should not resent the reminder that the level of enrollments must generally turn on public needs. They should also consider the fact that although they might now have to compete harder, at the beginning of their careers their lot was made significantly easier by taxpayer subsidy of their education.

3. Calling for reduction in enrollments solely to protect established practitioners violates the Golden Rule, which the *Principles* rightly declare to be among the fundamental moral tenets of the profession. A doctor who wants to shut the veterinary college door to qualified entrants is not recommending something he would want if he were an applicant. It is unfair and unseemly for someone who has had the advantage of a veterinary education to try to pull up the ladder because he was lucky enough to have gotten on board first.

4. In this society, neither the state nor the schools tell people how they must earn a living. Moreover, a veterinary school owes at least as much to those who are currently going through the program and are paying tuition as it does to alumni or nonalumni practitioners. We would not tolerate a school's pressuring alumni to change their career paths in order to make it easier for graduating seniors to compete for jobs. It can be no less wrong for a school to pressure current students to make career choices for the benefit of established doctors.

5. It is proper for the veterinary colleges to expose students to the wide range of practice opportunities. In order to do this well, they must be permitted by accrediting bodies and state boards to experiment with innovative and diversified curricula. Every veterinary educator has seen students who might choose a career in research, laboratory animal practice, pathology, public health, or government service if they could take significant course work in these areas. (We do not know how many talented people avoid veterinary school altogether because they do not want the standard private practice-oriented curriculum.) As long as all students must devote the overwhelming majority of their clinical time to dogs, cats, horses, and cows, the overwhelming majority of graduates inevitably will find their way into traditional private practices.

CRITICIZING COLLEAGUES

The Official Approach

The *Principles* devote considerable attention to the propriety of one doctor's criticizing another. Two sections of the code appear to encourage vigorous and prompt making of complaints before official and administrative bodies. It is stated that the profession "should safeguard the public and itself against veterinarians deficient in moral character or professional competence" (22). Moreover, members are told that they have a "duty" to report "illegal practices" to appropriate public authorities and the AVMA Executive Board (23). On the other hand, the code states that no member shall "belittle or injure the professional standing of another member of the profession or unnecessarily condemn the character of that person's professional acts" (24). "To criticize or disparage another veterinarian's service to a client is unethical;" if a colleague commits an act of incompetence, neglect, or abuse, one should call that behavior directly to the attention of the wrongdoer, or "if appropriate" to the state or local VMA or a public authority (25).

These sections do not seem entirely consistent. It is not clear, for example, how veterinarians can safeguard the public and the profession from incompetence or immorality without *ever* having to injure *any* doctor's professional standing. Nor is it clear whether the directive to report to the authorities any legal infraction (including, presumably, the most trivial or unlikely-to-be-repeated), is consistent with the prohibition against "unnecessarily" condemning a colleague's acts.

Most important, like many absolute rules that permit *no* exceptions, the principle that one may *never* criticize a colleague to or in front of a client fails to do justice under certain circumstances.

THE INTERESTS OF PRACTITIONERS

It is certainly in the best interests of most practitioners that they not be criticized in front of clients. A criticism, if strong enough, may lead a client to sue or make a complaint to the state board. The client might spread the bad word to other current or potential clients.

All these things can occur whether a criticism is correct or incorrect. These consequences can be especially unfair when a criticism is unjustified. And one of the major problems with quick criticism of a colleague is that it might well be unjustified. It is often difficult to know precisely what was presented to a previous doctor when he saw the patient. The client might now be confused or dishonest about what transpired. The second doctor might be incorrect in his approach and criticize a colleague who in fact acted properly. In many, perhaps in the overwhelming majority of cases, conferring with the previous doctor is necessary for getting the facts straight, avoiding unjustified criticism, and helping the patient.

THE INTERESTS OF CLIENTS AND PATIENTS

Unfortunately, it is not always in the interests of a patient, client, or the public for a doctor not to tell a client about the misdeeds of a colleague. Consider the following cases. They present situations that can and do occur.

Case 1: The first doctor (Dr. 1) has committed an act of negligence that the second doctor (Dr. 2) has every reason to believe will not be repeated. However, the law provides that a veterinarian is not entitled to a fee for negligent services. If Dr. 2 does not tell the client what happened, the client will never know that he paid Dr. 1's fee unnecessarily and is legally entitled to its return.

Case 2: Dr. 2, a specialist to whom the patient was referred by Dr. 1, knows that Dr. 1's approach to the patient was improper. He has also seen and heard of other examples of Dr. 1's incompetence and believes it is pointless to confront Dr. 1. Dr. 2 knows that if he does not say something to the client, the client will return to Dr. 1, thereby risking further injury to the patient.

Case 3: Dr. 2 concludes that Dr. 1 intentionally abused the animal and mistreated the client. When Dr. 2 confronts Dr. 1, Dr. 1 refuses to acknowledge his error and continues to heap abuse on the innocent client.

Case 4: Dr. 2 believes that Dr. 1 is frequently incompetent but will never be able to bring himself to lodge a complaint with the state VMA or board of registration. If Dr. 2 does not tell the client about Dr. 1's incompetence, there might never be any investigation of Dr. 1, and Dr. 1 will continue to harm animals and clients.

Case 5: The client comes to Dr. 2 suspecting that Dr. 1 injured his animal and asks Dr. 2 whether Dr. 1 was negligent. After reviewing the case and speaking with Dr. 1, Dr. 2 concludes that Dr. 1 was indeed negligent.

These situations are undoubtedly atypical. They also state as fact certain things (e.g., that Dr. 1 was negligent) that may often be far from clear. Yet, the cases illustrate circumstances in which a doctor's failing to tell the client that a colleague erred can harm the client, the patient, or both.

Case 1 refutes a claim I sometimes hear made by veterinarians, that when a second doctor can confront a previous doctor privately and can see to it the that former's mistake will not recur, no one is really harmed. However, even under these circumstances, the client *can* be harmed because he might be deprived of money that should have remained in his pocket. The animal might also have experienced unnecessary pain or illness.

In all the cases, a decision by the second doctor not to criticize the first can deprive the client of his legal and moral right to complain to somebody about the first doctor's behavior, for the client might not know that anything was amiss. In Cases 2 and 4, the second doctor's silence can threaten the health of the patient and other animals. And in Case 5, the second doctor's silence might entail his lying to the client and his failing to give the client a piece of information the client wants and is paying for.

Those who would insist that even in these five kinds of cases, the second doctor must *never* say anything bad about the first to the client are exhibiting an attitude that many clients would surely find disturbing – the view that a veterinarian does not work for the client who is paying the fee but rather for another veterinarian, whom he might not even know. Clients might well wonder whether such an attitude reflects the kind of loyalty to them and their animals they usually *assume* is part of the veterinarian-*client* and veterinarian-*patient* relationship.

I do not mean to suggest that even in these five cases, it is easy to decide how the second doctor should proceed. Nor am I arguing that these cases – or the general principle that a veterinarian works for the client who pays his fee – argue for liberal criticism of colleagues in less egregious situations. As a general rule, prudence and fairness do seem to require that one attempt to contact a colleague to ascertain the facts. It can be both dangerous and unfair to criticize a colleague. It might not be easy to find a satisfactory moral principle that does justice both to the interest of doctors in not being criticized unfairly and the interest of clients in knowing the truth and being able to pursue their legal rights. The problem with the approach of the *Principles* is that it appears to ignore these legitimate interests of clients, and their animals.

PROTECTING THE INTERESTS OF REFERRING DOCTORS

Good veterinary practice sometimes requires that a doctor refer a patient to a specialist, a practitioner with equipment or facilities not available to the referring doctor, or to a facility that operates during times the referring practice is closed.

In some cases, a receiving doctor might be tempted use the referral as an opportunity to win the client away from the referring doctor. Clearly, if this became a general practice, the legitimate interests of many clients and patients would be harmed. For then, doctors would stop making medically necessary referrals out of fear of losing their clients. Referring doctors would be harmed because of their inability to keep some of their clients satisfied, and receiving doctors would be harmed by not obtaining referrals.

In considering how receiving doctors ought to handle referrals, it is appropriate to distinguish two general kinds of cases: 1) the routine situation in which the receiving doctor has every reason to believe that the patient will obtain appropriate care upon return to the referring doctor, and 2) the unusual situation in which the receiving doctor concludes that returning to the referring doctor is not in the best interests of the patient or client.

In the first kind of case, it seems clear that the receiving doctor should encourage the client to return to the referring doctor for continuing care. Neither the interests of the patient or client require a change in doctors, and the receiving doctor has benefited from the referral. Difficulties arise, however, if the client *insists* upon using the receiving doctor in the future for care not related to the purposes of the referral. When the receiving doctor is a specialist in a very limited area (such as ophthalmology or cardiology) and does not practice with other doctors who can provide general continuing care, the answer might be easy: the receiving doctor cannot accept the patient on this basis because he is not equipped to provide the kind of care the patient will need. However, what ought to be done might not be so clear when a receiving doctor or other doctors in his practice can provide continuing care and the client wants him or his practice to take over care of the patient. If the receiving doctor agrees to do so, he probably will be violating the implicit understanding he had with the referring doctor that the case would be returned, and he might lose future referrals from that doctor. On the other hand, it is far from clear that the receiving doctor should automatically reject the wishes of a client who now insists on using his services. For clients do have the moral and legal right to decide how their animals should be treated, and what veterinarians they shall employ.

The situation becomes murkier, and potentially even less pleasant, when the receiving doctor believes that it is not in the best interests of the patient to return to the referring doctor. There are different possibilities here, ranging from the case in which the receiving doctor believes that the referring or original doctor will provide grossly inadequate care, to the case in which it might be just somewhat better for the patient to remain with the receiving doctor or to be seen by a third doctor.

Where the interests of a patient *clearly* would be harmed by its returning to the referring doctor, it seems to me that a strong argument can be made for the receiving doctor doing something to urge against such a return, provided that the receiving doctor has taken steps (by speaking with the referring doctor, for example) to assure himself that the patient would not be well-served by returning. Moreover, the desire of a client to choose his own veterinarian must always carry some weight on the scales of moral deliberation. Therefore, it can be argued that where the client comes to the receiving doctor already unhappy with the first doctor or simply wants to change doctors, the receiving doctor need find less deficiency in the referring doctor's performance to be absolved of his usual obligation to encourage the client to return to the referring doctor.

WHEN A CLIENT CHOOSES ANOTHER VETERINARIAN

However strongly he might object to a client's choice of another doctor, and however much he might hold the second veterinarian responsible for this choice, it is essential that a referring or original doctor not do anything to frustrate the wishes of the client or jeopardize the health of the animal. He must not refuse reasonable requests to provide copies of the patient's records to the client or a second doctor. Nor may he withhold essential information in order to make it more difficult for a second doctor to do his job or to motivate the client to return. Such actions could have serious legal consequences. The veterinary practice acts and regulations of many states require practitioners to furnish medical records when these are requested by the client or another veterinarian. In every state, a doctor can be held liable in a lawsuit by the client if his refusal to provide necessary information or records causes legally compensable harm to the patient or client. Moreover, it is morally wrong to hold the patient, who might need treatment and probably had nothing to do with the change in doctors, hostage to a doctor's dissatisfaction with a colleague's acquisition of the case.

The *Principles* agree with these recommendations, but with a twist that is worth noting. The code states that doctors should be willing to honor a client's request that the case be referred to another practitioner. The first doctor is said have to "an obligation *to other veterinarians* that the client may choose" to withdraw from the case and to forward the patient's medical records to another doctor who might request them (26). But in truth, the first doctor's moral obligation regarding forwarding of records is to the *client* and to the *animal*. If a subsequent doctor can be said to have a "right" to these records, it is only derivatively, because the client's wishes must be respected and because the animal can suffer if appropriate records are not made available. As it does elsewhere in its treatment of relations among doctors, once again the code seems to focus on the interests of veterinarians rather than on what is owed to clients and patients.

SPECIALIZATION AS A COMPETITIVE WEAPON

Specialists can be an enormous assistance to front-line general practitioners. However, some general practitioners are concerned about the potential use by specialists of their board certification as an unfair competitive weapon, i.e., as a means of attempting to convince the public that they will provide better care for an animal even when a general practitioner would be perfectly capable of handling the case.[a] Additionally, animosity has arisen between general practitioners and some specialists brought into communities by breed associations to conduct diagnostic clinics of purebred animals (27).

Any attempt by a specialist to convey the impression that he is ipso facto better qualified to care for a client's animals is unethical, and is already prohibited by official and administrative rules against false and misleading claims.

Such prohibitions have not had much effect on yellow pages advertisements. The typical yellow pages contain advertisements in which specialists proclaim their board certification, not to local practitioners, who already know of the specialists in the area, but to members of the public. It seems clear that some specialists place such advertisements with the precise intention of using their certification as a means of attracting clients, knowing full well that many potential clients will conclude incorrectly that a specialist must be better for *their* animals than a general practitioner. However, because board certification is a fact about a specialist, it might be extremely difficult to prove that a given specialist is publicizing his board certification with the intent to mislead or deceive. Moreover, the suggestion that specialists should not mention their

---

[a]The best known controversy regarding specialization as a possible competitive advantage involved a decision by the Canine Eye Registration Foundation to certify purebred dogs as free from hereditary eye disease only upon examination by a board-certified ophthalmologist. In 1979, four general practitioners sued the Foundation, the American College of Veterinary Ophthalmology (ACVO), the AVMA, and several board-certified ophthalmologists, charging them with violating the Sherman Antitrust Act. The defendants countersued. The plaintiffs' claims against the ACVO, the AVMA, and several of the veterinarian defendants, were dismissed. A federal magistrate found in favor of the remaining defendants on the complaint, which judgment was upheld on appeal. The court then issued summary judgment in favor of the defendants on their counterclaim. The plaintiffs were required to pay $416,893.99, which was then tripled in accordance with the Sherman Act. In 1986, the United States Supreme Court refused to review the lower court judgment, thus letting the award stand (28).

board certification in advertisements is likely to strike many specialists as an unfair attempt to restrict their ability to compete, and as an infringement of their moral and legal right to inform the public about their services.

REFERENCES

1. Wise JK: 1985 US veterinary practice income, expenses, and financial ratios. *J Am Vet Med Assoc* 190:1594-1598, 1987.
2. Wise JK: 1985 incomes of US veterinarians. *J Am Vet Med Assoc* 190:1334, 1987. These were the latest data available at the time of this writing.
3. Wise JK and Kushman JE: Synopsis of US Veterinary Medical Manpower Study: Demand and Supply from 1980 to 2000. *J Am Vet Med Assoc* 187:360.
4. 15 U.S.C. § 1.
5. 15 U.S.C. § 2.
6. 15 U.S.C. § 45(a)(1).
7. FTC Staff Lauds Veterinary Board's Ad Proposals. *BNA Antitrust & Trade Regulation Report* 50:694, 1986.
8. Bates v. State Bar of Arizona, 433 U.S. 350, 383-384 (1977).
9. Vakerics TV: *Antitrust Basics.* New York: Law Journal Seminars-Press, 1987, pp 6-27, 6-28.
10. Prosser WL and Keeton WP: *The Law of Torts.* ed 5. St. Paul, MN: West Publishing Co., 1984, p 967.
11. RESTATEMENT (SECOND) OF TORTS § 766 (1979).
12. See, Prosser WL and Keeton WP: *The Law of Torts.* ed 5. St. Paul, MN: West Publishing Co., 1984, pp 1005-1015.
13. RESTATEMENT (SECOND) OF TORTS § 559 (1979).
14. Virginia Beach Society for the Prevention of Cruelty to Animals v. South Hampton Roads Veterinary Association, 329 S.E.2d 10 (Va. 1985); see also, Dildine D: Silent Settlement Resolves Clinic Suit. *DVM* 13(1):1, 1982 (relating events regarding the Michigan VMA suit against the Macomb County Humane Society).
15. Animal Health Care Symposium Cosponsored by Veterinary Profession and Humane Groups. *J Am Vet Med Assoc* 183:393, 1983.
16. *1988 AVMA Directory,* p 468.
17. *1988 AVMA Directory,* p 469.
18. "Vaccination Clinics." *1988 AVMA Directory,* p 478.
19. Quoted in Clark R: *The Best of Ross Clark on Practice Management.* Lenexia, KS: Veterinary Medicine Publishing Co., 1985, p 102.
20. "Humane Organizations and Spay and Neuter Clinics: Examination and Surgical Sterilization of Pets." *1988 AVMA Directory,* p 478.
21. "Guidelines for Naming of Veterinary Facilities." *1988 AVMA Directory,* p 485.
22. "Principles of Veterinary Medical Ethics," Part 5. *1988 AVMA Directory,* p 474.
23. "Compliance with Law." *1988 AVMA Directory,* p 475.
24. "Deportment." *1988 AVMA Directory,* p 474.
25. "Professional Relationships with New Clients." *1988 AVMA Directory,* p 477. See also, "Consultations." *1988 AVMA Directory,* p 475; "Consultations." *1988 AVMA Directory,* p 476.

26. "Professional Relationships with New Clients." *1988 AVMA Directory*, p 477 emphasis added.
27. "Diagnostic Clinics, Guidelines for Conducting." *1988 AVMA Directory*, p 478.
28. Rickards v. Canine Eye Registration Foundation, Inc., 704 F.2d 1449 (9th Cir.), *cert. denied*, 104 S.Ct. 488 (1983); 783 F.2d 1328 (9th Cir.), *cert. denied*, 107 S.Ct. 180 (1986).

Chapter

— 19 —

Client Relations

Client relations is an extremely important subject for normative veterinary ethics. It might be fair to say that clients cause more ethical problems for veterinarians than patients. It is the client with whom the veterinarian must communicate, from whom he must receive payment, and by whom complaints are likely to be made. Moreover, because a client's interests or desires sometimes conflict with the interests of the patient, a veterinarian can be torn between serving the two.

There might be as many possible ethical issues relating to veterinarians' relations with clients as there are clients and doctors. This chapter discusses some of the more common ethical problems involving client relations that can often be considered apart from potential conflicts in interest between clients and patients. Chapter 20 will address problems that routinely can involve such conflicts. The reader must be reminded that because of the impossibility of addressing all the relevant issues here, and the difficulty and complexity of many of the issues that are discussed, these chapters are intended mainly as a stimulus for further thought and debate.

ACCEPTING NEW CLIENTS

As was explained in Chapter 4, a veterinarian may lawfully refuse to serve a client and his animal, provided that his reason for doing so is not one specifically prohibited by law, such as racial or religious discrimination. The law often requires far less of people than does morality. Our legal system and culture believe that people often ought to have the freedom to act morally or immorally if that is their choice.

The AVMA *Principles*, which is a document not of law but of ethics, appears to accept the minimal legal standard regarding freedom to choose clients as an *ethical* principle. "Veterinarians," the code states, "may choose whom they will serve" (1).

It is not difficult to appreciate why this is an unacceptable general ethical principle. Imagine a client who appears for the first time at a veterinarian's office when the doctor is free. The animal desperately needs a medication that the doctor can provide with minimal effort, and the client is willing to pay whatever the doctor wants. However, the doctor turns the client away after flipping a coin to decide whether he will take the case, or because the client is wearing a polyester leisure suit, or because the client is overweight. Surely, such a decision would be morally wrong. A veterinarian's job is to help clients and their animals, and these are not morally valid reasons for refusing to do this job. One cannot approach the issue of when one will accept or refuse clients with the simplistic maxim that "one may choose whom one will serve." Good reasons for turning away clients must be distinguished from bad.

The following discussion assumes that the doctor and his facility are qualified to handle a particular patient and are able to do so. Obviously, if either of these things is not the case, and the client can safely take the animal to a facility that is able to treat it, declining to accept the client is both a medical and an ethical imperative.

Questionable Payers

One legitimate reason for refusing to serve a new client can be a justified concern that the client is unable or unwilling to pay one's fee. The problem, of course, is that it can be extremely difficult to determine whether such a concern is justified regarding a client one has never seen before. Appearances can be deceiving. Moreover, many people who do not have a great deal of money have enormous regard for their animals and will make sacrifices elsewhere.

Veterinarians whose case load can accommodate new clients ought to presume that they will accept someone as a new client, and should accept new clients unless there is some good reason not to. This conclusion follows from the fundamental principle that it is the function of a practicing veterinarian to help people and their animals. There are ways of trying to assure reliable payment from new clients. One can accept credit cards, require a deposit before undertaking a procedure, or ask the client to specify his occupation and place of work or that of his spouse, which information can then be verified. One can have a frank talk with the potential client. Veterinarians, who are accustomed to counselling people concerning momentous decisions of life and death, can be very good at sensing the extent to which potential clients are committed to their animals and are prepared to be responsible for their treatment.

Disgruntled Clients of Other Doctors

Another kind of client one can sometimes be justified in turning away is the sort that comes to the office complaining about the services received from another doctor, or worse, from several veterinarians. Such people can be cantankerous and can make it impossible to treat the patient competently; they can attempt to embroil one in a dispute with another doctor; and they might be inclined to turn their complaints against *you*. There is nothing in a veterinarian's commitment to animals and clients that implies he must accept torture from clients, or that he must constantly fear a lawsuit.

To be sure, one must be sensitive and cautious before turning away a disgruntled client of another doctor. Dissatisfaction is sometimes justified. There might have been a personality conflict between the client and the former doctor for which the latter was partly responsible.

Strange or Potentially Troublesome Clients

Sometimes, even a brief encounter can indicate likely trouble from a potential client. Some people are so obviously obnoxious and demanding, or have such strange ideas about what should be done with the patient, that one can predict that a professional relationship would be a stormy one. Some potential clients bring the possibility of entanglement in activities unbefitting a veterinarian. For example, several practitioners tell me that they turn away people who appear to be using or breeding their animals for illegal dog fighting. Some veterinarians have had so much trouble catering to the demands and opinions of particular dog or cat breeders, that they find it preferable to decline to serve breeders who seek to become new clients.

The Relevance of the Patient's Condition

The condition of the patient is a relevant factor in determining how strongly other reasons (e.g., a potential client's obnoxiousness or financial condition) should count in the decision whether to accept a case. When the animal is not ill or does not need immediate care, the fact that the doctor knows he will not get along with the client or might have problems obtaining his fee will often seem sufficient to justify a decision to decline the case.

On the other hand, when a crucial need of the potential patient must be served immediately, lest it suffer or die, a veterinarian's commitment to animal health and welfare will exert great moral force in favor of accepting the case. Sometimes, this force will be sufficient to outweigh the veterinarian's legitimate qualms about the client. The fact that a client is obnoxious does not seem a sufficiently weighty reason for turning away an animal that needs immediate treatment to prevent it from dying. Sometimes, the force exerted by the animal's interests will not count in favor of taking the case. For example, where the animal requires an expensive procedure that the owner admits is beyond his means, a doctor might be compelled to decline the case, or to recommend euthanasia.

There are many possible different combinations of factors that can be relevant in deciding whether one is morally obligated to accept an ill animal. There are different conditions with different prognoses, perceived potential problems with clients, and conditions relating to the availability of care elsewhere. Sometimes there are alternative approaches a doctor can take to reconcile his own interests with those of the client and animal. It is sometimes possible to accept a patient on a temporary basis, until it recovers from a particular malady. Sometimes, it might be morally preferable to stabilize the patient so that it can be transferred to another doctor who is willing or able to accommodate the client's requirements.

The Problem of the Client-less Animal

Many small animal practitioners have faced the situation in which a stray animal or one whose owner is not yet known or present is brought into the office requiring emergency care. In the case of a stray, even if some governmental body will compensate the doctor, such payments might represent a small fraction of his costs. When the animal's owner is absent at the time of admission, the doctor might be uncertain about what the owner will find appropriate. He could face the prospect of suing for his fee.

Sometimes, alternative approaches are available that can make the situation less difficult. The laws of some jurisdictions permit a veterinarian to stabilize owner-absent animals and to recover all or part of the fee from the owner when he is located. Some doctors "budget" a certain amount for treatment of stray and owner-absent animals over given periods of time, and will absorb losses for such treatment, provided they remain under this level. A most admirable approach has been developed by Dr. Rodney Poling, a Massachusetts practitioner. Poling has established a stray animal fund to which civic organizations and individual clients contribute. When a stray or owner-absent animal is brought in for emergency treatment, the animal is automatically treated. If it is not possible to find the owner, the fund pays the practice for the animal's care. The animal is helped, and the practice does not suffer. Such an approach, if adopted throughout the country by individual doctors or groups of practices collectively, could end forever the terrible problem of whether to treat the stray or owner-absent animal.

WITHDRAWING FROM THE VETERINARIAN-CLIENT-PATIENT RELATIONSHIP

Clients can become financially unreliable, strange, or threatening after a professional relationship has begun. Under such circumstances, one sometimes will be morally justified in asking the client to find another veterinarian, for the same reasons that one would be justified in not accepting such a client in the first place.

However, withdrawing from the professional relationship can present special legal and moral problems.

Once a doctor has accepted an animal as a patient, the law obligates him not to withdraw from the case as long as the patient cannot be transferred without harm to another doctor, or until the client is given adequate notice of his intention to withdraw and adequate opportunity to obtain the services of another doctor. A veterinarian who fails in this obligation and terminates the veterinarian-client-patient relationship prematurely can be held liable to the client for abandonment, which is a form of negligence. Abandonment is a medical concept, based on the needs of the patient and not on the shortcomings of the client. Thus, even if a client is falling behind in his payments, or is making the doctor's life miserable, a doctor cannot unilaterally terminate treatment if the patient is in immediate need of it or if the client has not been given a reasonable opportunity to obtain treatment elsewhere. The legal obligation not to abandon a patient reflects the ethical principle that it is wrong to take out one's frustrations with a client upon a patient requiring immediate medical attention.

A doctor who wishes to terminate his professional relationship with a client also has the moral obligation (which all professionals have in their dealings with clients and the public) to use courtesy and tact. There is no need to inflict unnecessary guilt or bad feelings on a client or to risk oneself being made the target of an administrative complaint or lawsuit. It is important, however, that a doctor not tell falsehoods concerning the condition of the patient in order to make the parting easier. This could lead the client not to seek needed care, or cause him unnecessary distress or expense. Thus, it is wrong to try to get rid of a client whose animal requires continuing visits to a veterinarian by telling him that his animal is just fine and does not need further care. Nor is it fair to terminate the relationship by claiming that the animal really requires more extensive and expensive specialty care than one is able to provide, when in fact it does not.

FEES AND COLLECTION

The Ethical Dimensions of a Fair Fee

Some people believe that a fair or ethical fee is one that the market will bear. Just as a house or car, it is said, has no intrinsic "worth" apart from what people are willing to buy and sell it for, so, it is claimed, a "fair" fee or price is simply what a particular doctor can charge and receive. If someone is willing to pay $1,000 for a routine spay, who are we to say that the fee is unfair?

Certainly, a client's willingness to pay a proposed fee is an important factor in determining whether it is fair to him. Often, people will not be heard to complain that they have been treated unfairly if they have knowingly and voluntarily decided to pay what is requested by the provider of a service or product.

Nevertheless, "fairness" is not just another way of talking about what the market will bear. We believe that it is sometimes fair for a specialist who has invested years of time and money developing his skills to charge more than a general practitioner for his services, not because (or just because) clients might be willing to pay him more, but because his sacrifices and special skills *entitle* him to a higher fee. We believe that a doctor who travels to a farm in the middle of the night to attend a difficult case may fairly ask more than his usual fee for this service (if he can get it), not because the client will pay, but because the hardship and inconvenience entitle him to a higher fee. Likewise, we would say that a doctor who demands triple his usual fee from a client who rushes through the door with a dog just hit by an automobile is acting unfairly by taking advantage of a desperate situation.

Veterinarians have long recognized their ethical obligation to charge fees that are fair to both clients and themselves. However, the practice management literature regarding fees seems to give the issue of fairness minimal treatment – preferring instead to quickly settle on a "fair" profit percentage that is then used in formulae to translate costs, salaries, and time expended into fees. For example, one discussion states (2) that the actual percent of profit (after salaries and other costs) to be factored into a practice's fees "depends on items such as the amount of the veterinarian's investment in the practice, what fees are fair to the client, and what fees are to himself." These thoughts are incontestable. But the discussion then asserts, without further reasoning, that the profit figure "should be no less than 10% of gross income in a healthy practice," with higher percentages appropriate for practices with substantial investments in equipment or with specialized skills. One is not given a justification for the 10% figure. One is not told what factors are relevant in determining a figure that is fair.

The attempt to settle the issue of fairness by quickly choosing an intuitively attractive profit percentage figure is understandable. Most veterinarians need a simple and workable way of determining their fees. They have an interest in avoiding procedures that allow revenue to drip through the cracks or that force them into complex (and potentially costly) ethical deliberation about a fair fee each time they are confronted with a case that raises special ethical problems. Unfortunately, fairness does not always lend itself to mathematical computation or unvarying formulae. Fairness sometimes raises issues that have no clear answers. However, if fairness is to be taken seriously as a factor in establishing fees, both normative veterinary ethics and practice management must give it a good deal more attention than it has received thus far.

Some Considerations Regarding Fairness

The following thoughts are offered to stimulate the reader's further consideration of the issue of fairness in fees. As is the case with many suggestions offered in this text, their primary purpose is to probe and prod rather than to pass final judgment. One general statement can be asserted as a matter beyond argument: because of antitrust laws (see Chapter 18), any consideration of fairness in fees must presuppose that a decision about what fees to charge will rest with the individual practitioner deciding how ethical principles should affect his own independently-reached decisions.

1. One factor in determining a fair level of fees is one's educational background, training, and the nature of one's work. Veterinarians are more highly educated than tradespeople, and they deal with momentous matters of life, death, health, and happiness (both animal and human). Therefore, veterinarians should not assume that a level of profits normal for television repairmen or house painters is reasonable for them. If such tradespeople can earn a 10% profit in a given community, it would not be unfair for veterinarians to try to earn more.

2. It is incorrect to assume, as some practice management discussions do, that the issue of fairness arises only after one's overhead and salaries have been figured – that fairness simply means deciding upon an appropriate profit figure *after* costs. As shall be discussed in Chapter 22, one must ask whether one's own salary and those of one's associates and employees are fair. Moreover, there are sometimes ethical issues regarding overhead. If, for example, one is the only doctor in a community of people of modest means, and wants to purchase expensive equipment that will be used on a tiny fraction of one's patients, it can be asked whether it is fair to one's clients to buy this equipment if all of them will have to pay higher fees to cover the purchase.

3. The fee one asks of a client ought to bear some relationship to, and be connected with, the services one provides *that* client. It is appropriate to mark up certain items such as drugs in order to cover the general costs of the practice. For the mark-up that a client pays may enable the pharmacy to be properly stocked and the hospital to employ good technicians, all of which can inure directly to the benefit of that client and his animal. However, there can be an ethical problem with charging a client or a kind of client more in order to make up losses incurred because of service to other clients. Suppose, for example, that one charges 10% more for each comprehensive dental procedure because a competing mobile clinic has forced one to reduce fees for spays and neuters. A client whose animal needs dental work might rightly ask why he must subsidize the sterilization of other people's animals.

4. Although it will often be difficult to determine precisely at what point this might occur, at *some* point mark-ups or profit percentages can become so high as to be exorbitant or unconscionable. This can be the case for an item (such as a drug) that even after a mark-up, cannot be called expensive.

5. Because fees ought to be reasonably related to services provided, one should aim at charging all clients the same amount for the same procedures. This does not mean that exceptions cannot be made for people who might have difficulty with the bill. But it is wrong to charge wealthier clients more for the same procedure because they can more easily pay for it. This conveys the appearance – and involves the reality – of being paid a certain amount not because one's services are worth it, but because one can get away with charging it.

6. Many ethical questions regarding fees *can* be answered with the response that the client is not forced to pay a particular doctor's fees and can go elsewhere if he wants. Nevertheless, clients cannot always make completely knowing or voluntary choices regarding fees. First, clients are usually ignorant about what factors go into a doctor's fees. They might go elsewhere if they knew that their animal's root canal was subsidizing other patients' vaccinations, but they simply might not know. Second, there is often great pressure on clients to remain with a doctor even if they are uncomfortable about his fees: there might not be another veterinarian in the vicinity; the current doctor might be familiar with the animal and its medical needs; the client might find it difficult to refuse a service or product on the grounds that it is expensive after the doctor has recommended it; or the patient might require immediate care. It is a fact that very often clients do not have the same bargaining power with their veterinarians as consumers have with, say, a department store. One can usually live without a television set, and buying it later elsewhere will not be a great sacrifice. But finding, or even thinking about finding, another veterinarian when one's animal needs care can be much more difficult.

Veterinarians, therefore, should not take advantage of situations in which clients have a restricted choice of whether to accept their fees. If, for example, a course of treatment cannot be halted until it involves some expense, the client must be informed at the very start about the required fees and given the opportunity to decide whether they are acceptable. Under no circumstances should a doctor take advantage of an emergency situation to raise his fee or urge unnecessary procedures, for here, too, the client might be in a weakened state and easy prey to manipulation.

Making Exceptions for Certain Clients

The ideal situation, both from a management and an ethical standpoint, is to have in place a fee schedule that applies across the board to all clients and patients. If one's fees are generally fair, one can ask clients for them confidently and without guilt.

Sometimes, however, a doctor will find it impossible not to consider whether he should reduce the fee for a client unable to pay it. Clearly, if the usual fee for a service is fair, the doctor can first insist on exploring various ways of paying that fee. But sometimes, even this will be too burdensome for a client with an animal in need of one's services.

In considering the issue of reduced fees for certain clients, it is useful to keep in mind the distinction between obligations, actions one must morally do, and supererogatory acts, actions that are not obligatory but are morally praiseworthy (see Chapter 5). I do not want to suggest that veterinarians are never morally obligated to reduce a fee for a needy client. However, it seems to me that a much stronger general argument can be made for saying that reducing a fee can be a supererogatory act – and should be encouraged in certain kinds of circumstances without justifying moral condemnation if it is not done. Private practitioners are not charities, and many are far from wealthy. Reducing fees can be a sacrifice. But like other kinds of sacrifice, it can be morally praiseworthy. Moreover, there might sometimes be ways of reducing the sacrifice, such as budgeting a small amount for fee reduction, or instituting a fund to reduce fees in certain kinds of cases.

Legal and Official Approaches to Setting Fees

The law of most jurisdictions treats the matter of an appropriate fee differently, depending on whether there has been an agreement (either explicit or implicit) between a client and veterinarian that the client will pay the doctor's established fee. Where there is such an agreement, the doctor is usually free to charge as much or as little as he wants, except, perhaps, when there is an agreement to pay a fee that is so high or takes such advantage of the client's position that the law will call the fee unconscionable.

Where there has been no meeting of the minds about a fee, the law provides that the veterinarian is entitled to a *reasonable* fee. What is reasonable is an issue for a jury, and will depend on the doctor's training and skills, the nature of the work, the time and expense involved, and what other doctors in the area with similar qualifications would charge for similar services. In most jurisdictions, the client's wealth or ability to pay is not a relevant factor in determining the reasonableness of a fee, if there has not been an agreement about the fee. In this regard, the law reflects the ethical principle that the fee should be related to the work performed. However, the law does permit a doctor to take into account a client's ability to pay in determining a fee to which both parties then mutually agree.

The AVMA *Principles* state that in determining fees, veterinarians "may be *expected* to consider the nature of the condition, the time, the expense of other resources applicable to the case, and the client's ability to pay" (3).

Collections

Collecting one's fees is another area of practice that raises a myriad of difficult ethical problems. Different clients will present varying problems. What approach is morally appropriate often will depend on particular facts relating to the practice or doctor involved.

Among the many ethical questions that arise in the area of collections are the following:

- Does a veterinarian sometimes have a moral obligation to permit a client to be billed or to pay in installments?
- If postponed payment is permitted, may the doctor add a finance charge, and, if so, what is the measure of a fair charge?
- Can the use of credit cards be demeaning to the veterinarian-client relationship?
- If credit cards are accepted, is it fair to cash-paying clients to build the additional costs of credit card transactions into the fees of all clients?
- How far may a doctor attempt to intrude into the economic and personal life of a client before making a decision about extending credit?
- Should practitioners share information or impressions about the financial reliability of particular clients? Is it appropriate to circulate "deadbeat lists" containing the names of problem clients?
- Is it unseemly for a medical professional to accept items of personal property as collateral for payment? Are there moral limits to the kinds or value of property that may be accepted?
- Is a doctor ever morally obligated to treat a client's animal when the client already owes a certain amount and seems unable to pay it? To what extent are the kind of the animal, the gravity of its condition, and the amount of money still owed relevant factors in approaching this question?
- How many reminder statements is it appropriate to send to a delinquent client, and at what frequency?
- What are the moral limits to the kinds of language that may appropriately be included in such statements, or in other communications with the client intended to effect payment?
- Is it morally permissible to contact persons other than the client (such as family, friends, or employer) in order to effect collection?
- When is it appropriate to step outside the professional-client relationship and refer collections to a collection agency? Does a doctor have moral obligations regarding the choice of an agency to service his accounts?
- Is it morally appropriate to threaten a delinquent client with the sale or destruction of his animal? Is it morally appropriate to carry through such threats?

Threatening the Destruction or Sale of a Patient

In light of the current battle between more traditional conceptions of veterinary practice and the model of the veterinarian as a businessperson (see Chapter 15), one of the most interesting ethical issues regarding collections concerns whether veterinarians have more stringent moral obligations in the collection area than do ordinary commercial enterprises. Television repair shops and department stores routinely threaten delinquent customers with bad credit ratings, garnishment of paychecks, and other nasty actions by collection agencies or the courts. I would argue that because veterinarians should be viewed as medical professionals, certain kinds of actions are appropriate, if at all, far less often for them than for ordinary businesspeople.

The question of whether veterinarians may threaten clients with the sale or destruction of animals in their possession unless the bill is paid is especially important. The latter issue arose recently in a landmark decision of the Tennessee Supreme Court (4). A client brought her dog to the doctor after it had been hit by an automobile. The doctor accepted and treated the patient. However, according to the client, the doctor demanded that she pay the $155 bill "in cash and in full" by a specified date, and refused her request to pay in installments. The client alleged that she was telephoned repeatedly and was told that the hospital would "do away with the dog" as the doctor saw fit unless the bill was paid in full by the specified date.

The Court held that if the plaintiff could prove that her allegations were true, she would be entitled to a judgment for intentional infliction of emotional distress. The Court acknowledged the existence of a state statute permitting a veterinarian to turn over an animal to a humane society for disposal if a client does not fulfill his contractual obligations after a period of 10 days. But the Court pointed out that nothing in the statute justifies a veterinarian's *threatening* to do away with a client's animal. The Court held that the conduct alleged to have been committed by the veterinary hospital would be "outrageous and extreme and is not tolerable in a civilized society."

The Tennessee Court did not analogize the alleged behavior of the defendant to a human hospital's threatening to kill a baby in its care if the parents do not pay the bill. Nevertheless, clearly implicit in the Court's reasoning was a recognition that certain kinds of behavior that might be tolerated from ordinary commercial establishments concerning inanimate pieces of property would be unacceptable if done by a veterinarian. The Court appeared to recognize that it is profoundly immoral for anyone to taunt someone with threats to kill a beloved animal – and that this is even worse if done by a *veterinarian* with a general commitment to saving animal life and assisting animal owners.

The Court's distinction between disposing of a delinquent client's animal after giving the client notice of one's legal right to do so, and intentionally inflicting emotional distress by threatening such disposal is an important one. Even if the former might sometimes be morally (and legally) justified, the latter is not.

Equally important, however, is the issue of whether it is consistent with a veterinarian's commitment to patients and clients for him to kill, without threats, an animal wanted by a client. Some people would condemn such a course of action on the grounds that a veterinarian should never take the life of a wanted, healthy animal. (Some maintain that a veterinarian should never kill any healthy animal, be it wanted or unwanted.) However, one can often raise less radical arguments against killing the healthy animal of a delinquent client, as opposed to giving it to a shelter for adoption, or even returning it to the client. Killing the animal will usually accomplish very little for the doctor at potentially great cost to the client and animal. Charges might cease to accumulate, but this will itself not get the bill paid. Indeed, a client whose animal has been killed might be less willing to pay. Even if veterinarians are sometimes morally justified in killing a wanted animal, it does not seem terribly radical to suggest that if this is to occur, there must be at least some benefit in it for *someone*.

Sometimes, the only real rationale for killing a delinquent client's animal is a desire to punish the client or to prevent him from further enjoyment of the animal. But it is far from clear why taking the life of an innocent animal is an appropriate way of punishing or withholding satisfactions from an errant human being – or why a veterinarian who is generally committed to saving animal life should want to have any part of this kind of punishment.

The same sort of argument can also often be made against putting the animal of a delinquent client up for sale and applying the proceeds to the client's bill. The process often will not be in the doctor's interests. It can cost him a great deal of time, aggravation, and legal fees, and often will bring in less than the amount of the client's obligation. And selling the animal can involve a deprivation to an innocent creature that might more justly be imposed upon the real culprit through other means, such as reports to credit bureaus or legal action to collect the fee.

Legal Matters

Veterinarians contemplating various approaches toward collecting a fee must be attentive to applicable law. Federal and state statutes protect debtors against certain kinds of harassing behavior by or on behalf of creditors. Veterinarians who go overboard in criticizing delinquent clients or in pressuring them to pay, can find themselves liable for defamation of character or intentional infliction of emotional distress. Although a number of states do have laws permitting practitioners to sell or dispose of a delinquent client's animal under certain circumstances, these laws contain specific requirements regarding how long a bill must be unpaid before action can be taken, what kind of notice must be provided to the client, and precisely what the doctor must do. Failure to abide by these specific requirements can be disastrous. A veterinarian's scrupulous attention to the law might be the only protection he has against a judge's or jury's underlying opposition to his killing or selling the animal. To be sure, the fact that a doctor does follow the law in having a delinquent client's animal killed or sold does not guarantee the morality of his actions.

LOYALTY TO THE CLIENT

Fee-Splitting, Commissions, Rebates, and Kickbacks

As was explained in Chapter 13, a veterinarian has an obligation of loyalty to a client, which requires that he not compromise the interests of a client in favor of his own interests or those of other clients. It is therefore unethical, as the *Principles* (3, 5) and many state veterinary practice acts recognize, for veterinarians to split fees or to receive or give a commission, rebate, or kickback in connection with referrals. Nor should a doctor receive such moneys as a result of his recommendation that a client purchase nonveterinary goods or services, such as cremation, livestock supplies, and food.

A rebate, commission, or kickback is not restricted to the actual transfer of money. Many creative forms of kickbacks are possible. For example, a doctor who agrees with Company X to dispense its products instead of Company Y's in return for a special extra discount on the normal cost of certain Brand X products is accepting no less a monetary benefit than if Company X passed cash in a blank envelope.

Some doctors might object to a prohibition of kickbacks in circumstances in which they would make a certain referral or sell or prescribe a certain product anyway. In such a case, it might be argued, the only party that loses is the provider of the kickback. Such an approach is unsatisfactory because it raises unnecessary temptations that can intrude into doctors' independent exercise of their own best judgments on behalf of clients and animals. There may come a time when, for example, Company Y can provide a better product for certain patients. A doctor who is receiving a kickback from Company X has a strong motive for ignoring, or deluding himself about, the superiority of the better product. A client who comes to a veterinarian expecting his absolutely undivided loyalty should be able to rest assured that there is not present, even in the most remote nook of the doctor's psyche, the slightest temptation to abandon the dictates of independent professional judgment.

Pharmacy Issues

One controversy now facing medical ethics concerns the growing practice by physicians of selling prescription drugs. Opponents of this practice believe that physicians who sell drugs face a conflict of interest between the needs of their patients and their desire to profit from the sales. It is feared that physicians will choose drugs and brands that will bring them the greatest profits or that can be most conveniently kept in stock, rather than those that are best for patients (6).

Every veterinarian with whom I have spoken about the matter insists that he never chooses a drug for a patient because of its profitability. The AVMA *Principles* specifically state that "in the choice of drugs, biologics, or other treatments ... [veterinarians] are expected to use their professional judgment in the interests of the *patient*" (7). An AVMA policy statement also requires a veterinarian to offer prescriptions to clients who prefer to purchase a drug from someone other than the doctor (8). Nevertheless, the veterinarian's practice pharmacy, in which prices can be changed with the stroke of a pen, could provide some doctors a temptation to make decisions based primarily on their own monetary interests. The following reminders therefore seem in order:

1. Unlike most human medical patients, who still purchase pharmaceuticals at a drug store and can compare prices at different establishments, the majority of veterinary clients cannot or simply do not want to obtain a recommended drug other than from the doctor who has seen their animal. (Indeed, it would be negligent for a veterinarian to dispense a drug for an animal he has not examined.) Because these clients are at the mercy of their veterinarian, he must be especially careful to dispense an appropriate drug at a fair price.

2. It is proper to factor into decisions about what drugs and dosages to keep in stock the usual needs of one's patients as well as one's financial requirements. However, when the best drug for a patient is not one that can be stocked routinely, it is morally as well as medically wrong to dispense a less effective drug just because one has it and can turn a sale. In such cases, one's duty of loyalty to clients and patients requires one to obtain, or refer clients to a place where they can obtain, that drug. Sometimes a doctor may afford a client the choice between a drug in stock and one that must be ordered specially; but this should be done only when the drug in stock is adequate for the job and the client is permitted to make a fully informed and voluntary choice. Clients are by and large unsophisticated about drugs and biologics. They are likely to agree with whatever is suggested by a veterinarian.

In-practice Laboratory Testing

One service that is being recommended as a source of increased revenues (9), but which can sometimes create a conflict of interest for doctors, is in-practice laboratory testing. In-practice testing can offer enormous potential for taking unfair advantage of clients. Unnecessary, redundant, or overpriced testing is a violation of a veterinarian's obligation of loyalty to clients.

I believe that many veterinarians are not adequately explaining to clients why, for example, they must take additional x-rays or do further blood work after similar tests have already been done by a referring or previous doctor. Physicians and human hospitals have done a wonderful job convincing the public that laboratory tests are sometimes unnecessary, are frequently done to protect physicians rather than patients, and are always overpriced. Veterinary testing will come to be perceived in the same way unless practitioners recommend testing only when it is required medically, unless they explain the need for tests clearly, and unless they price the service fairly.

Pet Health Insurance

Although pet health insurance health plans appear to promise great benefits to many patients, clients, and practitioners, they can also create situations that test a doctor's loyalty to his clients. Although no insurance plan can guarantee that a subscriber will save money in the long run, the attraction of insurance is that by paying a premium now, one has a chance of saving money later. A veterinarian who runs his own pre-paid health plan must be careful to price options so that they give clients a fighting chance of saving money in the long run. Doctors would also compromise the best interests of clients if they took commissions or kickbacks in return for their participation in a company's plan or for their displaying its promotional literature. It would also be unfair to clients to raise fees just because insurance will now cover them. Ultimately, this will cost all subscribers more in premiums and out-of-pocket expenses than the legitimate worth of services provided would justify. In order to serve the interests of patients and clients, insurance programs must also permit referrals to and from other doctors (10).

Admitting Mistake or Fault

Another kind of situation in which a doctor's loyalty to a client can conflict with his own self-interest occurs when a mistake has been made. Clients are not legally obligated to pay for negligent services and are entitled to be compensated for certain kinds of damage caused by such services. Therefore, it will sometimes be in a client's interest to be told that a mistake was made or that an injury to the patient was the fault of the doctor or one of his employees. On the other hand, admitting mistake or fault is almost never in a doctor's interest, because it can result in loss of the fee, loss of the client, a complaint before a professional or government body, or a lawsuit.

TWO INAPPROPRIATE RESPONSES

One response to the issue of admitting fault that I have found expressed by some veterinarians is the claim that, at least when the patient is not injured or can be returned to the client in a healthy state, there is no issue regarding admission of fault. In such a case, it is said, the client is not harmed.

Aside from overlooking what might have happened to the unfortunate patient, this approach ignores the fact that clients are not legally obligated to pay for negligent or incompetent services. Therefore, failure to tell a client that a mistake was made can sometimes harm the client, if the fee is demanded or retained for incompetent services. Indeed, it can be argued that retention of a fee in such circumstances is tantamount to theft.

A second common response to the issue of admitting fault involves an attempt to insist that "the truth has been told." Suppose, for example, that a doctor performs an unnecessary intestinal biopsy upon an animal with digestive problems, that he performs this procedure in a negligent manner, and that his negligence causes peritonitis and death of the patient. The client asks what happened, and the doctor responds that the animal died from uncontrollable peritonitis. This was a real case, and I use it regularly to evoke the moral intuitions of my veterinary students. Some of them are inclined to say that this doctor need not worry about admitting fault because he is not *lying* to the client. He is not lying, it is claimed, because he was not asked whether he was at fault, and what he told the client was literally *true*. Such a response refuses to address the issue of whether fault ought to be admitted, and it does so by employing a questionable concept of "telling the truth."

ARGUMENTS FOR ADMITTING FAULT

There are very strong moral considerations that often appear to argue in favor of a veterinarian's admitting mistake or fault. First, if a doctor does not admit fault or indicate to the client that something was amiss, he sometimes will demand or retain a fee that he does not legally or morally deserve. Second, in failing to admit that a mistake was made, a doctor will sometimes be lying to the client, if the client inquires about what really happened or asks whether any mistake was made. Third, failing to admit fault will often be a violation of the Golden Rule and its admirable implication that veterinarians should treat clients as they would want to be treated if they were clients.

THE ARGUMENT AGAINST ADMITTING FAULT

The strongest argument against admitting mistake or fault is that doing so can have bad consequences for the doctor. To the doctor, this is an important consideration. But if one looks at the matter from an objective standpoint, it is far from clear why a client's interest in knowing the truth should be subordinated to a doctor's interest in keeping a fee or not being criticized or sued. For it is the client who is paying the fee, and for whom the doctor works.

MORALITY IN THE LIGHT OF PRUDENCE

Realistically, it is usually impossible to ask any professional person to admit a mistake or fault to a client. Therefore, the task of normative veterinary ethics in this area will probably be to formulate the best guidelines that can feasibly be put into action. The following are intended as suggestions toward this goal. These suggestions all presuppose that a doctor already knows a mistake has been made, something that might not always be obvious.

1. Sometimes, failing to admit mistake or fault will not result in retaining a fee to which one is not legally entitled. In the eyes of the law, a practitioner is entitled to his fee if he provides substantially the service for which the client agreed to pay. Moreover, a veterinarian's negligence alone does not excuse a client from his obligation to pay. Any negligence must also have been the cause of an injury that the law recognizes as compensable. Pain caused to an animal by a doctor's negligence is not among the kinds of compensable injury. In general, clients may recover only for physical or economic injury veterinary negligence has caused to them. Suppose that a doctor removes a tumor successfully, but carelessly leaves the patient with a minor cosmetic disfigurement. Moral considerations might argue in favor of reducing the fee. But in the eyes of the law, the doctor will be entitled to his fee and will not be liable for damages to the client, if the disfigurement does not cause the client economic damage (or the doctor did not guarantee there would be no disfigurement). If an error made by a veterinarian does not extinguish the client's obligation to pay the fee, where the doctor fails to admit such an error, at least he will not be retaining money that lawfully belongs to the client.

2. Even when a mistake is significant enough to affect a doctor's legal right to all or part of his fee, the doctor can sometimes employ means other than admitting fault to lessen the harm to the client. The fee can be reduced or waived, or the client can be offered lower cost or gratuitous services in the future. To be sure, such actions might not compensate the client for additional damage caused by one's mistakes, and failure to admit the mistake can prevent the client from taking appropriate action to obtain compensation for these losses. Moreover, reducing or waiving one's past or future fees will sometimes be a signal that something went amiss, and for that reason might not seem a feasible approach.

3. Even if a doctor is unable to admit a mistake to a client, he owes it to all his clients and patients to admit to *himself* when he or one of his staff erred or was at fault for injury to a patient. Every professional learns from mistakes. But such learning, and any consequent improvement in the quality of services one can provide to all patients and clients, is impossible if one engages in self-deception regarding one's own mistakes or those of one's staff.

Serving Clients with Conflicting or Potentially Conflicting Interests

A veterinarian's loyalty to clients can also be tested by situations in which he is asked to serve clients with conflicting or potentially conflicting interests. His loyalty to one client might provide temptations to compromise the interests of another. One example of such a situation is the case in which a doctor is asked by both the buyer and seller of an animal to examine it for soundness or some other feature of special interest in a transaction. Each party needs the doctor's complete loyalty. But if he is financially tied to both, he might not be completely honest with either, or both.

The *Principles* condemn as unethical accepting a fee from the seller of an animal when one is employed by the buyer to inspect it for soundness (11). However, the *Principles* do not discuss in general terms the issue of serving clients with conflicting or potentially conflicting economic interests. The following are but a few situations in which this issue can arise:

- Examining an animal to be purchased from a breeder by a member of the public when one's fee for the examination is paid by the breeder;
- Examining for a fee to be paid by the purchaser, an animal bought from a breeder who is a regular client, after the purchaser has been referred by the breeder;
- Providing regular veterinary services at a race track for owners whose animals compete against each other at that track;
- Serving two competing local show dog breeders;
- Providing theriogenology services for competing sellers of dairy cows.

In such situations, a doctor might sometimes be able to help one client at the expense of another, by revealing to the former some vital piece of information about, or indeed by doing something to, the latter's animals. Although he might strive conscientiously to be impartial, financial or personal considerations can sometimes make complete impartiality impossible. And even if he in fact remains impartial, if his clients have a falling out, he might find himself blamed or sued by one or both.

"Serving" two persons with potentially conflicting interests does not necessarily mean being paid by each. The following kind of situation, reported by a doctor who learned about conflicts between parties the hard way, is not uncommon. The seller of a horse informed a potential buyer that it had the heaves. The buyer stated that he did not wish to retain his own veterinarian. The seller told the buyer that he should feel free to talk to his veterinarian about the animal. The buyer called the seller's veterinarian after purchasing the horse and after the animal came down with a serious case of the heaves. The buyer then sued the seller to undo the sale, alleging that the seller did not disclose all the relevant facts about the animal. During the trial, the veterinarian was required to testify about what he said, or did not say, to both his regular client (the seller) and the buyer about the animal's condition.

It would be unrealistic to prohibit all veterinarians from ever serving clients with potentially conflicting interests. Sometimes, there are not enough veterinarians, or veterinarians qualified in a particular kind of practice, to go around. Sometimes, the service a doctor provides to competitors is so routine that it will not involve the opportunity to compromise any of them. Sometimes, a doctor's serving an owner in competition with an existing client might be necessary to save the life of an animal belonging to the former.

There is certainly a moral obligation, and one that is recognized by the *Principles* (12) and several state practice acts as well, to protect the professional confidences of clients unless one is required to reveal them by law or unless revealing them is necessary to protect the health or safety of animals or people.

However, although such a rule should be helpful in assuring confidentiality and loyalty to clients, the best way of promoting these values is usually to avoid situations in which they can be compromised. For his own safety and to assure the protection of his clients, as a general rule, a veterinarian ought to try to avoid serving clients with potentially conflicting economic interests. In the absence of an immediate medical emergency, he ought to avoid serving clients altogether when there is a substantial potential for his loyalty to one client being compromised by his loyalty to another. I would suggest that among the latter situations are the following: 1) being asked by both buyer and seller to examine an animal that is the subject of a sale; 2) serving competing clients after one client has asked for information regarding the animals or general business operations of another client; 3) serving competing clients after being exposed (even accidentally) to information that is essential to one client's competitive position and that could harm this client if revealed to the other client; 4) serving competing clients after being asked by one not to serve any of his competitors because of the confidential nature of information that might be obtained during the provision of veterinary services; and 5) serving clients who are, or are likely to be, opponents in a lawsuit concerning animals that have been or are likely to be examined or treated by the doctor.

COMMUNICATING WITH CLIENTS

Perhaps the most important area of client relations with ethical overtones is that of communication with clients. Often, a client's problems or dissatisfaction can be avoided or solved quickly by clear and respectful communication between the parties. If one has difficulty communicating with a client, it can be impossible to learn all the relevant facts that one must have in order to be able to decide on an approach that is medically and ethically proper.

Doctor-client communication is an area that has largely been ignored as a serious field of study by the profession and the veterinary schools. Students might pick up a few practical pointers from some of their instructors as they proceed through their clinics. However, such exposure tends to be spotty and inconsistent. Some of my students look at how differently their various instructors handle client communication – and conclude that the manner in which one deals with clients is just a feature of one's own personality, which is an individual matter and cannot be changed substantially.

Communication skills can, however, often be improved. Law schools routinely videotape students in simulated or actual settings with clients or judges, so that they can see how their physical mannerisms, tone of voice, and ability to listen and convey their ideas affect their capacity to serve clients. I believe that even some of the most experienced veterinarians would be astonished if they could view themselves on a tape replay as clients see them.

A serious discipline studying veterinarian-client communication does not yet exist (13). Nevertheless, one can say with confidence that the following virtues in a veterinarian can nurture respectful and effective communication:

- *Ability to listen*: A veterinarian must open his mind to what the client is saying. He should not be too busy formulating his own statements when he should be listening to the client.
- *Empathy*: It is often necessary to put oneself in a client's place. A client who is afraid of treating his pet with cancer chemotherapy might be transferring to the animal memories of cancer treatment of a relative or friend. A doctor must be able to understand why there might be such an impediment to the client's understanding of the treatment options. The doctor, who sees illness every day, must be able to appreciate how strange and frightening the illness of an animal can be to an owner accustomed to its good health.
- *Sympathy and compassion*: A veterinarian must try to be sympathetic regarding a client's worries or distress, even if he finds these concerns trivial or unreasonable.

- *Patience*: Veterinarians must understand that clients sometimes are unable or unwilling to comprehend the facts or treatment options. Clients must be given adequate time to appreciate the facts and to make decisions.
- *Sincerity*: Few things are more offensive than a practitioner whose behavior reflects insincerity, lack of interest, or downright hostility.
- *Clarity*: A veterinarian must be able to speak clearly in language that the client can understand, without treating the client in a condescending manner.
- *Tactfulness*: A practitioner must be able to be honest with clients while remaining tactful and courteous. Sometimes it might be necessary to make clear to a client that he is the reason the animal is ill or is not recovering. This often can be done in a way that is an encouragement rather than a criticism.
- *Professionalism in appearance and demeanor*: Effective communication requires that the client be able to confide in the veterinarian and trust his information and recommendations. This will be impossible if the client believes that the doctor is not concerned about him and his problems. Regard for personal appearance and demeanor is important in conveying to clients that one does care. Dirty or disheveled clothing, or coarse and disrespectful behavior toward or in the presence of clients, presents the impression that one does not care, and can create a wall between the veterinarian and client that makes communication impossible.

REFERENCES

1. "Principles of Veterinary Medical Ethics," Part 2. *1988 AVMA Directory*. p 474.
2. Hamlin F: Establishing Fees. In: Pratt PW: *Veterinary Practice Management*. Santa Barbara: American Veterinary Publications, 1979, pp 211-212.
3. "Fees for Service." *1988 AVMA Directory* p 475, emphasis added.
4. Lawrence v. Stanford, 665 S.W.2d 927 (Tenn. 1983).
5. "Commissions, Rebates, or Kickbacks." *1988 AVMA Directory*, p 475.
6. Robertson JD: Doctors vs. Pharmacists: Conflict of Interest. *Medical Malpractice Law & Strategy* 4(6):5, 1987.
7. "Drugs, Practitioner's Responsibility in the Choice of." *1988 AVMA Directory*, p 477, emphasis supplied.
8. "Prescription Writing." *1988 AVMA Directory*, p 486.
9. Roth DF: In-clinic Diagnosis Bring Profits and Client Appreciation. *Veterinary Economics* Apr 1986:45-52.
10. See, AVMA "Guidelines on Pet Health Insurance and Other 3rd Party Animal Health Plans." *1988 AVMA Directory*, p 486.
11. "Frauds." *1988 AVMA Directory*, p 474.
12. "Veterinarian-Client Relationships." *1988 AVMA Directory*, p 478.
13. For an eloquent argument for the establishment of such a discipline and its inclusion within the definition of veterinary practice see, Antelyes J: Empathy – innate gift or learnable skill? *J Am Vet Med Assoc* 192:1373-1375, 1988; and Antelyes J: Communication behavior vs communication. *J Am Vet Med Assoc* 193:178-180, 1988.

Chapter

—————— 20 ——————

Issues in Companion Animal Practice

One reason normative veterinary ethics is so interesting is that there is enormous variety in the value people place upon veterinary patients. Some are treated as members of the family for whom no effort or expense is to be spared. Others are destined for the dinner table.

This chapter considers several ethical issues in companion animal practice whose urgency and difficulty are attributable at least in part to the high regard many people have for companion animals. Although the discussion focuses on small animal practice, it must be understood that human-animal companionship (or the human-companion animal bond, which is not the same thing) is not limited to dogs, cats, and birds. Equine veterinarians, as well as other large animal doctors, can engage in what is rightly termed companion animal practice. Many of the issues developed here within the context of small animal practice are relevant to these veterinarians, and indeed to noncompanion animal practitioners as well.

EUTHANASIA

Appropriateness of the Terms "Euthanasia" and "Putting an Animal to Sleep"

Some people object to the routine use of such terms as "euthanasia," "putting an animal to sleep," or "putting an animal down." Philosopher Tom Regan points out that as the word is applied to human beings, "euthanasia" requires more than killing painlessly or with a minimum of suffering. If, Regan observes, I kill someone painlessly in order to inherit his money, that is not euthanasia, but murder. Regan asserts that the term "euthanasia" can be applied to people – or animals – only if killing them is in their interest. He objects to describing the killing of healthy animals with an interest in living as "euthanasia, properly conceived" (1). "To persist in referring to acts that culminate in the untimely death of these animals as 'euthanasia' is as inaccurate as the acts are regrettable" (2).

Regan is correct that the word "euthanasia" would not be applied to the killing of a healthy person for someone else's benefit. But his claim that it is therefore "improper" or "inaccurate" to speak of the euthanasia of a healthy animal for its owner's benefit is simply incorrect. For veterinarians and most other people do use the word "euthanasia" to refer to the process of killing an animal painlessly or with as little pain as possible – whether or not the animal is healthy or killing it can be said to be in its interest. This usage of the word is too widespread to be called improper; the usage reflects what the word "euthanasia" now means in our language when it is applied to animals.

Clearly, Regan is *recommending* a certain definition of the word "euthanasia" because he disapproves of many of the acts the word is currently used to describe. He would prefer a world in which the word "euthanasia" is applied to animals much as it is applied to human beings, because he believes that human beings and many animals are in certain respects equal in worth and value. However, it is one thing to argue for such equality (which Regan does), and another to accuse those who oppose it of speaking inaccurately.[a]

I have yet to find a veterinarian who does not know that euthanizing an animal involves killing it. I have yet to find a veterinarian who would not inquire about the morality of killing a patient, or who would take a certain position regarding killing it, *because* he uses the terms "euthanasia," "putting an animal to sleep," or "putting an animal down." It is also silly to suppose that only by enforced, unremitting use of the word "*Kill!*" will veterinarians or anyone else pay attention to moral issues concerning the killing of veterinary patients. If a mere word or phrase can insulate someone from these issues, surely, taking the word away will not cause him to engage in serious moral deliberation.

We all know what we are talking about: veterinarians sometimes kill their patients. The current way in which the word "euthanasia" is applied to animals reflects the fact that most people do not regard the painless killing of animals as akin to murder. Whether things ought to be otherwise is a matter for moral argument and not definition of terms. In this text, the term "euthanasia" will therefore be used regarding animals as it is by most persons, to mean killing painlessly or with minimal pain if such is necessary under the circumstances.[b]

---

[a]Another word whose use is criticized by many activists is "pet," which is supposed to demean animals. According to Ingrid Newkirk, national director of People for the Ethical Treatment of Animals, the word "pet" is "speciesist language." She views termination of this language as part of a larger program, which would include the abolition of companion animal breeds and the restriction of companion animals in the home to "refugees from the animal shelters and the streets. ... But as the surplus of dogs and cats (artificially engineered by centuries of forced breeding) declined, eventually companion animals would be phased out, and we would return to a more symbiotic relationship – enjoyment at a distance" (3). The assertion that all people who keep "pets" treat these animals in a condescending, demeaning, or disrespectful manner cannot be one that is based upon empirical observation. The facts simply prove otherwise. Rather, the assertion must be based upon metaphysical or philosophical claims that are held so deeply that they are impervious to the facts. How can one even begin to communicate with people who believe that our beloved companion animals would be better off existing (if they were permitted to exist at all) in some feral state – deprived of participation in human-animal bonds, in which they are loved, respected, and afforded effective veterinary care?

[b]The 1986 Report of the AVMA Panel on Euthanasia defines euthanasia as "the act of inducing painless death" (4). This is not an entirely satisfactory definition. It excludes situations in which a small amount of pain might be necessary to induce death, or when a painless death is not possible because the euthanasia must be performed in less than ideal surroundings. However, the Report does state that "whenever it becomes necessary to kill any animal for any reason whatsoever, death should be induced *as painlessly as possible*" (5).

"Active" versus "Passive" Euthanasia

In human medical ethics, a distinction is sometimes made between "active" euthanasia, the taking of actions to end a patient's life, and "passive" euthanasia, withholding treatment and thereby allowing the patient to die. This distinction is the subject of much controversy among philosophers and theologians. Some contend that there is no sensible distinction, because the aim and result are the same (6). Others maintain that only active euthanasia is morally prohibited, on the grounds, for example, that human life is a gift from God and must not be taken by man, or that physicians who commit active euthanasia will lose the confidence of patients if they cease to be viewed as vigorous battlers for life (7).

The options of not resuscitating an animal or withholding treatment must sometimes be considered by veterinarians and clients. Nevertheless, in veterinary medicine, the distinction between killing ("active" euthanasia) and letting die ("passive" euthanasia) is, at least at present, of much less importance than it is in human medicine. In veterinary medicine, euthanasia is characteristically active. Indeed, veterinarians typically do not apply the term "euthanasia" to letting a patient die as distinguished from taking its life.

One reason the distinction between active and passive euthanasia is so significant in human medicine is that many human patients can be kept alive long after they cease to enjoy a significant quality of life. Veterinary medicine is beginning to approach the abilities of human medicine in this respect, which may or may not prove to be a blessing. But at least at present, few veterinary clients have the inclination or financial means to prolong an animal's life when it has reached a vegetative state. Nor do most veterinary hospitals find doing this a reasonable utilization of limited resources.

It would be inaccurate to think that veterinarians euthanize desperately ill patients more frequently than do physicians solely because animals have traditionally been accorded less value than human beings. Many veterinary clients treasure their pets deeply but still choose quick, active euthanasia believing that this is the only way the interests of their animals can be *respected.*

Issues regarding the euthanasia of human patients are frightfully complex morally and socially. Moreover, it is not the case that veterinary ethics can illuminate moral issues regarding the euthanasia of people because "there is no clear-cut defensible gap between humans and animals from a moral point of view" (8). There *are* morally relevant differences between people and animals (see Chapter 11). These differences raise questions about the appropriateness of making euthanasia as available to physicians as it is to veterinarians.[c] Nevertheless, human medicine might learn much from veterinary medicine about how respect and love sometimes can be furthered by the compassionate termination of hopeless suffering.

---

[c]For example, because the life of a human being is more valuable than that of a pet, one can argue that a much stronger showing of the impossibility of recovery or improvement must be made regarding a person before active euthanasia can be contemplated as a possible option. Were euthanasia to be made as readily available to physicians as it is to veterinarians, there might well be much unjustifiable killing of people and a diminution in respect for human life.

The Choice of a Euthanizing Agent

The choice of a euthanizing agent can be an ethical as well as a technical decision. If an inappropriate agent is used, an animal can suffer needlessly, and ending its life might not be described properly as an instance of euthanasia.

The 1986 Report of the AVMA Panel on Euthanasia (9) surveys the most common euthanizing methods with regard to such factors as safety for personnel, ease of performance, rapidity of death, cost, efficacy, and species suitability. At least two aspects of the Report raise ethical questions.

First, although the Report indicates the expense of the various methods, it does not discuss explicitly the relevance of cost in the choice of a euthanizing agent. The Report does not consider, for example, whether the lower cost of one agent can justify its use, even though it might induce euthanasia less rapidly or with more potential side effects than a more expensive agent. I would argue that a patient, especially one that has suffered already, has a moral *right* in its final moments to as painless a death as possible. Therefore, the first consideration must always be inducing the quickest and least painful death. Given the fact that cost-effective euthanizing agents are available, choosing a euthanizing agent for utilitarian-economic reasons is appropriate only after it has been determined that there is more than one method that will meet the basic requirement of inducing as quick and painless a death as possible.

Another ethical issue arising from the Report concerns the euthanizing agent T-61® (American Hoechst Corp., Somerville, NJ). Many veterinarians appear to be enthusiastic about this product, which is not subject to the strict storage and reporting requirements of federal controlled substance laws. (Several doctors tell me that it is especially useful in euthanizing horses and other large animals.) On the other hand, T-61 has been attacked as inhumane by some animal welfare advocates and is not permitted in the United Kingdom (10). A recent survey of Massachusetts veterinarians (11) found that 44% had seen bad reactions (including muscle tremors, convulsions, agonal thrashing, and prolonged heart activity) when using the product, and that only 28.7% consider it a satisfactory euthanizing agent. The author of the study conceded that many respondents either liked or had no problem with the product, and that some of the reported bad results might have resulted from failure to follow the manufacturer's directions meticulously (11).

The Panel's response to this survey and other data questioning the appropriateness of T-61 was to call for "further controlled studies on the efficacy and humaneness" (12) of the product in several species. The Panel approved the use of T-61 "if barbiturates cannot be used ... but only when it is administered intravenously by a highly skilled person at recommended dosages and at proper injection rates" (13).

Given the lack of hard evidence proving the inhumaneness of T-61, the Panel's decision not to prohibit the product seems fair. Nevertheless, in my view, the Panel did not go far enough. Even if one assumes that a euthanizing agent is effective in theory, if in fact it is employed even in a small percentage of cases so as to cause unnecessary pain or discomfort, it is not a satisfactory euthanizing agent in practice. For veterinarians, the central question is not whether any bad reactions involved in the use of a euthanizing product should be attributed to some inherent defect in the product or to misuse of the product by practitioners. The first order of business must be protection of the animals. Because painless and affordable alternatives to T-61 already exist (at least for euthanizing dogs and cats), it is not fair to expect opponents of the product to prove that it is not humane. The fact that there is opposition to the product on the part of competent doctors surely shifts the burden of proof to supporters of T-61 to show that it *is* humane in practice.

In light of these considerations, it seems reasonable to give T-61 temporary approval for a specified period of time (say, 5 years). During that time, its advocates would be required to demonstrate that it can and will be employed as painlessly as any other available agent, under real conditions faced by actual practitioners. If such a showing cannot be made, approval of the product should be withdrawn for use in any species in which painless death cannot routinely be assured.

Euthanasia as a Focus of Conflicting Interests

There are few issues facing normative veterinary ethics that present more problems regarding the balancing of conflicting interests than euthanasia. It is not always in the common interests of the patient, client, and doctor that euthanasia be performed. Even when an animal is suffering desperately, and euthanasia seems in its interest, killing the animal can place tremendous burdens on its owner. The situation can become even less clear where the animal has a serious disease that diminishes its quality of life without causing constant suffering; in some of these cases, the client's interest in keeping his companion alive as long as possible might seem weightier than the animal's interest in a superb quality of life. There are cases in which a client mistakenly thinks that his animal's best interests would be served by euthanasia. Sometimes, the animal can do quite well, and euthanasia might be intended less as a favor to the animal than as a way of preventing the client from experiencing unpleasantness or inconvenience. At the other end of the spectrum are those clients who have little concern for their animals and want them killed simply to be rid of them.

The companion animal doctor is sometimes caught in the middle of these conflicts because he wants to serve both the client and patient. He also might have his own conflicting interests in approaching the situation. He might have an economic interest in euthanizing the patient if another doctor will do it if he does not. He might have an economic interest in convincing the client to proceed with treatment first, and a professional interest in attempting to see whether his skills are up to the patient's malady. His interest in serving and satisfying clients might incline him not to make too big a fuss if they suggest euthanasia. On the other hand, his interest in elevating his own professional status might be served by his encouraging a view of companion animals as beings that should not be killed until treatment alternatives are attempted.

Into this cauldron of competing interests must sometimes be stirred additional ethical, psychological, and social issues that go to the heart of how people view animals. For example, as was noted in Chapter 11, some people think that the only strong interest animals have is an interest in not experiencing "unnecessary" pain or discomfort. To these people, moral questions that assume animals can have an interest in a good life, or in life itself, will seem illusory. There is also the troubling question of when attachment to a sick animal might become unreasonable, or even pathological – so that keeping it alive cannot be viewed as a *legitimate* interest of its owner. Whether one finds a client's attachment to an animal reasonable will sometimes turn on whether one approves of certain kinds of attitudes toward animals. The person who views pets as filthy nuisances will find no amount of attachment to them reasonable. Some who value companion animals highly will find trying to hold on to a desperately ill pet understandable or even mandatory. Given the wide range of attitudes toward animals in our society, it sometimes will be difficult to reach agreement about whether a client's reluctance to have his animal killed is "unreasonable."

Euthanasia for Good Reasons:
General Considerations Regarding the Process of Euthanasia

In thinking about the morality of euthanizing veterinary patients, it is useful to begin with situations in which the end result of euthanasia is appropriate. In this way, one can appreciate that there are ethical considerations regarding the *process* of euthanasia. The weight of these considerations can differ, depending on the precise circumstances and justification for euthanasia. (For example, when an animal is already near death, questions regarding the proper time to mention euthanasia and the proper timing of euthanasia will probably be less difficult than when the patient is in the beginning stages of a debilitating disease.) Nevertheless, these considerations tend to apply in all cases of justifiable euthanasia. As the following discussion demonstrates, they can be as important ethically as the decision about whether euthanasia is justified.

Among cases of clearly justified euthanasia are those in which all of the following elements are present: 1) the patient is suffering from a condition for which veterinary medicine cannot offer a cure or solution at any price; 2) the condition is already causing the animal severe pain for which palliative measures short of inducing virtual unconsciousness are not available; 3) the client is psychologically able to make a voluntary and rational decision regarding euthanasia; and 4) the client is able to request euthanasia, understanding that the animal's interest in freedom from suffering ought to take precedence over his own impending grief or sense of loss. Euthanasia would be appropriate in such cases because putting the patient out of its misery clearly would be in the legitimate interests of the patient, client, and veterinarian. Nor could it harm the profession or other companion animals by encouraging an attitude of disrespect for, or lack of concern about, companion animals in general.

MENTIONING EUTHANASIA

Even when an animal is in desperate need of euthanasia, simply hearing the word "euthanasia" or being told about the option of ending the animal's life can be a terrible shock to a client. The client might not appreciate the seriousness of the animal's condition, or might have an initial (or continuing) resistance to the thought that euthanasia is really required.

Whenever possible, a doctor should not begin his conversation with a client by mentioning euthanasia. Rather, the animal's condition should be described and explained first, and the topic of euthanasia introduced only when the client appears ready to confront it. If the animal is in pain or is distressed, one might consider an analgesic or sedative when possible so as to afford the opportunity of introducing the subject of euthanasia with due regard for both animal and client. If a doctor is callous or inconsiderate in his first mention of the euthanasia option, the entire process of euthanasia can be a disaster for everyone.

PERMITTING THE CLIENT TO MAKE AND FEEL AS COMFORTABLE AS POSSIBLE ABOUT THE DECISION

Although there might be limited exceptions to this rule, generally a veterinarian must permit a client to make his own knowing and voluntary decision whether to proceed with euthanasia. The client has a moral right to make such a decision. It is his animal, and it is he who must live with the decision after it is carried out. A veterinarian who manipulates a client's decision toward euthanasia or who quickly accepts from a client the option of deciding what ought to be done is also risking the possibility of great aggravation for himself later. If the client has second thoughts, and appreciates that the doctor moved him forcibly to the decision, he might blame the doctor for making the wrong decision.

Allowing a client to make the decision requires that a doctor speak and act as objectively as possible. Even in cases when euthanasia is the only humane option, the likely results of prolonging life must not be dressed up in exaggerated or frightening terms.

Allowing a client to make the decision also requires providing him with an environment in which he can feel comfortable about the decision. In my view, although most veterinarians are extremely good in giving objective information and helpful advice regarding euthanasia, many provide their clients with terrible surroundings in which to make and reflect upon their decision. Some doctors remain in the examining room or hover over the client while he is supposed to make a decision, not realizing the kind of pressure such behavior can exert. Some veterinarians will indicate that the examining room must be used again soon, or disappear precipitously to another part of the hospital unaware of how difficult it can be for the client to search them out for further advice. The typical examining room, with its clean but stark environment, can itself be a terrible place to make a life and death decision.

Doctors are morally obligated to pay serious attention to the surroundings in which the euthanasia decision sometimes must be made. Ideally, there should be a place in which the client and members of his family can sit and think, unhurried and away from the hustle and bustle of the practice. The client should have access to a comfortable chair, a beverage, and the reassuring presence of support personnel or the doctor if needed. The client should be given the opportunity to be alone with his pet so that a final goodbye can be said. A comforting environment should also be available after euthanasia is completed.

Among the alternatives that should be discussed with the client is the option of being present during euthanasia. Some clients prefer this, but might feel uncomfortable about asking. What might be done with the animal after death may also appropriately be discussed before euthanasia is performed.

THE TIMING OF EUTHANASIA

One sometimes can assist clients to make the right decision by suggesting that the decision be postponed. When an animal is near death, this might not be possible. But sometimes it will be feasible to encourage the client to go out for a cup of coffee or to return home for a few hours or longer so that he has time to think. Sometimes, encouraging the client to take the animal home when this is possible can give the client further assurance of the wisdom of euthanasia and can allow him to begin to accept his impending loss.

PERFORMANCE OF EUTHANASIA

Dr. William Kay summarizes a doctor's ethical obligations regarding the performance of euthanasia succinctly: "the veterinarian and staff must respond with skill and concern" (14). As Dr. Kay explains, this can mean among other things 1) not allowing interruptions during the procedure; 2) discussing the client's decision to be present during or after the procedure; 3) making available to the client trained support personnel; 4) explaining the significance of body movements during euthanasia and emphasizing the absence of consciousness or pain; 5) providing a

quiet place where the client can remain with the body should he so desire; and
6) using an intravenous catheter where possible to assure a smooth, quick injection.

HANDLING THE BODY

The patient's body must be treated with dignity and respect. This must be done
not just in order to avoid unnecessary upset for the client but out of consideration for
the being that is no more. To respect a dead patient is to affirm and celebrate the
value of its life. This is why the companion animal doctor and his staff should treat
the remains in a dignified and solemn manner even if no one else will ever know of
it. Dr. Kay recommends that one close the eyes and place the tongue within the
mouth and clean the body carefully; that the body be wrapped in a clean blanket or
other suitable material; and that its condition be explained to the client if he wishes
to view the body after euthanasia.

DISPOSITION OF THE BODY

Doctors must never consider it a nuisance or something above and beyond the
call of duty to assist the client in the decision about how to dispose of the remains.
The doctor should assure that the client is aware of all the options available in the
community. The client must not be pressured into making a decision the doctor would
find preferable, and he must be given adequate time to make his decision. Even if
the doctor does not personally favor burial, he should accept and sympathize with a
client's choice of this option, and he should make every reasonable attempt to help
the client make burial arrangements.

COMFORTING AND COUNSELLING THE CLIENT

The doctor must stand ready to comfort the client before and after the animal is
euthanized. Reassuring the client of the correctness of the decision can be most
important. Telephoning, writing, or visiting the client after his pet's passing can
provide further support. When appropriate, the doctor may mention the possibility of
a replacement pet.

As Dr. Kay observes, many veterinarians feel uncomfortable about becoming
involved in the psychosocial dynamics of euthanasia. They "consider this role to be
outside their domain of knowledge, experience, influence, and responsibility" (15).
Veterinarians traditionally have not been trained to deal with these matters, and some
might prefer not getting involved to getting involved badly.

Nevertheless, veterinarians do have a moral obligation to offer comfort and
counsel to clients whose animals they euthanize.

First, there is usually no one else around but the veterinarian to provide support;
it is simply inhuman to end the life of a client's animal and then to bid a hasty
goodbye, leaving him hanging in mid-air with his grief.

Second, quite often the best comfort a client can receive is reassurance that
euthanasia was necessary for medical reasons. There is no one who has greater
knowledge of the medical necessity for euthanasia, or whose opinion will count more
with the client, than the doctor.

Finally, and most importantly, veterinarians are justified in defining veterinary
practice to include *ministering to the needs and interests of the patient's human
companions*. Physicians are as scientifically trained and devoted to their patients as

veterinarians. But few people would argue that physicians should not comfort the relatives or friends of a sick or dying patient. What makes the physician a *doctor* rather than just a "human disease expert" is (ideally) his concern for the entire life of the patient – which includes the people who are important to the patient. This is part of what it means to say that the physician is interested in the whole person and not just the mechanics of the patient's body.

Veterinarians would appear to have a stronger claim than physicians to be able to minister to their patients' close companions. For a veterinarian can never communicate with and comfort a patient to the exclusion of the patient's human companions. It has always been the patient's human companion with whom the companion animal doctor communicates and through whose eyes he sees much of the patient. Veterinarians who maintain that they cannot become involved in the psychosocial dynamics of their clients' emotions are fooling themselves. They are already involved. They might as well be involved skillfully and compassionately.[d]

SETTLING THE FEE

Doctors must avoid clumsy or insensitive requests for payment after euthanasia is completed. Some clients are not prepared to interrupt their grieving by stepping up to the receptionist's desk to write a check. Doing this can be even more difficult if the death of their pet was unexpected. On the other hand, a doctor sometimes will have a legitimate concern about whether his fee will be paid, especially if there are outstanding charges for services preceding the euthanasia and the client shows signs of dissatisfaction with these services. Although circumstances vary, doctors should try to be flexible in the manner in which the fee for euthanasia is settled. A polite indication from the receptionist that there is no need to worry about the bill now can go a long way in helping a distraught client through his ordeal. He might remember this thoughtfulness when it comes time to seek veterinary care for another animal.

Issues Concerning the Appropriateness of Euthanasia

Even when a doctor feels comfortable about euthanizing a particular patient, it can be a major effort to pay sufficient regard to his moral obligations to patient and

---

[d]A few large veterinary hospitals employ social workers to counsel clients. Some of these people undoubtedly do much good (16). Some clients might benefit from a referral to an outside mental health practitioner. Some veterinarians might benefit from expert instruction about how to approach upset or bereaved clients. Nevertheless, questions must be asked before veterinarians relinquish one of their most important functions to others. Will routine assignment of client counselling to social workers encourage veterinarians to define themselves as technical experts, whose function is to deal only with the mechanics of the patient's body? Will veterinarians who rely routinely on social workers be less sensitive to clients' interests when medical options are discussed? Can the availability of a social worker provide an easy justification for not engaging in difficult ethical deliberation, and for quickly moving on to the next appointment? Are social workers really better at counselling clients than veterinarians who could take the time to do so? Do social workers possess special expertise in dealing with the many *ethical* issues that can arise when clients must contemplate various alternatives for their animals? Will the images of the veterinarian as a healer and friend (see Chapter 15) be helped or undercut by the notion that veterinarians require another profession to assist them in approaching patients and clients? In general, would the routine use of social workers encourage, or discourage, veterinarians from viewing attention to ethics and client relations as part of *their* professional role?

client. The situation can be complicated substantially when it is not clear whether euthanasia is appropriate, or when one disagrees with a client's decision or the client's reasons for that decision.

The following discussion presents typical situations in which questions about the justification of euthanasia must also be raised. In all these situations – as indeed always in his approach to clients – a veterinarian must not confuse the question of what would be best for patient and client with the issue of who has the moral right to make the decision (*see* Chapter 10).

WHEN A CLIENT MISTAKENLY BELIEVES EUTHANASIA IS NECESSARY FOR THE ANIMAL'S WELFARE

Sometimes a client will request euthanasia with the intention of serving the animal's interests, but is mistaken in believing that euthanasia is necessary for this purpose. This can be a relatively easy kind of case to handle, if in fact the client has only the animal's interests in mind. For example, some clients believe that euthanasia of their dog is preferable to amputation of one leg because they think that a three-legged dog cannot be active and happy. Likewise, some clients assume that a pet that has lost its eyesight is necessarily condemned to a life of misery. In many such cases, one can serve the interests of both the patient and client by explaining that such animals sometimes do quite well with a bit of patience and effort from their owners. The doctor might not have to challenge the preferences of the client because he might be able to provide information that will permit the client to satisfy his underlying preferences.

WHEN THE ANIMAL IS AT THE BEGINNING STAGES OF A PROGRESSIVE ILLNESS OR CAN LIVE COMFORTABLY FOR SOME PERIOD OF TIME

Clients sometimes want to consider euthanasia when an animal is at the beginning stages of a progressively debilitating illness or has a condition that is not yet distressing the animal or with which it can live comfortably at least for some period of time. Once again, if the client's sole concern is the animal's welfare, one sometimes will be able to point out that euthanasia might be advisable some time in the future, but is not yet necessary. The situation becomes stickier when part of the client's motivation for preferring euthanasia is his own fear of seeing the animal grow progressively worse, or his reluctance to experience sadness and grief as the animal deteriorates. Although it would be presumptuous for a doctor to underestimate or belittle such emotions, there sometimes is a role for him in assisting the client in making sure that euthanasia would indeed serve the client's underlying preferences. For example, one might be able to determine that the client is really afraid of watching the animal suffer, and in some cases, one will be able to show the client that this need not happen in the short term and can be addressed appropriately later. Or, the client might be overestimating the amount of effort required on his part to maintain the animal.

The doctor can also often further the client's own preferences and assist the patient at the same time by being sensitive to any anthropormorphizing that might be responsible for a misapprehension of the facts. If the client is trying to put himself in his pet's position, and is imagining how he would feel if he knew he had a terminal illness, the doctor should be able to point out that the animal will have no such understanding, and in the short term at least, might do quite well. Sometimes this is exactly what a client wants to hear.

WHEN KEEPING THE ANIMAL ALIVE WILL CAUSE UNWANTED INCONVENIENCE

The situation can be extremely difficult where a client wants his animal euthanized because taking care of it will be an unwanted inconvenience. There is a wide range of possibilities here. The client might be ill or infirm himself, so that caring for the animal will be a major burden. At the other end of the spectrum are people for whom more than opening a can of food is a major inconvenience. Even if one supposes that a veterinarian should serve patients as well as clients, it is sometimes far from clear that euthanasia is the wrong approach. Where a client is infirm or incapable of taking proper care of the animal, and the animal cannot be placed elsewhere or would do poorly if placed with another owner, the argument that keeping the animal alive is in its best interests might not be very strong. Where the client has little concern for the animal, it might be questionable whether he can ever be persuaded to give the animal what it needs for a satisfactory life.

I would suggest that the profession take two general approaches to clients whose animals can live a decent life but who prefer euthanasia to inconvenience.

In the long term, veterinarians can encourage a more caring attitude toward pets. Clients must be educated about not only the pleasures of animal ownership but also its responsibilities. The profession should not be bashful about proclaiming that companion animals are beings of great worth *entitled* to love, respect, and first-class veterinary care. As such an attitude becomes more prevalent, veterinarians should see fewer clients for whom inconvenience is a reason for euthanasia.

In the short term, a doctor can approach clients who prefer euthanasia to inconvenience by doing what he can. Where appropriate, one can point out that the inconvenience might not be so great. Perhaps the client will take the animal home for a while to see how things work out. One can also explore the possibility of placing the patient elsewhere, perhaps with a relative, and perhaps on a temporary basis until the client is capable of caring for it. Some veterinarians tell me that they would like to suggest such things but are afraid of appearing too pushy. If a client cannot at least understand why a *veterinarian* would want to suggest ways of saving an animal's life, that person will probably never be worth a great deal in monetary terms to the practice.

WHEN AN ALTERNATIVE TO EUTHANASIA WILL COST THE CLIENT MORE THAN HE IS WILLING OR ABLE TO PAY

There is no doubt that adequate care is sometimes beyond the economic abilities of some clients. However, ethical analysis is not served unless one speaks carefully before asserting that a client is "unable" to pay for or "cannot afford" treatment. In our society, many people purchase goods and services for which they cannot pay in full at the time of purchase. Yet, they can "afford" to purchase these things because they undertake to purchase them. Many clients who state, or have convinced themselves, that they "cannot afford" an alternative to euthanasia can afford it in the sense in which they would literally be able to pay for it if they made financial arrangements to do so. What they really mean is that they do not regard saving the animal as *worth* the economic burden.

There surely are clients who cannot afford an alternative to euthanasia, or who are justified in concluding that they should not undergo the economic sacrifice helping their animal would entail. Nevertheless, in tailoring their approach to the issue of euthanizing animals capable of being helped, doctors must distinguish clearly between cases of true economic inability and of unwillingness to pay. This is so for the following reasons:

1. Because the problem is often unwillingness to pay, and because such an attitude is often beyond the ability of a doctor to change when he has a client in the office, the most effective way of challenging the attitude that a pet is not worth the economic sacrifice might be to prevent this attitude from forming in the first place. And the best way of accomplishing this might be to promote throughout society the view of the companion animal as a member of the family entitled to first-class medical care.

2. The profession might be less motivated to fight for such a view of companion animals if doctors overestimate the occurrences of cases of true inability to afford treatment.

3. Doctors might have a greater chance of saving an animal whose owner's thinking can be changed by refusing to agree with the owner that he cannot afford an alternative to euthanasia when in fact he can. Although veterinarians generally must avoid coercing or pressuring clients into making decisions, they are not obligated to lift the burden of decisions from clients' shoulders. When a client wants to euthanize his animal because treating it is not worth it to him, the client should know that this is the reason behind the decision. Some clients could care less about such a realization, but it might stimulate others to rethink their choices. When a doctor suspects that the decision is not really one of affordability, it is not inappropriate for him to say to the client politely, but firmly, "Mr. Jones, we have medical means of saving this animal. It might take us some time to figure out how we can do this consistent with your cash flow situation. But I want you to know that I think we can do it, and I am willing to sit down with you and try if you are willing." If such a client chooses euthanasia, at least he will know it is his choice and not the doctor's.

4. Because clients will tend to conclude that they "cannot afford" an alternative to euthanasia the higher the cost of the alternative, if the profession wishes to reduce the number of medically unnecessary euthanasias, it must try to help clients reduce the burden of cost (though not necessarily the cost) of treatment options as much as possible. Many veterinarians extend credit when doing so is necessary to save a patient's life. Pet health insurance programs could prove an effective means of reducing the number of euthanasias performed because of client inability or unwillingness to pay for treatment.

5. Sometimes, it will be morally appropriate to refuse to euthanize a patient. Suppose an animal could be brought back to health for just a few dollars more than it would cost to euthanize it and the client requests euthanasia to save the money. Here, a veterinarian would be within his rights to tell the client that his personal and professional values prohibit him from killing animals that can be helped with minimal additional expense, and that he considers euthanasia under such circumstances to be no different from killing a perfectly healthy animal simply because its owner wants to be rid of it. I do not mean to minimize the problems that can arise once one concedes the appropriateness of refusing to euthanize because one considers that the financial burden to the client does not justify it; for then, one must think about how high a financial burden may be expected of a client. Nevertheless, it seems clear that companion animal doctors who include among their values the saving of animal life and the promotion of animal health, must at least be open to the possibility of refusing to kill an animal when this is requested for trivial reasons.

EUTHANASIA OF HEALTHY, WELL-BEHAVED PATIENTS

Although many veterinarians do euthanize animals simply because their owners no longer want them, there are strong moral objections to this practice.

Not in the interests of the profession. First, it is not in the general interest of the profession to perpetuate an image of itself as willing to kill any companion animal on demand. As I have argued in this text, companion animal doctors will be able to meet their full earning potential only if society comes to view companion animals as beings entitled to love, respect, and first-rate veterinary care. Veterinarians who kill on demand are sending a message to clients and the public that their patients are not worth much at all. Clients will not believe the pleas of the profession that their animals are worth first-class and sometimes costly care if individual doctors do not endorse this attitude themselves.

In order to promote an image of their patients as beings of importance, veterinarians need not always oppose the euthanasia of unwanted animals. Sadly, euthanasia often seems the only way of dealing with such animals. What I am urging is that *veterinarians* should not be involved in their private practices in this tragic process – except in the most unusual and compelling kinds of cases (such as when it is clear that a client will kill an animal himself if the doctor does not do it). Doctors can tell clients that it is against their ideals to kill healthy, well-behaved animals on demand. They can tell clients that they believe in the value of their patients' lives and they believe that if a healthy animal is not wanted, at least it should be given a chance at being adopted. They can tell clients who insist on euthanasia that it must be done at an animal shelter or humane society, not by the doctor.

Some veterinarians will protest that economic pressures compel them to euthanize a healthy animal when a client requests it, because if they do not do it, someone else will, and they will lose the fee. This attitude is shortsighted. In the long run, this approach prevents the community of companion animal doctors from meeting the economic challenges of the day with the most potent weapon at its disposal – the image of the kind and compassionate healer dedicated to the interests of his valued patients.

Not in the interests of clients. It often is not even in the interests of clients to have their unwanted animals killed by a veterinarian. For this can cost the client more than surrendering the animal to a shelter, which usually costs nothing. To be sure, some clients might prefer to have a veterinarian euthanize their animal because they might view this as approval by the doctor of their decision. Although veterinarians should not be discourteous to owners who seek euthanasia for healthy animals, they have no obligation to make these people feel comfortable about such a decision.

Not in the interests of the patient. It is not in the interest of a healthy companion animal that could do well with another owner to be killed. But neither is it in the interest of companion animals in general. For it is in the interest of all companion animals to be afforded good veterinary care by their owners. Insofar as the killing of healthy animals by veterinarians hinders the full development of the image of the companion animal as a being entitled to respect and care, the killing of individual healthy animals will have some effect in preventing members of the public from giving the very best veterinary care to their animals.

WHEN EUTHANASIA IS CONTEMPLATED BECAUSE OF BEHAVIORAL PROBLEMS

It has been estimated that 40% of pet owners who are not satisfied with their animals are unhappy about perceived behavioral problems, and that between 35 and 50% of all euthanasias of companion animals are performed because of behavioral problems (17).

Euthanasia for behavioral reasons presents difficult ethical and technical issues for the profession. It sometimes is the case that an animal's behavioral problems are attributable at least in part to its owner. Nevertheless, even when this is so, the animal can be so vicious or intractable that returning it to the owner's home or placing it elsewhere is unfeasible. Doctors are sometimes faced with the apparently unfair, but unavoidable, situation of having to kill an animal because of the misdeeds of its owner.

Technically, the profession in general is not yet equipped to stem the tide of medically unnecessary euthanasias resulting from behavioral problems. Important work is being done by some veterinarians and behavioral scientists to establish verifiable empirical knowledge in the area of companion animal behavior (18). However, the typical pet owner who seeks advice about behavioral matters from his veterinarian is likely to receive the same kinds of homespun suggestions he can obtain from friends, relatives, or a local book store. Most veterinary schools still regard behavior as a "soft" subject that merits at best a sprinkling of (usually elective) class hours when students desire some diversion from the rigors of the "real" curriculum.

As is the case when a client inclines towards euthanasia because he believes keeping his animal will be too inconvenient or costly, a veterinarian can perform a useful function in clarifying for the client his own preferences – by making it clear if a behavioral or combination of a behavioral and a medical approach might solve the problem. Likewise, the doctor can tell the client when, in his view, euthanasia is unjustified or at least premature, and he may refuse to euthanize when he believes that the animal might be helped or placed elsewhere.

Nevertheless, it seems clear that if the number of euthanasias of pets with behavioral problems is to be reduced significantly, the profession as a whole must wage a two-front attack. It must place in the hands of doctors as much useful knowledge as is available regarding approaches to behavioral problems. The profession must also promote better education of pet owners about the causes of common behavioral disturbances and about the personalities and behavioral problems of various kinds and breeds of animals. If clients can be educated about behavioral matters before they bring a pet into their homes, the likelihood of certain kinds of predictable problems will be reduced.

A major burden rests squarely on the shoulders of the veterinary schools. They must place on their faculties behavioral experts who will do research applicable to situations faced by practicing doctors. Students must be required to take meaningful course work in behavioral issues. Behavioral studies – like ethics – must be recognized as a legitimate intellectual endeavor of crucial importance to the mission of the veterinary schools.

WHEN THE ALTERNATIVE TO EUTHANASIA MIGHT CAUSE THE PATIENT TO SUFFER OR TO EXPERIENCE A DIMINISHED QUALITY OF LIFE

The most complex ethical issues regarding euthanasia tend to arise when the alternative to ending the patient's life can involve its suffering pain or experiencing a diminished quality of life. In such situations, the interest of the patient in a continued life can conflict with its interest in not suffering and in not living a life of greatly reduced quality. The client might have an interest in keeping the animal alive that can conflict with his desire that it not suffer, as well as with his interest in not undergoing undue inconvenience and expense. The veterinarian can be torn between his desire to serve the patient and his desire to serve the client. All this can be complicated by that fact that it is sometimes unclear what the results of a given noneuthanasia approach will be. The client must sometimes weigh the *uncertainty* of the success of a treatment option against the potential benefits and harms to the animal and himself.

In considering how to approach situations in which alternatives to euthanasia might cause problems for the patient, it is useful to appreciate the variety of possible different kinds of cases. This can be done by listing some of the more important morally relevant considerations and the possible different permutations of these factors. Clearly, the following are among the morally relevant considerations: 1) the probability that a given approach will meet with success; 2) the nature of such "success" in terms of the likely quality of life to be experienced by the patient; 3) the probable duration of this quality of life before grave illness occurs and euthanasia must be considered again; 4) the likely amount of pain or discomfort that will be experienced by the patient as a result of the approach; 5) the likely upset or inconvenience the approach will cause the client; and 6) the likely expense of the approach.

Table 20.1 presents several possible ways of categorizing these considerations, and can be used to generate a large number of possible permutations taking just these factors into account. The table also lists four of the possible situations. A doctor should want to consider with the client all feasible noneuthanasia approaches. These approaches should then be compared with euthanasia in terms of their effects on the patient and client.

Table 20.1

Some Morally Relevant Considerations Bearing on the Appropriateness of Euthanasia

PROBABILITY OF REACHING INTENDED QUALITY OF LIFE IF GIVEN NON-EUTHANASIA APPROACH IS TAKEN	INTENDED QUALITY OF LIFE	PROBABLE DURATION OF INTENDED QUALITY OF LIFE	LIKELY PAIN OR DIS-COMFORT TO ANIMAL RESULTING FROM APPROACH	LIKELY UPSET OR INCON-VENIENCE TO CLIENT OF TREATMENT AND CONTINUING CARE	LIKELY EXPENSE TO CLIENT OF TREATMENT AND CONTINUING CARE
high	excellent	long	great	great	great
moderate	good	medium	moderate	moderate	moderate
low	fair	short	minimal	minimal	minimal
uncertain	poor	uncertain	uncertain	uncertain	uncertain

Selected possibilities:

- A treatment (or nontreatment) alternative to euthanasia has a high probability of giving the animal a long and excellent quality of life. The animal likely will experience minimal pain, and there likely will be minimal upset and expense to the client.
- A treatment (or nontreatment) alternative to euthanasia has a low probability of giving the animal a short and fair quality of life. The animal likely will experience moderate pain, and there likely will be minimal upset and expense to the client.
- A treatment (or nontreatment) alternative to euthanasia has a low probability of giving the animal a short and fair quality of life. The animal likely will experience moderate pain, and there likely will be great upset and expense to the client.
- A treatment (or nontreatment) alternative to euthanasia has an uncertain probability of giving the animal a good but short quality of life. The animal likely will experience moderate pain, and there likely will be great upset and expense to the client.

Because of the large number of possibilities, it is difficult to propose brief guidelines that will do justice to all possible situations. However, the following suggestions emerge from the table and the realities it reflects:

1. Because there are, in the abstract, so many different possibilities, one important ethical function of the doctor is to *provide the client with accurate information*. Each medically feasible noneuthanasia approach and its likely effects on the patient and client must be presented clearly. The doctor must view it as the first order of business to help the client restrict the universe of discourse to arguably appropriate choices by making sure that the client understands the *facts* about each medically feasible alternative.

2. A doctor has a moral obligation to treat a client as an intelligent adult capable of understanding all sides of the situation. Some doctors find it helpful to put themselves, in turn, in the place of the client and the animal. For example, suppose the alternative to euthanasia involves loss of the patient's ability to urinate. The doctor can describe how the animal is likely to live, and then explain what its continued life would entail for the client. There is great potential in relating the facts to abuse one's position of trust. It is one thing to explain to a client what it is to express an animal's bladder. It is quite another to twist one's face into a contorted appearance and exclaim with great horror, "Do you know what you will have to do day in and day out? You really don't want *that*, do you?"

3. Part of a doctor's obligation to present the facts is to make sure that the client understands the facts. Some clients will try to insulate themselves from the discomfort their animals are suffering by leaving them in the hospital, unvisited, until the worst is over. The doctor must make it clear to the client how the animal is doing. This will sometimes require insisting that the client see what is happening.

4. A doctor's general obligation to permit a client to make the decision about care for his animal does not preclude the doctor from presenting himself as an advocate for the animal and offering on its behalf arguments against the apparent tendencies of the client. Although the client must be presumed more knowledgeable about himself and his own needs, the veterinarian is more knowledgeable about what is likely to happen to the patient. It is sometimes appropriate for a doctor to state, for example, that in his view it is inhumane and unfair to keep the patient alive. At times, it will be appropriate to state that if the client insists on keeping the animal alive, he must take it to another doctor. One problem with this approach is that it can be so forceful that it might exert undue influence on the client's ability to make his own voluntary decision.

5. One possible way of dealing with the situation in which a client insists on a course of treatment that is clearly not in the patient's interest is to suggest that the client consult another veterinarian for a second opinion (perhaps, another doctor in the practice, and at no additional charge). This can sometimes help to convince the client that the requested approach is indeed inappropriate. Suggesting a consultation with another doctor can also help when the client is under the misapprehension that a perfectly appropriate procedure (such as amputation of a leg or cancer surgery that might leave cosmetic defects) will ruin the animal or its relations with the client.

6. Just as speaking up for the patient will sometimes mean presenting the arguments for euthanasia, so will it sometimes mean advising against euthanasia. As is the case when a client is inclined toward euthanasia for reasons of inconvenience or expense, even when treatment might entail some discomfort for the animal, a companion animal doctor should try whenever possible to think life rather than death. Getting into the habit of agreeing to clients' requests for euthanasia can put one in a *frame of mind* in which alternatives might not be explored vigorously.

Making a Difference

Some of my veterinary students become extremely upset when clients choose euthanasia because they do not want to incur the inconvenience or cost of treatment, or because they are just tired of their animals. These students wonder if it makes sense to study for years to learn how to save life if they are going to be asked time and again to take life.

I suggest to them that it is far better to be depressed about such situations than unfeeling, because those who feel nothing are unlikely to work for change. On the other hand, one cannot take upon oneself the burden of the world's mistakes. One must realize that we live in a society in which many companion animals die needlessly. Yet, change is possible. Slowly but surely, as the profession promotes the value of companion animals and individual doctors make sure that clients understand when treatment is available, fewer medically unnecessary euthanasias will be performed.

It is sometimes easy to lose sight of how much attitudes toward companion animals have already changed. To my students who despair of the possibility of change, I quote an 1897 decision of the United States Supreme Court. In that case, the Court expressed strong reservations about dogs, and indeed about other animals we now treasure deeply. According to the Justices, dogs cannot be

> considered as being upon the same plane with horses, cattle, sheep and other domesticated animals, but rather in the category of cats, monkeys, singing birds and similar animals kept for pleasure, curiosity or caprice. ... Unlike other domestic animals, they are useful neither as beasts of burden, for draught (except for a limited extent), nor for food. They are peculiar in the fact that they differ among themselves more widely than any class of animals, and can hardly be said to have a characteristic common to the entire race. While the higher breeds rank among the noblest representatives of the animal kingdom, and are justly esteemed for their intelligence, sagacity, fidelity, watchfulness, affection, and, above all for their natural companionship with man, others are afflicted with such serious infirmities of temper as to be little better than a public nuisance. All are more or less subject to attacks of hydrophilic madness (19).

Today, this view of the dog, cat, and "singing bird" seems a curious reflection of a time long gone. (And, of course, one reason this view is gone is that veterinary medicine can now provide effective medical care for these animals.) Some day, a client who requests euthanasia when his pet can be helped might be no less a thing of the past. In the meantime, practitioners committed to health and life may do what they can to urge against every unjustifiable euthanasia. In the course of a lifetime of practice, that can add up to many lives saved.

DEALING WITH A CLIENT WHO IS UNABLE TO MAKE A RATIONAL DECISION

As I have argued, whether or not one of the alternatives to be considered includes euthanasia, a veterinarian should always strive to permit a client to make his own informed, rational, and voluntary decision about what is to be done with his animal. Sometimes, however, a client might be unable to make such a decision. He might be physically or psychologically infirm. He might be unable to understand the facts and options the doctor is attempting to relate. He might be so emotionally overwrought that he cannot understand the nature and consequences of treatment options or appreciate what some of these options could do to him or his animal.

Some doctors tell me that in such cases they believe they are justified in forcefully guiding the client toward a particular decision, especially when failure to make that decision will cause the animal to suffer. (This might be done by bullying the client into a decision, or more subtly, by shading the truth or characterizing the alternatives so as to make the option decided upon by the doctor the inevitable "choice" of the client.)

In my view, such approaches might sometimes be appropriate, especially when immediate action is required to prevent or alleviate suffering by the patient. However, as a general approach, forcing one's own decision upon an infirm or irrational client confuses the moral right of a veterinarian to speak up for the patient with the right to speak for the client as well. Veterinarians rarely have better knowledge about their clients than clients possess about themselves. Moreover, even in instances in which a doctor might know more about a client's needs than the client, there usually will be other people who not only know more than the doctor about the client but have a much stronger moral claim to speak on the client's behalf. I am referring to relatives of the client, who do have a moral right that supersedes that of someone outside the family to step in and make a decision for a loved one when a decision must be made for him. Others who have a stronger moral claim to speak on a client's behalf than the veterinarian are close friends of the client.

It follows from these considerations that when a client does not appear able to make a voluntary and rational choice regarding care for his animal, and when the animal's condition allows time for postponing an immediate decision, the doctor should attempt to contact a family member or friend who can assist the client in making a decision. Ideally, such a person should come to the practice to confer with both the client and doctor. This approach will not only assure that the client's needs will be spoken for. It can help to protect the doctor against a potential legal claim that the doctor violated the client's right to make the decision regarding treatment of his animal.

PROTECTING A PATIENT FROM AN IGNORANT, NEGLECTFUL, OR ABUSIVE CLIENT

Practitioners sometimes see clients whose decision about a particular treatment, or whose general care for their animal, is harmful to the animal. In such situations, a doctor's inclination to speak out in the animal's behalf can conflict with his desire to keep the client, or the realization that his chances of changing the client's behavior are remote.

Veterinarians occupy a different position in circumstances involving abuse or neglect of patients than do physicians. In many cases, state laws require physicians to report to public health or law enforcement authorities injuries or conditions that appear to have resulted from neglect, abuse, or certain kinds of criminal activity. This can afford physicians protection from complaints by patients, because they can respond that they were compelled by the law to report a problem. Veterinarians, on the other hand, in most states are rarely, if ever, required by law to report cases of abuse of their patients, even those so serious as to amount to the crime of animal cruelty. Moreover, there is often no assurance that an abused animal will be cared for properly when abuse is reported to the authorities; some government agencies and humane societies are more likely to euthanize such animals than to try to rehabilitate or place them.

In short, in many cases in which a client is harming his animal, the only person who will be able to speak up for that animal is the veterinarian – and if the doctor does speak out, there probably will be no one to shield him from the consequences.

The range of possible responses to cases of ignorance, neglect, or abuse vary widely. When a client seems genuinely concerned about his animal, but is harming it out of ignorance, the doctor can make a significant contribution to the interests of both the animal and client by educating the client. In such cases, contacting the client periodically or scheduling regular follow-up visits can often be helpful. When the problem is laziness on the client's part to attend to his animal's needs, some enthusiastic exhortation and encouragement might do the trick. The difficulties become greater when a client has a downright bad or abusive attitude toward the animal. In some cases, careful criticism of the client's behavior might be possible, but criticism can be pointless when a client seems incapable of really caring for the patient. Some doctors will suggest that a client think about giving up the animal for adoption, or will volunteer to take it from the client to assure that adoption will be attempted. In extreme cases, sparing the animal further suffering might require reporting the matter to the local government body authorized to deal with animal cruelty.

Sometimes, the only self-respecting and ethical approach will be to oppose the client's requests and to insist on a particular course of action if the client wants to retain one's services. In one case, a client came to the hospital with a desperately ill and suffering cat. The client was about to leave for a weekend trip with his family. He understood that his animal faced certain agony if permitted to live a moment longer without pain-deadening drugs. But he did not want to ruin the weekend for himself and his family by having the animal euthanized right away, and asked the doctor to keep the animal going under intensive care, no expense spared, until the following Monday when the family returned and could cope with the situation. There seemed to the doctor only two humane approaches: to agree to the client's request, euthanize the animal, and tell the client that it died of natural causes over the weekend; or to advise the client that keeping the animal alive was wrong and to use all means at his disposal to persuade the client to agree to prompt euthanasia. The former approach would bring the advantages of a larger fee and the possibility of retaining the client. The latter approach would be consistent with the high moral ideals that motivated the doctor's dissatisfaction with the client's request in the first place.

LYING TO BENEFIT PATIENTS OR CLIENTS

The last example raises another issue of concern to normative veterinary ethics: under what circumstances a veterinarian might be justified in lying to clients to protect the interests of patients or clients.

Lying is a controversial subject among philosophers in general and biomedical ethicists in particular. Some maintain that one should never lie, whatever the consequences (20). Others hold that we have a strong obligation to tell the truth, but that this obligation is sometimes outweighed by an obligation not to hurt people unnecessarily or to help them (21). Still others recommend liberal use of lying in the medical context in order to benefit patients (22).

The following are among the kinds of lies that veterinarians can tell to clients in order to protect the interests of patients:

• Telling the client that the animal's suffering is much worse than it is, in order to induce the client to agree to euthanasia, so that the patient will not suffer needlessly;

- Telling a client who asks if there is a noneuthanasia alternative that there is no such alternative when in fact there is, in order to induce the client to choose euthanasia rather than the alternative, which will cause the animal to suffer and has a low probability of success;
- Telling a client that one will euthanize his healthy animal when in fact one has no such intention and will attempt to place the animal in a suitable home;
- Deliberately underestimating the cost of a proposed procedure, in order to get the client committed to the procedure to a point where he will feel obligated to pay the additional costs once they become necessary;
- Deliberately overestimating the cost of a noneuthanasia alternative that is not likely to succeed in order to induce the client to choose euthanasia.

The following are some of the kinds of lies a doctor can tell to clients in an attempt to benefit them:

- Telling a client that his animal passed away peacefully and without suffering, when in fact it suffered considerably;
- Assuring a client who chose euthanasia prematurely that putting the animal to sleep was medically necessary at the time;
- Telling a client that there are no alternatives to euthanasia when in fact there are, in order to spare the client the considerable upset or expense such an alternative would entail;
- Deliberately overestimating the costs or underestimating the probability of success of a noneuthanasia alternative, in order to spare the client the upset or expense of such an alternative;
- Assuring a client that his animal died from unavoidable natural causes, when in fact its death was caused by the owner's neglect or abuse.

It is beyond the scope of this text to offer a theory of lying in the veterinary context. The following observations are offered to assist the reader in formulating his own approach to the issue:

1. To lie is to make an assertion that one knows to be false with the purpose of inducing someone else to believe that it is true. Lying is thus only one form of deception, and the fact that a deception might not be termed a lie does not make it morally correct. Failing to tell a client that a member of his staff was responsible for the patient's death might not be properly called "lying." But whatever one calls it, it certainly can be a deception that raises moral issues; for it can involve withholding information from a client with the intention of preventing him from knowing some fact he might want to know. Sometimes, the moral issue for a veterinarian will be whether it is justifiable to withhold or manipulate information even though these actions might not, strictly speaking, be termed "lying."

2. One must avoid any temptation to think that lying is justified if it produces more happiness than unhappiness for all concerned. Lying is inherently evil. It involves a manipulation, indeed in a very real sense, a possession of the person to whom one lies. This is so even when a lie is intended to benefit the person who is told the lie. As Charles Fried explains, lying

> violates the principle of respect [for persons], for I must affirm that the mind of another person is available to me in a way in which I cannot agree my mind would be available to him – for if I do so agree, then I would not expect my lie to be believed. ... When I do intentional physical harm, I say that your body, your person, is available for my purposes. When I lie, I lay claim to your mind (23).

When a veterinarian lies to a client, he violates the implicit understanding between the two that the doctor serves the client, who is an autonomous adult capable of making his own choices. Therefore, if lying to a client is ever justified, it can only be justified for the gravest of reasons, and only in the most extreme and infrequent of circumstances.

3. As Fried argues (24), a case can be made for lying when one is being forced into either lying or violating a very important moral duty, and lying to a potential wrongdoer is the only way of acting in accordance with the duty. Fried imagines a situation in which someone is forced by an assassin to tell the whereabouts of the assassin's would-be victim. In such a case, Fried maintains, lying is justified because the assassin has no right to the truth, telling the truth would violate one's duty not to cause great harm, and the lie would be told to someone attempting to perpetrate a greater wrong. Although lying normally involves great disrespect for the person who is told the lie, the assassin in Fried's example forfeits the right to this respect because he is attempting to use the institution of truth-telling to enable him to act in a way that is fundamentally disrespectful of others.

Fried's principle does not justify lying when it would result on balance in more happiness than unhappiness. A veterinarian might be able to maximize utility (see Chapter 5) by telling a client that he will euthanize a healthy patient intending all the while to give it to someone else, or by lying to a client about the availability of treatment in order to spare the client unnecessary upset or expense. But such clients would not be forcing the doctor into a choice between lying or causing great harm. In these, and many other kinds of cases, the doctor is not being asked to lie, and even if he were, he could continue to tell the truth knowing that he is not responsible for the fact that someone would be more upset by the truth than a lie.

On the other hand, one can imagine circumstances in which a client's demand for the truth would put a veterinarian in a position in which he must lie in order to avoid being an integral part of a heinous moral offense. Suppose a race horse will suffer irreparable injury and great pain if it is run, the client requests a medication that the doctor knows will enable it to run, but the client makes it clear that the horse will be scratched only if the doctor (and no one else) says it will break down if it is run under any circumstances. Here, I would argue, the veterinarian may lie about the horse's ability to run because he is placed in an unavoidable position in which his telling the truth would be part of a great moral wrong.

To be sure, this last example is somewhat fanciful – a fact that illustrates that Fried's principle justifies lying by a veterinarian (or anyone else) only in the most unusual circumstances. For if the doctor in the example knows that he routinely must lie in order to spare the client's animals great suffering, he will probably be able to extricate himself from the professional relationship. When this is possible (as it often is), or when there is another doctor who will do a client's unsavory bidding, it is difficult to characterize the situation as one in which the veterinarian is being coerced by the client into a choice of either lying or doing great harm.

VETERINARIANS AND BREED STANDARDS

The standards of breed associations can raise ethical problems for a companion animal doctor. He might be asked to euthanize a healthy animal whose only "failing" is that it does not meet such standards. Veterinarians routinely perform surgical procedures required by certain breed standards. Some doctors are asked to remove or conceal breed standard "defects."

A Professional Approach to Breed Standards

To a large extent, the existence of these problems stems from the breed standards themselves. If standards were more inclusive, there would be fewer animals for whom euthanasia or fraudulent cosmetic procedures are sought.

Breed standards can play an important role in assisting people to choose an appropriate animal. Different breeds provide different physical and psychological characteristics, which can be matched to the needs and proclivities of owners. Additionally, the various appearances and personalities of the breeds are often intrinsically interesting and pleasing. Although breed standards are all, to a certain extent, accidents of history, given the breeds as they have emerged, some standards can make esthetic and behavioral sense and need not in themselves involve a denigration of the value of the animal. For example, it is not unreasonable to restrict show quality Yorkshire Terriers to a weight of 7 pounds and their distinctive range of colors (25). A 15-pound Yorkie is quite a different kind of critter. There seems nothing wrong, given the way this breed has developed, to ask that people who prefer a small, white dog consider the Maltese, which has its own delightful appearance and personality.

Unfortunately, some breed standards make no sense from an esthetic standpoint. Yorkies are "disqualified" if they have an albino toenail, even though it usually takes some effort to find any nails under all the hair. Some breed standards cause animals discomfort because they require the surgical procedure of ear cropping. Other standards involve or have resulted in physical characteristics or genetic predispositions that range from the uncomfortable, as in the case of the many-wrinkled Shar-pei prone to skin problems (26), to the fatal, as in the case of the Manx cat which has a high incidence of spinal and neurological anomalies (27). As one text notes, "with many breed standards, undesirable features unfortunately are often associated with anatomic features the breed standard prescribes" (26).

There are several reasons why veterinarians must take an active interest in the promotion of rational breed standards.

First, the profession already plays an important role in supporting breed standards: some veterinarians euthanize or sterilize animals that do not meet these standards, and they often acquiesce in the judgments of breed associations that certain animals are only "pet quality." If veterinarians are supporting breed standards, they might as well support standards that are morally defensible.

Second, as healers and protectors of companion animals, veterinarians should not tolerate standards that cause such animals significant pain, discomfort, or disease for no other reason than that some people find traits associated with these problems pleasing.

Third, as professionals who serve the interests of their clients, veterinarians have a moral obligation to help clients avoid unnecessary expense and emotional distress. Some esthetically foolish breed standards translate into vastly higher prices owners must pay for "acceptable" animals. Other standards can bring clients significant heartache and veterinary bills when the time comes to cope with a breed-associated disorder.

Finally, as we have seen, veterinarians have a strong self-interest in elevating the image of their companion animal patients. Clearly, some breed standards degrade and devalue companion animals. An animal is not regarded as something of great value if it is subjected to painful procedures or can suffer a debilitating disease simply because some people find a certain trait esthetically pleasing.

It follows from these considerations that the profession should, at the very least, work to eliminate breed standards that 1) are esthetically superfluous given the general appearance of a breed and are used as a justification for the killing of healthy animals; 2) require veterinary procedures that cause significant discomfort to patients and expense to clients; and 3) are associated with discomfort or disease.

The AVMA has recognized in principle the legitimacy of efforts by the profession to promote rational breed standards. Its official position on ear trimming recommends "that action be taken to delete mention of cropped or trimmed ears from breed standards for dogs and to prohibit the showing of dogs with cropped or trimmed ears if such animals were born after some reasonable date" (28). To be sure, many questions can be asked about what breed standards violate moral requirements, and about what veterinarians and their professional associations should do to eliminate such standards.

Euthanasia and Sterilization of "Defective" Animals

As I have argued, it is a denigration of the value of companion animal patients, and of the image of the veterinarian as a medical professional, to kill healthy companion animals that can make good and loving pets. Killing healthy animals that can make wonderful pets but that deviate from purely esthetic breed standards is no less a devaluation of the patient and doctor, whether or not these standards are defensible from an esthetic standpoint.

It is certainly better to sterilize a "defective" healthy animal than to kill it. However, if a particular standard is one that veterinarians ought to oppose, sterilizing animals that do not meet this standard to "protect the breed" is to engage in the support of an improper standard. Nevertheless, a doctor who can convince a client who wants a so-called "defective" animal killed to sell it as "pet quality" on condition that it be sterilized has done a good deed given the world as it is. Surrender of a "defective" pure-bred animal to a shelter can often allay a client's fear that the breed will be "polluted" as well as save the animal's life, because many shelters require sterilization of adopted animals.

Ear Cropping and Tail Docking

In recommending the elimination of ear cropping, the AVMA has determined that whatever benefits might result from the process do not merit the costs to patients and clients. The correctness of this judgment is, I submit, beyond dispute. The procedure requires general anesthesia, as well as substantial knowledge of the surgical technique and meticulous attention to detail. Even then, it is associated with hemorrhage, difficulty in keeping supporting braces in place, self-trauma, and adverse psychological effects. These problems tend to be worse when the procedure is done on older animals (29). Commonly, the ears fail to stand, necessitating further intervention (30).

One veterinarian notes in his discussion showing doctors how to trim ears that some veterinarians are opposed to the procedure. He justifies his discussion by claiming that if veterinarians "refuse to do it ... others who are less qualified will do it much less humanely" (31). This is a terrible argument. The fact that some people might treat animals more inhumanely than veterinarians does not justify their being treated inhumanely. Indeed, if anything, it is worse that veterinarians treat them inhumanely, because veterinarians presumably are committed to the prevention of unjustifiable animal suffering.

Some animal welfare advocates also call for elimination of docked tails from breed standards on the grounds that this is an immoral mutilation or "disfigurement" (32). These terms are not so much an argument as a conclusion, and in the case of tail docking they are highly overblown. Few people would argue that sterilizing an animal for the convenience of its owner or to prevent unwanted strays is a "mutilation," even though it involves invasive surgery and will probably be of no direct benefit to the animal. The question is whether the possible detriments are serious enough to outweigh the benefits. Dogs with trimmed tails appear "disfigured" only to those who prefer the natural tail, and many people do not prefer the natural tail. The esthetic enjoyment of a short tail is, to be sure, not a momentously important benefit. But the detriments of the procedure need not be serious either. When performed early in a puppy's life, tail trimming can be accomplished quickly, without anesthesia, and does not appear to cause great or long-lasting distress (33). Given the impact on the animal, the procedure does not seem morally prohibited. On the other hand, a respectable argument can be made that, because tail docking is useless and not of significant benefit to either patient or client, it would be *better* if veterinarians did not do it.

Concealment of Breed Defects

One approach to sensible *or* indefensible breed standards that is not acceptable is concealment of traits that violate these standards. To do this is to deceive or defraud those for whom buying, breeding, or showing animals with genuine traits is important. Doctors who find certain breed "defects" to be unsupportable, or who do not regard sterilization of animals with such traits to be reasonable, can behave ethically by opposing the relevant standards openly, instead of engaging in behavior that could deceive someone down the line.

DECLAWING AND "DEBARKING"

The removal of the claws of domestic cats raises serious ethical issues, because the procedure can have a definite negative impact on the animals. There is the discomfort and normal risks associated with the surgery, and the fact that a declawed cat can suffer serious injury or lose its life if it escapes from the house and cannot defend itself. The AVMA has attempted to strike a balance between the problems this procedure can cause for the animals and the fact that for some owners, declawing is necessary to prevent destruction of their possessions. The AVMA has concluded that "declawing of domestic cats is justifiable when the cat *cannot* be trained to refrain from using its claws destructively" (34).

There are probably few pronouncements of official veterinary ethics ignored more frequently than this one. By all accounts, declawing is a very common procedure (35). It is, surely, far more common than the number of cats that cannot be trained to refrain from destructive use of their claws. If doctors are to follow the official standard and pay due regard to the interests of feline patients, they must attempt to help clients address the problem of destructiveness by all available nonsurgical means. If declawing still appears to be necessary, clients must be informed clearly about what must be done to safeguard the animal.

According to one veterinarian, surgery on the vocal cords to suppress barking is "often done when dogs are kept alone in apartments during the day or whenever their barking becomes a nuisance" (36). Like the declawing of cats, this procedure poses significant risks to the animal. It is associated with long-term complications that are difficult to correct, including stricture or webbing of the glottus (37). Routinely, the animal continues to make a noise that is described by the author quoted above as "a coughlike sound."

Some veterinarians chastise objections to debarking as unscientific and sentimental. The dogs, these doctors claim, do not know the difference, and people who criticize the procedure are merely imagining the unhappiness they would experience if they were unable to talk.

Whether debarked dogs experience frustration or unhappiness is not the only issue. Most dogs make an enormously wide range of sounds. Barking and more subtle kinds of vocalizations can be used to ask for or demand food or a walk, to gain an owner's attention, warn off intruders, signal that the dog does not wish to be annoyed, express anger or frustration, and in play. Clearly, to take such behaviors away is to prevent the great majority of dogs from doing many things they would ordinarily do. Their lives and experiences will be less. Indeed, because barking seems to be so much a part of the nature of most breeds, many people would be inclined to say that debarking these animals makes them less of a dog.

Moreover, although we have limited access to the canine mind, there seems greater reason to conclude that dogs do feel frustrated by being unable to bark than that they do not. Dogs are sophisticated in their mental apparatus, which is constructed in most of them to include a good deal of vocalization. Few things that are so much a part of such a being's life would not cause discomfort or frustration if removed or severely restricted. I have seen debarked dogs that appeared to be trying in vain to warn their owners of an approaching stranger. They seemed to know that they were not quite making it work. To dismiss this interpretation as sentimental is to close one's eyes to the facts.

Given the potential medical complications of debarking, its clear deprivation of a range of behaviors, and its likely result of frustration or discomfort, there must be very strong reasons for debarking a dog. It is not enough that the barking is a nuisance to the owner or his neighbors. It is not enough that addressing the problem by nonsurgical means would require behavioral training or expense. Surely, no weaker showing should be made for debarking a dog than for declawing a cat. If one were to apply the AVMA's position on declawing to debarking, one would have to insist that before debarking is justified, the problem must be serious enough to be called *destructive*, and behavioral or other nonsurgical means *cannot* work. Veterinarians who perform this procedure just because a client finds his dog's barking to be a nuisance are participating in a serious denigration of the value of their canine patients and of their profession.

THE KEEPING AND TREATMENT OF WILD OR EXOTIC SPECIES

Since 1973, the AVMA has endorsed a policy opposing the keeping of wild or exotic animals as pets and demanding that "all commercial traffic of these animals for such purposes should be prohibited." This policy is justified on the grounds that 1) people "acquire skunks, raccoons, monkeys, alligators, and other exotic species because they like to possess unusual pets or regard them as status symbols;" 2) exotic species create "disease, diet, and exercise problems" different from those in dogs and cats; and 3) disposing of such animals "can be a traumatic experience, with difficulty in relocating such animals" (38). The AVMA has held firm to this policy, even in the face of substantial opposition by veterinarians who treat wild species, especially ferrets (39).

The issues of whether it is morally appropriate for veterinarians to treat wild pets and whether the organized profession should oppose such treatment must be distinguished clearly from the question of whether it is morally permissible for veterinarians to treat certain species of wild animals in states where doing so is illegal. As I argued in Chapter 4, doctors who disobey questionable wildlife laws might disobey reasonable ones as well, and could be responsible for injuries or zoonoses caused by animals that should not be possessed by private citizens. Every state in this country permits people to keep a wide range of wild and domestic animals as pets. If people cannot lawfully have a ferret, for example, they still may choose from among many other kinds of animals. It is therefore difficult to maintain that a client's desire to keep or a veterinarian's desire to treat a particular prohibited species are sufficiently important to justify risking the consequences of disobeying the law.

The AVMA policy against the possession of wild animals as pets is intended to prevent unnecessary suffering by animals and people. Nevertheless, some of the claims raised in support of the policy are patently false and do not appear to reflect a willingness to consider all sides of the story.

For example, there are surely too many different kinds of wild and exotic[e] species to make it possible to brand *all* equally as inappropriate pets. Surely, there are *some* exotic animals that can be kept healthy and safe by *some* knowledgeable and careful owners. If this were not the case, all states would prohibit the possession of all wild species. Moreover, although there undoubtedly are some people who acquire certain wild animals as status symbols or for certain strange psychological reasons, the same is true of some people who own dogs or cats.

Moreover, the AVMA's position regarding the dangerousness of *all* wild pets seems highly exaggerated. It is claimed that ferrets, for example, "have severely bitten many people, especially inflicting mutilating bites to infants," that they "are susceptible to and could transmit rabies" and that there is "no licensed rabies vaccine for use in ferrets" (40). However, what one wants to know is how the rate of bites by pet ferrets compares with the rate of bites by pet dogs and cats. One wants to know the extent to which ferret bites are attributable to owner negligence rather than some feature inherent to the species. One wants to know the actual incidence of rabies in pet ferrets that are receiving good veterinary care. According to the federal Centers for Disease Control, the likelihood of rabies in ferrets that have not been in contact with wildlife or that have been vaccinated with modified live virus rabies vaccine is "extremely remote" (41). The fact that there is no licensed ferret rabies vaccine is a function of a lack of adequate research data (42) – a situation that might well change as the animal gains greater acceptance. It is impossible to believe that practitioners who speak enthusiastically about ferrets as pets and about their ability to provide these animals good veterinary care, are all ignorant or incompetent.

There are many reasons why the organized profession should reconsider its opposition to the keeping of wild and exotic species as pets.

First, opposing private ownership of all wild species is like banning the consumption of alcoholic beverages. It simply will not work (43). Given the fact that

---

[e]The law defines a "wild" species as one that is not domesticated, i.e., one that has not been bred or tamed for economic uses, or generally and typically does not live in very close association with man. The legal definitions of the "wild" and "domestic" are not entirely biologically based. Although a few courts and legal scholars would have it otherwise, whether a particular animal will be classified as wild or domestic generally does not turn on whether it has been tamed, but on whether it belongs to a *species* that is wild or domestic relative to a given area. For example, a trained and gentle elephant that is located in the United States is classified as a wild animal; but the law will regard the same elephant when it is located in India as a domestic animal, because in that country elephants are commonly used as beasts of burden. An "exotic" species can be defined as a wild species not native to a particular area. Some veterinarians maintain that ferrets are not wild animals because they cannot fend for themselves in the wild, or because there are countries in which they are considered domestic animals. These are not relevant considerations. In the eyes of the law, ferrets, parrots, budgerigars, cockatoos, rabbits, and lizards located in the United States are all wild animals.

many such animals are in homes around the country (and are there lawfully), the interests of these animals and their owners would be served by the availability of first-rate veterinary care. A policy discouraging practitioners from treating these animals can only drive owners to seek medical advice from less qualified pet store operators and self-styled lay "experts."

Second, a blanket policy against the keeping of all wild animals as pets prevents the articulation and promotion of discriminating policies regarding these animals. The public and government undoubtedly need guidance about what species can make good pets, and about what owners must do to care for them properly. However, the organized profession will play no role in the determination of rational distinctions and standards if it opposes the keeping of all such animals.

Third, the organized profession will not be able to exert its influence to assure technical competence and ethical behavior on the part of those veterinarians who are treating wild or exotic pets, if its approach to the keeping of these animals is opposition.

Finally, encouragement of veterinary care for species that do make good pets can provide another source of practice revenues. Accomplishing this might not be easy. Some doctors will need further training before they can competently treat some of these species. Already overburdened veterinary students will be required to learn about even more kinds of animals. Undoubtedly, certain species must remain off-limits to owners and veterinarians alike. But for reasons I have already discussed, it is far better for veterinarians to address the revenue problem by increasing the range of patients for which they can provide competent medical care than by turning to the merchandising of nonprofessional goods and services.

REFERENCES

1. Regan T: *The Case for Animal Rights.* Berkeley: University of California Press, 1983 p 109.
2. *Id.*, 119.
3. Just Like Us? *Harper's Magazine* 277:50, Aug 1988.
4. 1986 Report of the AVMA Panel on Euthanasia. *J Am Vet Med Assoc* 188:253, 1986.
5. *Id.*, 267, emphasis supplied.
6. Rachels J: Active and Passive Euthanasia. *N Engl J Med* 292:78-80, 1975.
7. Louisell D: Euthanasia and Bioeuthanasia. *Linacre Quarterly* 40:307, 1973.
8. Rollin BE: *Animal Rights and Human Morality.* Buffalo: Prometheus Books, 1981, p 60.
9. Report of the AVMA Panel on Euthanasia. *J Am Vet Med Assoc* 188:252-268, 1986.
10. E.g., Fox MW: Editor's commentary. In Fox MW and Mickley LD (eds): *Advances in Animal Welfare Science - 1985.* Boston: Martinus Nijhoff, 1986, pp 85-86.
11. Rowan AN: T-61 use in the euthanasia of domestic animals: A survey. In Fox MW and Mickley LD (eds.). *Advances in Animal Welfare Science - 1985.* Boston: Martinus Nijhoff, 1986, pp 79-84.
12. Report of the AVMA Panel on Euthanasia. *J Am Vet Med Assoc* 188:262, 1986.
13. *Id.*, 263.
14. Kay WJ: Euthanasia. *Trends* 1(5):52-54, 1986. This wise essay deserves the study of all veterinarians.
15. *Id.*, 52.

16. See, Cohen SP: The Role of Social Work in a Veterinary Hospital Setting. *Vet Clin North Am Small Anim Pract* 15:355-363, 1985.

17. Schwabe CW: *Veterinary Medicine and Human Health*, ed 3. Baltimore: Williams & Wilkins, 1984, p 624.

18. E.g., Hart BL: *Behavior of Domestic Animals*. San Francisco: Freeman, 1983; Voith V: Behavioral Disorders. In Ettinger SJ (ed): *Textbook of Internal Veterinary Medicine*, ed. 2. Philadelphia: W.B. Saunders Co., 1983, pp 208-227.

19. Sentell v. New Orleans and Carrollton Railroad Co., 166 U.S. 698, 701 (1897).

20. E.g., Kant I: *The Doctrine of Virtue*. Gregor MJ (trans). Philadelphia: University of Pennsylvania Press, 1964, pp 428-430.

21. E.g., Beauchamp TL and Childress JF: Principles of Biomedical Ethics. ed 2. New York: Oxford University Press, 1982, p 223.

22. E.g., Leslie A: Ethics and the practice of placebo therapy. In Reiser SJ, Dyck AJ, and Curran WJ (eds): *Ethics in Medicine*. Cambridge, Mass.: MIT Press, 1979, p 242 (stating that "deception is completely moral when it is used for the welfare of the patient"); Collins J: Should doctors tell the truth? In Reiser *et al.*, p 221 (maintaining that "every physician should cultivate lying as a fine art").

23. Fried C: *Right and Wrong*. Cambridge: Harvard University Press, 1978, pp 69-78.

24. *Id.*, 67.

25. Munday E: *The Yorkshire Terrier*. New York: Arco Publishing Co., 1967, p 17.

26. Muller GH, Kirk RW, and Scott DW: *Small Animal Dermatology*. ed 3. Philadelphia: W.B. Saunders Co., 1983, p 204.

27. Bailey CS and Morgan JP: Diseases of the Spinal Cord. In Ettinger SJ (ed): *Textbook of Internal Veterinary Medicine*. ed 2. Philadelphia: W.B. Saunders Co., 1983, pp 555-556.

28. The Veterinarian's Role in Companion Animal Welfare. Schaumburg, IL: American Veterinary Association, undated, unpaginated.

29. Smith KW: Cosmetic Ear Trimming. In Bojrab MJ (ed): *Current Techniques in Small Animal Surgery*. ed 2. Philadelphia: Lea & Febiger, 1983, pp 90-93.

30. Smith KW: Surgical Correction for Faulty Carriage of Trimmed Ears. In Bojrab MJ (ed): *Current Techniques in Small Animal Surgery*. ed 2. Philadelphia: Lea & Febiger, 1983, pp 93-96.

31. Smith KW: Cosmetic Ear Trimming. In Bojrab MJ (ed): *Current Techniques in Small Animal Surgery*. ed 2. Philadelphia: Lea & Febiger, 1983, p 90.

32. Cosmetic Surgery or Surgery to Correct "Vices." *Position Statements*. Greenwich, CT: Association of Veterinarians for Animal Rights, undated, unpaginated.

33. Cawley AJ and Archibald J. Plastic Surgery. In Archibald J (ed): *Canine Surgery*, ed 2. Santa Barbara: American Veterinary Publications, 1974, p 139.

34. *The Veterinarian's Role in Companion Animal Welfare*. Schaumburg, IL: American Veterinary Medical Association, undated, unpaginated, emphasis supplied.

35. See, e.g., Herron MR: Feline Onychectomy. In Bojrab MJ (ed): *Current Techniques in Small Animal Surgery*. ed 2. Philadelphia: Lea & Febiger, 1983, pp 420-422 (stating that the "veterinary clinician is often called upon to declaw cats").

36. Leighton RL: Soft Tissues, Tonsils, Pharynx, Larynx, and Trachea. In Archibald J (ed): *Canine Surgery*. ed 2. Santa Barbara: American Veterinary Publications, 1974, p 350.

37. Kagan K: Devocalization Procedures. In Bojrab MJ (ed): *Current Techniques in Small Animal Surgery.* ed 2. Philadelphia: Lea & Febiger, 1983, p 264.
38. Wild or Exotic Animals as Pets. *1988 AVMA Directory,* p 489.
39. Ferret as Pets. *J Am Vet Med Assoc* 189:17, 1986.
40. Ferret Controversy. *J Am Vet Med Assoc* 190:261, 1987 (adoption by the AVMA Council on Public Health and Regulatory Veterinary Medicine of language of the National Association of State Public Health Veterinarians).
41. Viral Diseases: Pet Ferrets and Rabies. *Veterinary Public Health Notes.* Atlanta: Centers for Disease Control, Oct 1980.
42. *The Merck Veterinary Manual.* ed 6. Rahway, NJ: Merck & Co., 1986, p 1015.
43. See, e.g., Petzke D: The Pet of the Year Isn't a Pimp or a Pup But It is Just as Cute. *Wall Street Journal* Apr 4, 1986:1 (estimating 400,000 ferret owners in the United States).

Chapter

21

Farm, Food, and Sport Animal Practice: The New Frontier of Normative Veterinary Ethics

Normative veterinary ethics can rely on a growing consensus regarding the nature of companion animals and their importance to clients. The increasing appreciation of the value of these animals prompts many of the questions that must be asked about companion animal practice and points the way to certain answers.

In contrast, there is as yet no emerging consensus about the nature or value of typical farm, food, or sport animals. The overwhelming majority of people believe that it is morally permissible to use certain animals for food, draft, fiber and other products, and in sporting events. However, few people know very much about the lives and experiences of these animals. It is far from obvious what they would say about ethical issues relating to agricultural and sport animals if these animals were accorded greater public attention. Indeed, there is significant uncertainty and disagreement among those who study and work with agricultural and sport animals about what scientific and ethical principles should govern our behavior towards them.

The very fact that companion animals can be so highly regarded raises difficult issues for agricultural and sport animal doctors. Some farm and sport animals are not markedly different in their mental capacities from companion animals. At a time the profession seeks to promote companion animals as valued beings, to what extent must it also advocate the interests of its food, farm, and sport animal patients? In general, what should be the role of practitioners who serve economic interests of agricultural and sport clients, in a profession whose increasing number of companion animal doctors has a strong stake in the promotion of *animal* interests?

These issues are complicated by the fact that many large animal doctors are under severe economic pressure. Normative veterinary ethics must recognize the legitimate interests of doctors and their clients. Nevertheless, due regard also must be given to the interests of the animals and the public. There can be no guarantees that ethical deliberation will always make life easier for already beleaguered agricultural and sport animal practitioners.

The primary aim of this chapter is to identify important issues relevant to assessing the profession's moral obligations regarding agricultural and sport animals.

the central thesis of the chapter is that normative veterinary ethics stands barely at the frontier of serious consideration of many issues raised by food, farm, and sport animal practice. There is need for much scientific and ethical investigation. In the meantime, one must avoid premature and superficial responses to hard questions.

SETTLING UPON BASIC PREMISES

One task for an acceptable approach to ethical issues in agricultural or sport animal practice is to establish certain basic premises from which practical moral deliberation can proceed. The following are offered as examples of such principles.

1. People may use and benefit from agricultural and sport animals.

One fundamental premise upon which all farm and sport animal practice rests is that people may sometimes use animals for purposes such as food, fiber, and entertainment. This view is so widely and deeply held in our society that one can assert it not just as a correct moral principle, but as a fact of life that any realistic approach to normative veterinary ethics must accept as a given.

To be sure, there are those who believe that it is inherently immoral for human beings to use animals for our own ends. Some of these people may think that they are owed a demonstration of why the human use of animals is permissible. Several arguments for weighting human interests more heavily than animal interests are presented in Chapter 11. But for us to engage here in an attempt to refute animal use abolitionism would be a hopeless task. Those who endorse abolitionism are no more likely to accept refutations of their point of view than the rest of us would be disposed to agree that an animal farmer is the moral equivalent of a slave owner, or that a meat-eater is no better than a human cannibal.

Articulating the objections to animal use abolitionism is a legitimate task for animal ethics, which as a branch of philosophical ethics seeks theoretical completeness. However, for the veterinary profession, its clients, and the great majority of the public, abolitionism is a fringe position espoused by a hardy, but nevertheless tiny few. It has almost always been so. This is not just a historical fact, but important moral evidence. Through the centuries, in diverse places and cultures, the overwhelming majority of mankind have consulted their basic moral intuitions – and have concluded that it is proper to use animals for food, fiber, draft, entertainment, and companionship. Abolitionists may prefer to think that this belief has been a giant, horrible prejudice. However, the fact that most people who have lived and toiled on this earth have arrived at the same general conclusion is itself powerful evidence of its correctness.

2. Agricultural and sport animal clients are entitled to a fair profit and may factor economic considerations into management decisions.

Because people may morally have certain animal products and services, producers of these goods and services are entitled to a fair profit. Otherwise, these items could not be provided. Because producers are entitled to a profit, they may sometimes factor economic considerations into decisions about what will be done with their animals, even though such decisions sometimes might have a negative impact on the animals. This is not the end of the matter. For the animals too have legitimate needs and interests, which place limitations upon how they may be used or treated.

3. The role of public demand in the determination of how agricultural and sport animals are treated must not be underestimated.

People who are critical of the treatment of agricultural and sport animals tend to focus on owners, veterinarians, and others involved in the production process as the source of alleged problems. In fact, the ways in which agricultural and sport animals are treated rarely flow from some immutable value system or mind-set of producers or veterinarians. The *public* is the pre-eminent force in the determination of how agricultural and sport animals are used. I have met few producers who would object to more extensive facilities for swine, or greater growing space for broilers, or spending the resources to try to save every sick animal – if consumers were willing to pay the higher prices that such measures would require. The fact that producers cannot make a living unless they provide what the public wants at an acceptable price does not, of course, make all means toward this end morally acceptable. Moreover, producers can be mistaken in thinking that a given husbandry method is more profitable than others that might be better for the animals. Nevertheless, it is public expectation that sets many of the boundaries within which deliberations about agricultural and sport animal welfare operate. Success in promoting the welfare of these animals will depend substantially upon an educated and compassionate public.

4. Agricultural and sport animals have interests that must be taken into account.

Although animal interests need not always prevail when a farm or sport client is faced with a management question, these interests exist nevertheless and must be given the attention and weight they deserve. This seems obvious. Nevertheless, discussions devoid of attention to animal interests are appearing with increasing frequency in the literature espousing the model of the veterinarian as an economic herd manager (see Chapter 15).

Profit is not enough. One of the claims of this emerging literature is that maximization of profit should be the overriding aim of producers and that noneconomic concerns may be considered only after the likelihood of maximum profit is assured. One discussion recommends computing the "expected value" of each alternative approach to an animal health question by

> weighing the value (in dollars) of each potential outcome with the probability that the outcome will occur, given a particular decision, and then summing the weighted values for all potential outcomes for a given branch of the decision tree. If the decision maker chooses the branch with the highest expected value, then he can expect to maximize his profits over a series of such choices (1).

To illustrate this method, the authors ask whether a dairy cow in early lactation with a left displaced abomasum should be given an omentopexy or should be rolled. They calculate that the probable net profit for the operation exceeds that for rolling and therefore recommend the operation. On the other hand, the probable outcomes for omentopexy and percutaneous fixation using a bar suture are calculated as identical. "Since the expected values are equivalent," the authors conclude, "the decision about which approach to use can be made on other than economic grounds" (2). The discussion does not mention the animal's present or future welfare as a relevant consideration in decision-making.

A recent study (3) of the effects of *post partum* disease on milk production in dairy cows reports that certain conditions (e.g., cystic follicles and milk fever) are associated with increased production, while other diseases appear to diminish production. The study sets forth *post partum* disease incidence rates, goals and "action levels" for a number of common diseases. It is stated, for example, that there should be a goal of less than 3% of lactations affected by milk fever, and action to address the disease should commence when this level rises to 10%.

The study does not identify the actual or potential discomfort experienced by the animals as an independent variable in determining whether or at what point veterinary treatment ought to be administered. "Veterinary service" is included as a cost to be factored into the farmer's decision. However, there is no indication that animal pain or distress – insofar as these are evils for the *animals themselves*, as distinguished from potential problems for producers – are relevant to determining the need for veterinary care. It is urged that "(b)efore making recommendations regarding nutrition, disease prevention, or reproduction, the veterinarian should compare the losses incurred from the disease problem with the cost of reducing or alleviating that problem" (4). Such a statement need not be objectionable, provided attention is given *somewhere* to the animals as objects of concern in their own right. Instead, the authors state (4) that "the cost" of disease

> may include the following major components: (1) decreased milk production, (2) milk withheld from market following antibiotic therapy, (3) direct veterinary services, (4) medications, (5) reproductive inefficiency, (6) extra labor, (7) disease preventive and control programs, and (8) loss of animals by death or involuntary culling.

Detriments to the animals are not included explicitly as an independent "cost" of disease or relevant criterion in decisionmaking.

The concept of an ethical cost. The notion that all management decisions can be made solely on the basis of probable maximization of profit is unacceptable. Sometimes, profit may appropriately be the deciding factor. If, for example, two approaches to animal husbandry are equally acceptable from a moral point of view (say, because neither causes more distress to the animals than the other), a farmer might be justified in choosing the more profitable approach. Sometimes, economic considerations may justify a somewhat diminished level of animal welfare, provided that at least an acceptable welfare level is maintained (see below).

However, one should not assert as a general principle that noneconomic considerations can be entertained only after probable profit maximization is calculated. Farm and sport animals are not machines or plants, but sentient beings. As we saw in Chapter 11, all animals capable of experiencing negative mental states have an interest in not experiencing such states. They also have other interests. One must *always* give some consideration to the impact upon these interests of any production method or course of veterinary care. This is owed to farm and sport animals in return for what is taken from them.

An "ethical cost" can be defined as a detriment, not solely expressible by or reducible to monetary terms, of some behavior or enterprise, that must be considered in determining the moral appropriateness of that behavior or enterprise. Ethical costs are not restricted to (although they may sometimes include) such negative mental states as pain, suffering, distress, or discomfort. An ethical cost of a certain course of action can be the fact that it would violate a moral right not reducible to utilitarian cost-benefit analysis. Ethical costs in veterinary practice are not limited to detriments to animals. Among the potential ethical costs of certain ways of treating animals may be the failure of certain animals to experience positive goods. Ethical costs can also include human noneconomic costs, such as insensitivity to animal welfare that can result from certain ways of treating animals.

It does not follow from the concept of an ethical cost that profit may never justify animal distress. The concept of an ethical cost does not preclude taking into consideration quantifiable economic costs that might be associated with attempting to lessen or remove some ethical cost. The concept of an ethical cost is consistent with deciding not to provide a certain kind of veterinary care in the name of general herd productivity, if ethical analysis should determine that such an approach is morally justified under given circumstances. It may be difficult to identify relevant ethical costs in herd management practices and to assign these costs their proper weight. But moral behavior in agricultural or sport animal practice requires that ethical costs be considered together with economic costs and benefits.

Is due regard for animal interests consistent with a completely quantitative approach to herd management? Many discussions of cost-benefit analysis in herd management appear to assume that making decisions can be reduced to calculating and comparing numbers. However, if – as is morally obligatory – animal interests must also be factored into decision-making, it is doubtful whether completely quantitative approaches are achievable either in theory or in practice.

Animal mental states, like human mental states, are not precisely quantifiable. Although some researchers are attempting to find measurable behavioral or physiological signs of states such as stress (5), the states themselves are not capable of exact measurement. We do not have, and we surely will never have, units of pain so that we can say that one animal is experiencing, say, twice the pain as another – although we can often determine that one appears to be in more or less pain than another. (We do not even have precise pain units for people, who can communicate their mental states to others.) Nor is it clear how we should quantify and compare across different mental states. Does an hour of moderate discomfort equal 5 minutes of moderate pain in the same animal? In different animals of the same species? In animals of different species? I do not mean to suggest that it is foolish to try to estimate and compare animal pain or distress. It is sometimes necessary to do so, and it is often possible to do it in a rough way. Rather, the point is that it seems impossible to engage in *precise* quantification of the sort that mathematical models of herd management would require in order to place animal interests into their formulae.

Moreover, even when one can reach an intuitively plausible comparison involving animal mental states, there will often remain an independent ethical element not reducible to quantitative comparison that must be factored into the decision about how one ought to act. Suppose it seems plausible to say that by raising veal calves in total confinement in 60 cm-wide crates a farmer can achieve a certain level of profit and can produce a level of satisfaction in the public that taken together "exceeds" any pain or distress experienced by the animals. There still remains the question of whether the profit and public satisfaction provide sufficient moral *justification* for the practice. Sometimes, simply comparing benefits with detriments might seem appropriate. But it will not always be so.

Verbal maneuvers: redefining "disease." Some advocates of the model of the veterinarian as economic manager admit that they will tolerate disease under certain circumstances to promote productivity (6). However, other proponents of this model want to redefine the concept of disease so that a dilemma between choosing between productivity and health will not arise. Dr. Thomas Stein suggests that disease should not identified by the presence of such things as fever, diarrhea, or cough in individual animals.

> Rather, problems are identified as inadequate performance. In dairy herds this might be measured by calving-to-conception interval, days in milk at first breeding, or rolling average for annual milk production. ... Disease in populations describes a deviation between what is *happening* and what is *expected* to happen ...
> This redefinition of disease implies that health and production are identical (7).

In other words, one should not speak of "disease" in, or the "health" of, individual members of a herd or population. The presence of individual animals with cough and fever caused by some microorganism would not indicate the presence of "disease" if the whole herd or population functions as a whole to maximize expected profitability.

It is not surprising why such a redefinition of disease might appeal to some veterinarians. As I suggested in Chapter 15, many people would doubt whether someone who always subordinates decisions about disease to questions of economic productivity ought to be called a "doctor," or a practitioner of veterinary *medicine*. By redefining health and disease in terms of productivity, some proponents of the model of the veterinarian as economic manager may be asserting that they are rightly classified as veterinary doctors.

In any event, Stein's proposed redefinition has little to recommend it. Few veterinarians or clients are likely to accept it. His definition certainly would have a hard time coexisting with the concept of disease utilized in companion animal practice, in which disease is a condition of individual animals, and productivity is rarely an issue, much less considered synonymous with absence of disease. Most important, the ethical issue is not whether something called "disease" may be tolerated in order to maximize production. The issue is whether or to what extent some of the physical states currently seen as components or signs of disease (such as fever, diarrhea, and cough), and the mental accompaniments of these states, may be tolerated in order to promote production. This question will not disappear if the word "disease" is redefined to mean lack of expected productivity.[a]

Thought substitution: "Animal welfare goes without saying." When one challenges producers and veterinarians who do not include explicit reference to animal welfare in their discussions, one often receives the response that "*of course,* animal welfare goes without saying." This is so, it is claimed, because those methods that are productive are also good for the animals. Productivity and animal welfare, it is said, are necessary and invariable correlates: "A productive animal is a happy animal."

There is impressive evidence that productivity is often associated with animal welfare. Certain husbandry practices clearly protect animals from the vagaries of the weather, disease, predators, and themselves. From a pragmatic point of view, the frequent link between productivity and welfare may be the most important tool veterinarians and animal welfare advocates possess to improve the lot of farm and sport animals. The argument that profits can be improved by attention to animal welfare should be one that producers can accept readily.

However, there are several reasons why it is obvious that productivity and welfare need not always go hand in hand.

First, as Professor Stanley Curtis observes, animal welfare is not an absolute. One can often say that there are different possible *levels* of welfare, ranging from

---

[a]Stein cites with approval another proposed redefinition of health as "the level of production that the animal's owners have set as their objective and which is consistent with humane practices" (8). This definition, too, errs in making productivity part of the very essence or definition of health. Nor is it helpful to include reference to humane practices in a definition of health. To ask whether some husbandry practice is "humane" is to ask whether it is, all things considered, morally appropriate (see below). Neither medical diagnosis nor ethical analysis will be served by putting off all decisions regarding whether an animal or group of animals is "healthy" until after one has answered the ethical question whether they are being treated properly.

conditions so slightly beneficial that one would want to say there is a minimal level of welfare, to conditions that approach or constitute optimal welfare (9). Although certain methods of production may yield minimal welfare, or may yield a higher level of welfare than other methods, they may still be far from producing *optimal* welfare. This does not necessarily make such conditions wrong. The judgment must sometimes be made to sacrifice some degree of welfare in order to achieve a certain level of productivity. However, once one recognizes that this is sometimes a possible choice (even if it can be a correct choice), one cannot simply assume that productivity and welfare always converge. One must at least entertain the possibility that they diverge so that one can then justify an approach that does not yield optimal welfare, or that yields a lower level welfare than another possible approach.

Second, economic forces that determine what is profitable often have nothing to do with animal welfare. The fact that consumers may refuse to pay more than a certain amount for pork, or want lamb or turkey during certain holiday seasons, puts economic pressure on producers to institute certain kinds and schedules of production. But there is no reason in principle why such economically-induced husbandry methods must also result in any particular level of welfare.

Third, it is simply beyond question that some production methods will sometimes either cause animals to experience some distress or produce a level of welfare at least somewhat lower than optimal. Among common examples are dehorning calves without anesthesia, total indoor husbandry of swine, and intensive battery cage confinement of laying hens. It is worth emphasizing again that a given husbandry method is not rendered impermissible simply in virtue of the fact that it might not produce optimal welfare. However, the issue of whether a given level of welfare is morally justified cannot be raised at all if one blindly proclaims an identity between productivity and welfare.

I am not maintaining that economic cost is an irrelevant or unimportant consideration in determining what producers and veterinarians may do. My target is the view that attention to animal interests is irrelevant, or is relevant only insofar as it is a means of furthering the interests of farmers, veterinarians, or the public. Economic analysis of food and farm animal management is still in its infancy. It is premature to conclude that no mathematically rigorous decision procedures can be found that will seem morally as well as economically acceptable for certain kinds of management situations. Nevertheless, there is a growing theme in the herd management literature that attention to animal interests is old-fashioned, soft-headed, and ignorant of the facts of life (10). Animal interests, and moral obligations in veterinary practice that reflect the existence and importance of these interests, are as much unavoidable facts of life as anything else. Animal welfare is too important to "go without saying."

5. Individual animals count.

Another basic premise for normative veterinary ethics is that individual agricultural and sport animals count. Herds or groups do not feel pain or undergo distress, individual animals do. Therefore, even insofar as we might be allowed to apply utilitarian considerations to animals in herds, we must still pay attention to the mental states of individual animals. Individual animals also count in the sense that the interests of one or of a few can take precedence over some interest of producers, veterinarians, or the public. This can happen when the price of bringing trivial enjoyments to a large number of people is the imposition of grave suffering upon a smaller number of animals. Individual agricultural and sport animals also count in the sense that pain, distress, and discomfort can be as much an evil to them as it can be to other kinds of animals.

6. Agricultural and sport animals have some basic moral rights.

Animal interests sometimes are sufficiently weighty to rise to the level of moral rights (see Chapter 12). Because agricultural and sport animals are sentient beings, it is undeniable that they must have *some* basic moral rights. For it is simply impossible to suppose that they may be subjected to the most severe pain or the most deprived conditions even if this would bring great pleasure to someone or a large number of people. At *some* point, the line of permissible treatment will be overstepped.

It is considerably easier to say that agricultural and sport animals have some moral rights than to demonstrate what rights they have, or to determine the strength of these rights relative to human interests and rights. Perhaps normative veterinary and animal ethics can suggest preliminary or interim principles regarding the rights of agricultural and sport animals, while further necessary ethical and scientific investigation proceeds. One famous statement of minimal basic animal rights was offered by the British "Brambell Committee" to Enquire into the Welfare of Animals Kept under Intensive Livestock Husbandry Systems. The Committee proposed "five freedoms" for agricultural animals: "sufficient freedom of movement for an animal (1) to get up; (2) lie down; (3) groom normally; (4) turn around; and (5) stretch its limbs" (11). These demands relate not just to the fact that animals deprived of certain basic natural movements are likely to experience negative mental states. The "freedoms" reflect the intuitively appealing notion that certain aspects of an animal's nature are entitled to at least a modicum of respect.

The relevance of domestication. Dr. Fred Jacobs argues (12) that domesticated animals cannot have moral rights. He states that they "have been created by man rather than by nature and hence are, through necessity, subject to the control of man from cradle to grave. Were man to relinquish control of these animals, both man and the domestic animals would suffer catastrophe as biological species." Jacobs criticizes those who think that domesticated animals have "inalienable rights to a perfect existence," or a "right to existence," or must be left free to "roam the countryside and backwoods and damage the environment."

Jacobs' objections to obviously extreme positions are reasonable, but his objections do not count against the view that domesticated animals have moral rights. As was explained in Chapter 12, the concept of animal rights does not entail any particular claim about what rights animals have. To say that animals have rights is to say that they have some very strong interests and claims upon people whose weight cannot be reduced to utilitarian calculation of detriments versus benefits.

The fact that certain characteristics of farm and sport animals, including parts of their temperaments, have been affected by domestication is a relevant consideration in determining the nature and weight of their interests. It also seems plausible to argue that producers have a moral obligation not only to improve husbandry methods to reduce animal stress but also to try to change animals to reduce the kinds of objectionable experiences they can have (13). Yet even such an argument may have its limits. In *Brave New World*, the novelist Aldous Huxley imagined a society that genetically engineers its people to have varying levels of intelligence, so as to enhance the productivity and happiness of the whole. This fictional society is fundamentally disrespectful to human beings. It makes many of them less than what people can be, even if some are too stupid to know it. (Significantly, even Huxley's imagined world must resort to drugs and other forms of psychological manipulation to extinguish unhappiness and anxiety.) Farm animals are beings of some worth and value in part because of their ability to receive their environment. They are lucky, compared with plants, amoebae, and earthworms, because there is so much more of the world that they are capable of taking in. It is therefore not altogether foolish to ask whether too much engineering to extract out distressful mental states would make of agricultural animals less than we ought to allow them to remain. The creation of supermoronic farm animals capable of little more than ingestion, excretion, and production might not be a bother to these animals. But it would say something about the regard one has for these creatures, and, perhaps, for others as well. This may not be a view of animals veterinarians should want to encourage.

At least at present, domesticated animals are capable of experiencing pain and distress. They also have other interests domestication has not extinguished. Moreover, as Jacobs concedes, the fact that domestication often produces animals that cannot fend for themselves obligates people to protect them from conditions they cannot handle without human help.

7. Although assessment of mental states is an important consideration in the determination of animal interests, one must avoid exaggerated claims about these states.

One of the most difficult tasks faced by animal welfare science is determining what mental states animals do experience. Strict behaviorists either deny the existence of animal mental states or refuse to talk about these states because they cannot be observed and measured "objectively." Such behaviorists have little to contribute to animal welfare discussions, which proceed from the eminently reasonable view that animals do have sensations and experiences. On the other hand, there is no shortage of grossly exaggerated attributions of sophisticated mental states to animals.

If one underestimates or overestimates the mental lives of animals, one cannot assign proper moral weight to their interests. Even a cursory look at the literature regarding the assessment of animal mental states reveals that there remains a great deal of conceptual and scientific work to be done before we can fashion a morally satisfactory approach to animal interests.

Mental states and physiological processes. A number of investigators proceed on the assumption that if certain chemicals or physiological processes are associated with specified mental states in human beings, the presence of such chemicals or processes in animals would demonstrate the existence of the *same* mental states in the animals (14). One problem with such a methodology is that it may involve redefinition of the concepts we now apply to human beings, thus resulting in attribution of something quite different to the animals. For example, "fear" as people ordinarily speak of it, involves not just an unpleasant mental state, but the perception of an *object* or state of affairs (that which is feared) that is seen *as* dangerous or threatening. If chemical or physiological process X were to be found in the brains of human beings when they experience fear and in the brains of cows when these animals appear to be avoiding or reacting negatively to some condition, it would not follow that the cows are experiencing fear. For it is far from clear that cows are sophisticated enough to perceive something *as* an object distinct from themselves and to perceive it *as* dangerous or threatening – although we may be able to say that they have some kind of negative mental experience akin or analogous to fear. Nor does the mere presence of a chemical or physiological process in an animal's brain seem sufficient evidence of such mental activity, except to someone who is already disposed to ignore the criteria people normally demand before we say that someone or some being is experiencing fear.

The dangers of premature definition. In 1987, the AVMA organized a Colloquium on the Recognition and Alleviation of Animal Pain and Distress. The Proceedings of the Colloquium (15) demonstrate that the profession stands ready to take the lead in the scientific study of animal pain. But there was also evidence of a tendency of some investigators to engage in hurried and superficial definitions of extremely complex mentalistic concepts.

A Colloquium Panel Report offered definitions of the terms "pain," "anxiety," "fear," "stress," "suffering," "comfort," "discomfort," and "injury." "Anxiety," for example, was defined as "an emotional state involving increased arousal and alertness prompted by an unknown danger that may be present in the immediate environment." It was asserted that fear "can be defined similarly, except that fear would refer to an experienced or known danger in the immediate environment." The Report surmised that a dog trembling in a veterinarian's office during its first visit may be experiencing anxiety while such behavior during the second visit may better be described as "fear of a remembered event" (16).

These definitions of "anxiety" and "fear" depart from what people ordinarily mean by these terms. They also reflect substantive views of animal mental states that are, at the very least, premature. People commonly speak of fear of the unknown, and of anxiety about a known event that is distant from the "immediate environment" temporally or spatially. One can also feel anxious about a past event (e.g., about whether a relative was harmed in a natural disaster), provided there is something one does not yet know about that event. It is also incorrect to refer to either anxiety or fear as "an" emotional state. Our concepts of these states include ranges of different, but related experiences. Anxiety can involve feelings of uncertainty, fear or dread about one's self. To say that you are anxious about your veterinary licensing exams or an impending hospitalization is to say that you see *yourself*, your plans, your happiness, your state of mind threatened by some event or contingency. Experiences of anxiety often require a highly developed sense of the future, because being anxious typically involves an appreciation that one does not know what *the future* will bring. The term "anxiety" is frequently applied to deep and brooding uncertainty relating to life's more important experiences.

It has been determined that receptors for benzodiazepines are found in all vertebrates except the cartilaginous species (17), and that such substances appear to have calming effects on animals, as well as people we would describe as anxious (18). Yet, it simply does not follow from these facts that dogs that tremble in veterinarians' offices – much less cows, sheep, chickens, or laboratory animals – have a sufficient sense of self or of the future, or are capable of sufficient dread about their own predicaments, to justify the attribution of anxiety.

I submit that the very act of defining anxiety and other mental states without including the sophisticated experiences these concepts ordinarily encompass, will lead some people to think that the task of describing animal mental states is much easier than it is. These people may find (some may be assuming this from the beginning) that animals are more like human beings than they really are. They may conclude that the presence in animals of some chemical or some *part* of the complex behavior we view as evidence of certain mental states shows that animals, too, experience these very same states. And they may conclude this not because scientific evidence demonstrates that animals experience these states, but because *new concepts* are being employed that can be applied more easily to animals.[b]

---

[b]Some of the AVMA Panel's definitions seem to eliminate the internal, subjective components of certain mental states. "Comfort," for example, is defined as "a state of physiologic and behavioral homeostasis in which the animal has adapted to its environment and has normal feeding, drinking, activity, sleep/wake cycles, reproduction and social behavior" (21). "Stress" is defined as "the effect of physical, physiologic, or emotional factors (stressors) that induce an alteration in the animal's homeostasis or adaptive state" (22).

As the AVMA Panel recognized, it is important that investigators have some commonality of definition, lest they talk and argue about different things. However, the fact that animals have real mental experiences does not justify going overboard in ascribing mentalistic concepts to them. These concepts have important moral implications. For example, if a certain husbandry method really causes cows to experience *anxiety*, the argument against this method would be stronger than if it merely causes slight discomfort. If we do not apply these concepts with care, we risk mischaracterizing both the mental lives and moral claims of the animals whose welfare we seek to promote.

One suggested methodology. Stanley Curtis suggests a way of assisting investigators to take animal interests into account while they await further progress in the description and evaluation of animal mental states. Curtis argues that "(a)ssessment of well-being in agricultural animals cannot include an estimate of any mental suffering because we still are unable to do such an evaluation." He recommends that we search for all physiological, behavioral, and performance indicators "of stress and distress. Meanwhile, health, reproductive, and productive traits continue to be the most reliable farm-level indicators of fit between agricultural animals and their environments" (19).

Curtis' warning about facile attribution of mental states to agricultural animals is well-taken, but his statement requires some qualification.

First, one must be careful not to assume an identity, as Curtis apparently does, between animal well-being and absence of stress or distress. Intuitively, it seems clear that some animals have interests in positive states or conditions. For example, Curtis notes that sows and growing pigs direct their attention to, and try to manipulate, objects suspended in front of them. He suggests that these animals might be "'hungry' for external stimulation in general" (20). This formulation accords with Curtis' definition of animal well-being as fulfillment of needs. For the frustration of "needs," as people ordinarily use this term, does typically lead to feelings of distress or unhappiness. (Ordinarily, we think of a "need" as a physiological or psychological requirement, deprivation of which threatens continued existence, good health, or psychological equilibrium.) However, it is far from clear that pigs must suffer or experience distress if they are not provided with external stimulation. Yet it still may be plausible to conclude that they are *better off* having such stimulation – and that providing them with it will therefore raise their level of *welfare*.

Second, it is incorrect to say that we cannot yet attribute suffering to animals. We make such judgments frequently. We often feel compelled to make them because avoidance of mental states such as pain and suffering is an important component of animal welfare.

Curtis is surely correct in insisting that we must be careful about our concepts and evidence before attributing to animals sophisticated mental states we readily attribute to human beings. Sometimes, this may mean inability to describe with our usual vocabulary precisely what mental states might be present. Some animals exhibit quite different behavior and physiological responses from those we see in human beings (23). The barrier of understanding nature has erected between ourselves and many animals can complicate the task of assessing animal welfare. We often may be unable to say precisely how unpleasant or pleasant the animals' experiences are. However, the difficulty of the task does not make it illegitimate.

8. *All other things being equal, a husbandry method or course of veterinary care that causes animals less pain, suffering, distress, or discomfort is preferable to one that causes them more.*

Some pain or distress is beneficial, either as a way of assisting an animal to protect itself or to counter other negative states (24). Nevertheless, all other things being equal, pain and other negative states are bad for animals just as they are for people. Therefore, it seems correct to assert that if several alternative approaches are equally profitable, but one would cause the animals less pain, suffering, distress, or discomfort than the others, it would be wrong not to pursue the less painful (distressful, etc.) approach. To do otherwise would be to cause the animals unnecessary pain or distress, something even the anticruelty position (see Chapter 11) regards as wrong.

9.   All other things being equal, a husbandry method or course of veterinary care that gives animals more positive mental states or greater well-being is preferable to one that gives them less.

As I observed in Chapter 11, many people believe that animals are entitled to freedom from "unnecessary" negative states and conditions, but that they are not entitled to positive benefits such as pleasure, happiness, or general well-being. Nevertheless, it does not seem terribly controversial to suggest that if several management or veterinary approaches are equally profitable, but one would bring more positive benefits to the animals than the others, the more beneficial approach ought to be chosen. Doing otherwise would be ungenerous and uncharitable for no apparent reason. The premise that, all things being equal, one ought to promote animal benefit is far from trivial. It requires farmers, the profession, and animal behavior scientists to support efforts to determine how positive animal mental states might be promoted.

10. It is often unhelpful to maintain that animals should be spared "unnecessary" pain, suffering, distress, or discomfort, or that they should be treated "humanely."

"Necessity." As we saw in Chapter 11, typically, to claim that a given amount or kind of animal pain or distress is "necessary" is to make two judgments: 1) that a human aim for which the pain (distress, etc.) is imposed is legitimate or is sufficiently important to justify the pain; and 2) that the amount or kind of pain in question is in fact required for the achievement of that aim.

For example, some veterinarians, farmers, and animal welfare advocates argue about whether total confinement rearing of veal calves is really "necessary." (This husbandry method is discussed in greater detail below.) Although they seem to be discussing the same thing, they may be talking about two quite different matters. Some will assume the legitimacy of tender, white veal meat as a goal and are arguing about the possibility of a confinement method that will produce such meat, but that will not cause the animals undue distress. For others, the issue is whether such meat is a legitimate goal to begin with, or is sufficiently important a goal to justify any amount of animal distress.

Debates about the "necessity" of a given kind of animal treatment often bog down in confusion and disagreement. One reason this can occur is that people arguing about "necessary" pain or distress tend to shift back and forth between the issues of the legitimacy of the goal and whether a given means toward that goal is in fact required for achieving it. When agreement seems possible about whether a certain amount of animal pain is in fact required for a certain goal, suddenly there will be disagreement about whether that goal is legitimate or is sufficiently valuable to justify the animal pain. And if agreement about the legitimacy of a goal seems likely, someone will ask whether a proposed treatment of animals is really required in order to achieve that goal. This process of shifting between the two very different questions encompassed by the notion of "necessity" can repeat itself endlessly. The notion of "necessity" contributes to this process, because those engaged in argument may think that they are still discussing only one issue, namely the "necessity" of some animal pain, distress, or discomfort.

The best way of avoiding such confusion is to stop talking about the "necessity" of pain or distress associated with various ways of using or treating animals. It is far better to address directly the two questions encompassed by the current notion of "necessity:" 1) whether a human aim for which some animal pain or distress is imposed is legitimate or is sufficiently valuable to justify the pain; and 2) whether the amount or kind of pain in question is in fact required for the achievement of that human aim. Such issues can be difficult enough. The chances of resolving them will only be diminished by the ambiguous and distracting concept of "necessity."

"Humaneness." It is difficult to object to the assertion that people ought to treat animals humanely. For as most people ordinarily use the term, treating animals "humanely" means treating them as they ought to be treated, in accordance with the moral obligations we human beings have regarding them. Thus, saying that people should treat animals "humanely" is like saying that people should act rightly. Each statement is obviously correct. But by itself, each tells us nothing. We need to know what, more precisely, it *is* to act rightly or to treat animals humanely. An animal farmer and an animal use abolitionist will almost certainly agree that "all animals ought to be treated humanely." However, to the farmer, humane treatment is consistent with raising animals for food, while to the abolitionist it is not. They will disagree about what constitutes the humane treatment of animals because they disagree about how animals ought to be treated.

There is nothing inherently wrong with applying the terms "humane" or "inhumane" to various ways of treating animals. But to assert that a given way of treating them is humane or inhumane typically is to express one's conclusion about whether such treatment is or is not morally appropriate. Statements about "humaneness" and "inhumaneness" therefore belong at the very end of arguments, after reasons for one's conclusions have already been provided.

THE IMMENSITY OF THE TASK

The 10 basic principles developed above cut against some views regarding how agricultural and sport animals may be treated. However, these principles only lay preliminary groundwork for many difficult questions.

A Host of Conceptual, Empirical, and Ethical Issues

Some of these issues are conceptual: they involve the definition of terminology used in factual and ethical claims about animals. Among the concepts that require further analysis before normative veterinary ethics can make substantial progress in the farm and sport animal area are "animal welfare," "pain," "suffering," "distress," "discomfort," "pleasure," and "benefit."

Other difficult issues are empirical in nature: their resolution requires investigation into factual matters. Among such issues are those concerning what mental states farm and sport animals do experience, what husbandry methods promote or hinder such states, and whether certain methods promote productivity as well as animal welfare.

Empirical investigations can also raise ethical questions. For example, two people might agree that pigs do in fact experience boredom and are happier with external stimulation. Yet they may still disagree about whether a producer has a moral obligation to make his pigs happier. Another important ethical issue concerns the extent to which diminutions in levels of animal welfare can be justified by the interests of producers and the public.

What Is Animal Welfare?

One critical conceptual task faced by normative veterinary ethics is defining animal welfare, in general or in specific kinds of contexts.

The literature on farm animal welfare reflects significant disagreements about how to measure and promote animal welfare. There are some who argue for productivity as the primary index of animal welfare, and others who disagree. Such things as the animals' self-choice, fulfillment of the innate "telos" or nature of a species or breed, the absence of stress-related chemicals, the presence of normal behavior, the absence of disease, and reproductive success all have their adherents and detractors as candidates for indicia of animal welfare.

These controversies are made more difficult by the fact that not all the disputants appear to conceive of "animal welfare" in the same way. The following are just a few of the different definitions or characterizations of animal welfare that can be found in the literature:

"a state of complete mental and physical health where the animal is in complete harmony with its environment" (25).

"a condition of physical and psychological harmony in the animal itself and of the animal with its environment. The indications of well-being are good health and behaviour which is entirely normal" (26).

"the degree to which [animals] can adapt without suffering to the environments designated by man" (27).

absence of "methods for handling and management [that] are so extreme as to induce stress or its overt symptoms, distress, on animals. Stress is understood to mean extensive physiological and behavioral disturbance in the animal resulting from noxious environmental factors" (28).

absence of "suffering" (29).

"mental well-being," which is identified with the absence of "suffering"(30). Suffering is defined as "a wide range of unpleasant emotional states" including "fear, pain, frustration and exhaustion" and other mental states "such as those caused by loss of social companions" (31).

freedom from pain and suffering. "Pain" is defined as "aversive stimulation of the central nervous system (CNS) originating from the damage of tissues and, or, organs either by disease, injury or functional disorder." "Suffering" is defined as "aversive stimulation of the CNS originating from behavioural and physiological conflicts with the environment" (32).

"well-being," characterized as the fulfillment of "needs" (33).

Each of these definitions differs in substantial respects from the others, and some of them are incompatible. Such definitions are typically set forth as truisms, without supporting arguments. These definitions typically occur at or near the beginning of discussions. Claims are then made about whether a given practice promotes "welfare" already defined. But many of these definitions are far from self-evident. Some point investigators down roads that exclude certain kinds of empirical and ethical research. For example, someone who defines welfare as the absence of suffering has *already* excluded as irrelevant, research directed toward the promotion of positive mental states. Those who define welfare as the absence of suffering in environments designated by man have already presumed the propriety of certain human practices. Someone who defines welfare in terms of basic animal needs has already decided not to take into account (except as evidence of needs) what might more appropriately be described as animal wants rather than needs.

Because many investigators appear to be employing different concepts of animal welfare, it is often far from clear that their disagreements are really just factual ones about whether some given practice promotes the same endpoint, i.e., animal welfare. For example, welfare advocates like Dr. Michael W. Fox who urge respect for certain aspects of a farm animal's innate nature or "telos" sometimes are concerned not just about unpleasant mental states that frustration of "telos" might cause, or pleasurable states fulfillment of "telos" would enable. They also see fulfillment of "telos" as a good in itself. This is an ethical judgment. Those who do not share it may find certain investigations or positions incorrect or even incomprehensible.

As more is learned about animals and the effects upon them of various methods of husbandry and management, our views about how they may or must be treated will develop. This in turn may affect how we define or conceive of their "welfare." At this early stage in the development of animal welfare science, investigators should be wary of definitions of welfare that could limit important empirical research by making unexamined or debatable moral assumptions.

AGRICULTURAL ANIMALS: WELFARE ISSUES

There are many reasons why normative veterinary ethics should concern itself with moral issues in farm animal welfare. Veterinarians are involved in many management techniques, either directly or as advisors to producers. Moreover, as the AVMA has recognized, even when veterinarians do not participate in certain management practices, it is their responsibility as general advocates of animal welfare to "encourage humane practices by education and advice" (34). Dr. Franklin Loew is surely correct when he observes that "animal welfare is *the* most important veterinary issue of the late 20th century" (35).

Current Welfare Issues in Husbandry and Production

Tables 21.1 and 21.2 present an overview of welfare issues arising out of food animal husbandry. Table 21.1 focuses on swine and presents (without supporting arguments) some of the major issues and claims made for or against certain practices. Table 21.2 presents several current debates relating to the welfare of other species. Many of the positions taken regarding these issues are similar to those that are raised in discussions about swine.

Table 21.1

Some Animal Welfare Issues Relating to the Production and Care of Swine

MANAGEMENT METHOD	CLAIMED BENEFITS	CLAIMED PROBLEMS
Total confinement rearing (in enclosed buildings)	productivity disease control protection from weather management efficiency	joint diseases decreased weight gain infertility improper ventilation leading to discomfort disease management inefficiency violation of "telos"
Concrete flooring	improved sanitation durability	joint disorders violation of "telos"
Slatted flooring	eliminates need for bedding improved sanitation improved disease control efficient waste management	injuries, lameness, arthritis (concrete slats) decreased weight gain nipple necrosis
High stocking density during finishing	reduces heating expense management efficiency	insufficient ventilation "social confusion" aggressiveness, injuries infection build-up
Dark or semi-dark lighting conditions	reduced aggression decreased expense	depression stress boredom inspection/supervision problems violation of "telos"
Nonpelletized (dry, sandy) feed	reduced expense	esophogastric ulcers
Accelerated fattening (e.g., ad libitum feeding)	meat productivity	joint and leg weakness
"Skip" (alternate day) feeding of sows	obesity prevention	hunger, discomfort violation of "telos"

Table 21.1 – *continued*

MANAGEMENT METHOD	CLAIMED BENEFITS	CLAIMED PROBLEMS
Tail-docking	prevents cannibalism, injuries	unnecessary mutilation ignores underlying causes of aggression
Castration	eliminates meat odor offensive to some consumers	great expense, no real benefit unnecessary mutilation
Continuous tethering/ confinement of sows	efficient use of floor space efficient monitoring	lameness behavioral problems violation of "telos"
Farrowing stalls/ crates	efficient use of floor space improved waste management protection of piglets	increased disease longer labors, dystocia greater incidence of stillborn and mummified piglets nipple necrosis abnormal behavior, stress violation of "telos"
Early weaning of piglets	quicker breeding of sows improves dietary management	growth delay violation of "telos"
Raising of piglets in raised battery cages	efficiency improved waste management protection of piglets	inferior health of piglets contamination by dropping wastes violation of "telos"
Subtherapeutic antibiotics in feed	prevents disease promotes growth	masks underlying causes of disease
Long-distance transportation to slaughter	necessary in some areas	dramatic "shrinkage" in body weight stress

Table 21.2

Some Animal Welfare Issues Regarding the Production and Care of Ruminants and Poultry

Dairy Cows and Calves

Open (outdoor) feed-lot rearing
Separation of calves from cows 1 to 3 days following birth
Tying of calves to barn walls
Rearing of calves in single-animal pens
Housing of cows in "comfort stalls" restrained by neck chain without freedom
to enter or leave at will
Total indoor confinement of cows and calves
Flooring in indoor systems (e.g., slatted
versus nonslatted; hard flooring without bedding;
elevated metal-rod flooring for calves)
Dehorning without anesthesia
Surgical alteration of bull penis to aid in estrus detection

Veal Calves

Single-animal stalls or crates
Flooring (slatted versus nonslatted; oak versus other materials)
Cleanliness of stalls or crates, waste removal
Ventilation, light
Feeding of low-iron, low-fiber liquid diets
Use of antibiotics in feed

Beef Production

Open (outdoor) feed-lots
Total (indoor) confinement systems
Stressful transition of animals to feed-lot
Proper density of animals in feed-lots and enclosed barns
"Bulling" of males by other males in feed-lots
Dehorning without anesthesia
Castration without anesthesia
Hot-iron (versus freeze) branding
Use of subtherapeutic antibiotics, growth stimulants,
and reproductive regulators
Methods of shipment to slaughterhouses
Humane handling of animals in slaughter plants
Ritual (kosher) slaughter

Table 21.2 – *continued*

Sheep Production

Total (indoor) confinement systems
Outdoor feed-lots lacking shelter or windbreaks
Early shearing to stimulate appetite
Use of subtherapeutic doses of antibiotics
Castration without anesthesia
Tail-docking without anesthesia
Allegedly cruel, ineffective methods of predator control

Broiler Chickens

Cage (versus floor) systems
Stocking densities
Low illumination systems
Heat, ventilation, removal of ammonia and other air pollutants
Killing of unwanted chicks, poults, and pipped eggs by suffocation, grinding,
volatile liquids, or simple disposal
Beak trimming
Concentrated, low-fiber diet
Use of vaccinations and medicated feeds
Losses and injuries during catching and loading of poultry for shipment
Effectiveness of electrical stunning prior to killing

Laying Hens

Intensive battery cages (stocking density per cage,
degree of cage slope, wire-bottomed cages)
Size of colony
Forced moulting (use of starvation/water deprivation, lighting reduction,
or low-sodium/calcium diets)
Beak trimming
Declawing
Enriching the internal environment to prevent "boredom" and "boredom"-related vices
Dubbing (partial removal of comb)
Extension of laying periods through manipulation of lighting
Heat, ventilation, removal of ammonia and other air pollutants
Killing of unwanted chicks by suffocation, grinding,
volatile liquids, or simple disposal

Turkeys

Use of slatted floors (versus deep litter)
Stocking densities
Proposed cage systems for breeder hens
Control of lighting to regulate egg production
Heat and ventilation
Desnooding
Wing clipping
Toe clipping

The tables illustrate many (but by no means all) of the questions that currently occupy the attention of producers, veterinarians, and animal welfare advocates. Inclusion on the tables does not indicate a view on my part that an issue points to major deficiencies in current husbandry methods. Nor am I suggesting that the opposing sides on each of these issues always have equal credibility. In the interest of brevity, many of the topics in the tables are presented in a general way. For example, it is not enough to talk about "concrete flooring" for swine. There are different kinds of concrete, and some concrete floors can be coated or padded so as to change their effects on the animals. A number of investigators believe that great improvements in animal welfare can sometimes be achieved not by abandoning a general kind of technique, but by subtle modifications of it (36). Nor is the presentation by Table 21.1 of conflicting arguments in terms of claimed benefits and problems intended to suggest that these issues should be resolved by utilitarian "cost-benefit" analysis.

The tables illustrate the formidable task faced by normative veterinary ethics and animal welfare science in assessing and promoting farm animal welfare. For embedded in many of the issues are hard conceptual, empirical, and ethical questions only the surface of which has yet been scratched. What mental states do these animals experience? How should we conceive of varying levels of welfare for them? How are their interests in these levels to be weighed against legitimate human interests? What methods of production and veterinary care might now improve welfare while having minimal impact on productivity, so that animal welfare can be enhanced while animal welfare science goes about determining how welfare can be promoted in the long term? To what extent must profits be decreased so that certain levels of welfare can be assured? What is an animal's nature or "telos" and to what extent and for what reasons might it be entitled to respect? To what extent should the law attempt to assure certain levels of animal welfare? What, more precisely, should be the role of the veterinary profession in advocating farm animal welfare?

Dehorning Cattle without Anesthesia

One of the central arguments of this chapter is that in approaching agricultural and sport animal practice, normative veterinary ethics and animal welfare science should avoid premature conclusions that are not justified by current factual and ethical knowledge. Nevertheless, I want to illustrate the application of principles developed in the text to some specific issues. I shall discuss briefly (and by no means exhaustively) two of the more controversial topics in agricultural animal welfare: the dehorning of dairy and beef cattle without the use of anesthesia and total confinement rearing of so-called "milk-fed" veal.

Some people condemn the dehorning of calves without anesthesia because the practice causes the animals pain. The fact that pain is imposed certainly provides moral weight in opposition to the practice. However, there are important considerations on the other side. On balance, these considerations show that although dehorning young calves with anesthesia might be an ideal, it is still not the case that all farmers who dehorn these animals without anesthesia are acting wrongly.

Dehorning often is required to prevent the animals from injuring themselves and their human handlers (37). When performed properly on younger animals, dehorning without anesthesia does not appear to cause long-lasting pain or discomfort. The anesthesia process may itself cause some distress, because it requires the injection of a nerve-blocking agent, which prolongs the length of the entire procedure. Finally, dehorning with anesthesia can be time-consuming and expensive. For many farmers, anesthesia of calves would cause a major drain on already scarce resources. This would compromise their ability to provide the animals with more important things, including veterinary care to prevent or cure serious illness.

Although dehorning young calves without performing a nerve block often seems justifiable, dehorning adult animals without anesthesia is another matter. This practice can not only impede productivity (of lactating dairy cows, for example), but also results in pain that appears to be much greater and longer-lasting than that experienced by calves dehorned without anesthesia. Here, I would urge, one crosses the line between what can be imposed on animals in the name of economic cost.

An important moral ideal of veterinarians is to spare all patients as much pain as possible. Accordingly, the AVMA supports "the use of procedures that reduce or eliminate the pain of dehorning and castrating cattle and recommends completion of these procedures at the earliest possible age" (34). The AVMA also wants research to develop "improved techniques for painless, humane castration and dehorning" of cattle (34). If cost-effective ways of painlessly dehorning calves become available, their use will no longer be praiseworthy, but morally obligatory.

Total Confinement Raising of "Milk-fed" Veal

Total confinement production of formula-fed veal often involves calves "chained in single stalls 56–61 cm x 1.5 m on raised wooden slats to facilitate cleaning. No bedding or freedom of movement is provided. The calves can neither turn nor lie down with ease in these stalls" (38). They are also fed a liquid low-fiber, low-iron diet that, together with the restrictions in locomotion, are said to produce the characteristic light-colored meat.

INTERESTS OF THE PUBLIC

It is difficult to maintain that the public has a strong interest in the kind of pale meat that results from this sort of husbandry practice. It is not clear that most people can discern any difference between the color of "milk-fed" and non "milk-fed" veal, once it is cooked (39). Some proponents of milk-fed veal argue that a large proportion of the product is consumed by Jews who observe kosher dietary laws (40). In fact, there is nothing in Jewish law that requires consumption of veal, much less formula-fed veal. Milk-fed veal is an expensive, luxury product. It is substantially different from dairy products, eggs, chicken, pork, and beef, which are staples of the American diet. A significant decrease in the supply or increase in the price of these products would cause great hardship across the economic spectrum.

INTERESTS OF THE ANIMALS

It is beyond question that some veal calves are subjected to terrible conditions. There exist facilities (which, producers often say, are smaller, less profitable operations) that are filthy, smelly, dark, and are constructed of materials on which the animals can injure themselves. But there are problems even with more "modern" facilities. In many, there is continuous medication with antibiotics to suppress infection and illness. The low iron and roughage diet has led to cases of general weakness, excessive sucking and licking, and fur balls resulting from licking of the coat to obtain roughage (41).

Additionally, there is the inability of the animals to move about in a variety of ways normal to the species, and to come in contact with other animals. Aside from the common-sense conclusion that such confinement must be distressing (and evidence that it sometimes is), these animals are being deprived of certain freedoms that impartial reason declares they have a great interest in experiencing. Part of the problem with confining veal calves in small enclosures for the whole of their existence is that they are deprived in their short lives of a semblance of what it is like to be themselves. This problem remains even if the animals do not experience significant pain, suffering, or distress.

Objecting to total confinement and formula-feeding of veal calves does not imply condemnation of all husbandry methods that restrict animal movement or diet. Each kind of case must be considered on its own terms, with due regard for the importance of the public's interest in inexpensive and safe food products. The problem with total confinement of veal calves is that it serves such an inessential human interest at such an enormous cost to the animals.

THE INTERESTS OF PRODUCERS

The raising of formula-fed veal constitutes a major industry and a significant proportion of total veal production. According to USDA figures, 1,021,639 formula-fed veal calves were slaughtered in fiscal year 1987. The figures were 1,288,891 for "bob" veal, 186,163 for nonformula veal, and 379,797 for calves over 400 pounds (42).

Some producers argue that it is possible to produce satisfactory veal at a profit with far less deprivation to the animals than that associated with total confinement methods (43). If correct, such contentions provide a strong argument against more restrictive methods. However, that total confinement raising of veal calves is profitable, or may be more profitable than other methods, is not a conclusive argument in its favor. The fact that one can make money at some enterprise, or that elimination of the enterprise would bring great hardship to those already engaged in it, does not render it morally acceptable. Likewise, there is little force to the claim that producing "milk-fed" veal provides a market for dried skim milk that would otherwise go into government stockpiles (44). The underlying problem is government policy supporting irrational overproduction of milk. It hardly seems fair to address this problem by causing misery or deprivation to innocent animals. Another argument often raised in favor of total confinement husbandry is that it provides an outlet for many unwanted dairy calves that would otherwise simply be killed. This may provide an argument in favor of some use of these animals, but it does not demonstrate the appropriateness of total confinement veal production. Moreover, we sometimes think it is better to end the lives of certain animals (such as unadoptable stray dogs and cats) than to permit them to suffer or live under terrible conditions.

THE INTERESTS OF THE FARM COMMUNITY AND VETERINARIANS

I have found that many farmers and veterinarians who are not engaged in veal production express support for total confinement husbandry because they view opposition as the first stage of a general attack on animal agriculture. Some animal rights activists do hope that abolition of total confinement raising of veal calves will lead to ending the use of animals for food. However, opposition to certain husbandry methods does not entail opposition to animal agriculture. Nor does the fact that certain people take a stance against a husbandry method make that stance wrong or unworthy of support by veterinarians. Opposing certain reforms because activists endorse them can only harm farmers and the veterinary profession in the long run, because it assists opponents of animal agriculture to present themselves to the public as the only people who care about the animals.

THE OFFICIAL POSITION

The AVMA's official view is that "veal calf production is well established, can be humane, and can improve the welfare of calves" (45). Its Guide for Veal Calf Care and Production (46) permits confinement rearing, with limitations. For example, "animals should be able to stretch, stand, and lie down comfortably and naturally." It is also urged that "veal calves kept in total confinement be kept on oak slatted floors" to permit ease of movement, ventilation, and waste removal. The Guide counsels proper construction materials and the seeking of professional advice in the event of injury or distress. The Guide's recommendations are clearly well-intentioned, and would improve the lot of many animals. As a document of official veterinary ethics, it is not surprising that the Guide attempts to reconcile existing competing interests. However, the Guide seems to miss the intuitive appeal of the argument that agricultural animals have an interest in certain basic goods, such as the ability to walk around and to have some contact with other animals, and that this interest can be overridden, if at all, only by a very important human interest or need. Opposition to total confinement husbandry of calves appears to be growing among the public and veterinarians in the rest of the world (47). At present, the formula-fed industry in this country does seem "well established." But things can change. Time will tell whether organized veterinary medicine some day will be judged to have missed an important opportunity to establish its credibility in the farm animal welfare area.

Some Other Welfare Issues in Veterinary Care

TO TREAT OR NOT TO TREAT?

One issue with animal welfare ramifications often faced by agricultural practitioners is whether to treat a sick or injured animal (as opposed to recommending that it be killed or shipped for slaughter) when treatment may be economically unwise for the client.

Among the relevant considerations are, of course, the probable economic costs of treatment, slaughter, or immediate euthanasia. However, due regard must also be paid to animal welfare. This can mean among other things: 1) not delaying a decision whether to treat when delay would cause the animal unnecessary suffering; 2) taking into account the relative likely suffering as well as the relative expense associated with various treatment options; and 3) not permitting an animal to suffer for a prolonged period of time. Often the most cost-effective and humane course of action will be euthanasia or expeditious shipment.

An important issue in agricultural practice concerns the role of the doctor in the making of a client's decisions. Some large animal practitioners tell me that they are quite aggressive in recommending euthanasia or slaughter when one of these approaches is in the client's economic interest. They are especially forceful when a client balks at making a decision because of emotional attachment to an animal. It is surely appropriate for a veterinarian to point out economic aspects of various alternatives. Nevertheless, if a client makes a decision that the doctor finds economically imprudent, it is still the client's decision to make.

Another important aspect of the decision whether to treat concerns the administration of drugs that will keep an animal alive long enough to be shipped. Several veterinarians have admitted to me that they administer drugs even when not completely confident that at the time of slaughter the legally required withdrawal time will have passed. Among the justifications offered for such an approach are that it is the responsibility of a slaughterhouse inspector to condemn an animal that is too sick or drugged, and that any drug residues in a particular animal will be "diluted" by other meat when it reaches the consumer's table. As shall be discussed below, veterinarians can have legitimate, good-faith differences with government authorities about the proper use of drugs in food animals. But if a practitioner *knows* that an animal may contain drug residues at slaughter and pushes the determination on to someone else who may or may not make it, he is committing a great moral wrong upon the public. He also risks exposing the profession as a whole to condemnation for reckless drug use and to more vigorous government regulation than might be necessary.

ADVOCATING ANIMAL INTERESTS

A veterinarian's status as a medical professional puts him in a unique position to speak for the interests of his patients. The following are among the kinds of information that veterinarians can provide to clients when animal welfare considerations must be factored into decision-making:

• Whether an animal is being overworked to the extent that it is threatened with acute or chronic injury or disease, and whether resting, euthanasia, or shipment for slaughter is the only feasible way of preventing short- or long-term suffering;
• Whether an animal is too injured or broken down to be used for breeding without causing suffering or discomfort;
• Whether an animal needs special nutritional treatment or care;
• Whether a condition suffered by one or several members of a herd is likely to spread to other animals unless action is taken;
• Whether animals require professional care to be maintained at an adequate level of welfare.

UNDERUTILIZATION OF VETERINARY SERVICES

Many veterinarians and animal welfare advocates agree that there is far less utilization of veterinary services by farmers than animal welfare and productivity require (48). The recent AVMA *Report on the US Market for Food Animal Veterinary Medical Services* states that in 1985, beef producers spent 62% of their total animal health care expenditures with a veterinarian; dairy producers 75%; hog producers 47%; and sheep producers 54% (49).

The AVMA *Report* suggests that the solution for veterinarian underutilization is the model of the agricultural doctor as economic manager (see Chapter 15). According to the *Report*, the veterinarian is the "logical person" to deliver advice focused on the entire "financial performance of the livestock enterprise." The *Report* is quite certain that the "fundamental task" for food animal doctors is to shift to providing such services (50).

However, it is far from obvious that the profession should rush quickly to promote the model of the economic manager for all farm animal practitioners. The AVMA *Report* concedes that few veterinary students receive serious training in agricultural economics (51), and that producers consider private practitioners less knowledgeable about agribusiness and economics than they themselves or agricultural extension agents (52). The *Report* also admits that the "feasibility of improving veterinarians' knowledge and cost-effectiveness relative to other suppliers of information is a *critical question*" from veterinary educational and marketing standpoints (53).

Descriptive veterinary ethics should determine how many practitioners and students are suited – intellectually, aesthetically, and morally – to the model of the veterinarian as economic manager. Many veterinarians, surely, gravitate toward farm animal practice because they like the kind of life it traditionally has provided, including opportunities for hands-on interaction with large animals and farmers. Many agricultural doctors have an abiding concern for the welfare of farm animals. Before the veterinary schools and professional associations set out to refashion the image of the agricultural doctor, it might be wise to determine how many present and future veterinarians are interested in such a transformation. The profession should also consider more fully how due regard for animal welfare can be maintained by those veterinarians who might want to function as economic managers. Also relevant are the potential effects of management-oriented approaches upon the public's image of agricultural practitioners and the profession as a whole.

AGRICULTURAL ANIMALS: MIXED WELFARE AND PUBLIC HEALTH ISSUES

Lay Administration of Drugs; Prescription versus Over-the-Counter Products

The AVMA *Report* on the market for food animal veterinary services states that in 1985 only 24% of the total $949.4 million sales of food animal veterinary pharmaceuticals and biologicals (excluding feed additives) was made by veterinarians. Based on manufacturers' prices, it was estimated that veterinarians accounted for only 9% of the total $1,779.2 million sales of pharmaceuticals, biologics, and feed additives (54). The *Report* documents (55) widespread dissatisfaction among agricultural doctors about the following: administration of drugs by farmers; sales of drugs and vaccines by feed and animal supply stores; dispensing of drug advice by lay feed and drug salesmen; aggressive marketing techniques by lay drug sales operations; roving lay salesmen who dispense from trucks; and mail order operations conducted by laymen or veterinarians.

As the reactions of the practitioners related in the AVMA *Report* make clear, all this lay use and advice concerning drugs, vaccines, and biologicals is not only hurting veterinary business, but is harming many animals as well. Many farmers and self-styled "experts" do not know what they are doing. Animals suffer. Veterinarians sometimes are called when problems become so bad that laymen can no longer pretend to be able to deal with them. At a time when government is increasingly concerned with misuse of antibiotics in food animals, the health and safety of the public may also be threatened by widespread administration of antibiotics by laymen.

Unfortunately, some veterinarians appear to be playing a role in the indiscriminate medicating of animals. In 1987, the FDA reported the results of an undercover investigation of 50 veterinary clinics and 7 veterinary drug distributors in Maryland (56). FDA agents posing as prospective clients were successful in making purchases of requested veterinary prescription drugs at 23 of the clinics but at none of the drug distributors. In most cases, the purchases were made from people who appeared to be clerks and not from doctors. The drugs purchased included Dexamethasone and Flumethasone. The FDA expressed its concern that the "very loose controls over the sales of prescription veterinary drugs" followed by their use by laymen "poses the risk of injury to treated animals as well as the potential exposure of humans to hazardous drug residues in meat and other food products."

Reliable data are needed regarding the effects of lay administration of various drugs and biologics on animal welfare, productivity, and public health. It would be unrealistic to require that all drugs always be administered by or under the direct supervision of veterinarians. In many cases, there are both economic and welfare justifications for administration of drugs by farmers. But because it is clear that there is far too much medication of animals by laymen, the profession need not fear research into welfare and productivity aspects of this practice. Whatever is learned cannot help but strengthen the economic position of agricultural doctors.

If factual analysis of the effects of lay medication warrants, the appropriate government authorities ought to consider requiring some form of veterinary participation in the medication of food animals. At the very least, the states ought to prosecute laymen who are engaging in the unlawful practice of veterinary medicine as currently defined in these jurisdictions.

State boards of veterinary medicine and professional associations should move decisively against veterinarians who are involved in the indiscriminate supply of drugs to farmers, without adequate knowledge about the animals that receive them.

Finally, both federal and state governments must enact and enforce strict and consistent laws to prevent misuse of drugs deleterious to animal welfare and public health. Congress and the FDA should address conscientiously the issue of what drugs and biologicals ought never to be permitted to be sold over-the-counter. In 1988, Congress finally passed a law that would place a separate category of veterinary prescription drugs into the federal Food, Drug and Cosmetic Act. (Previously, the notion of "veterinary prescription drugs" was only a regulatory creation of the FDA.) Government must do more than examine particular drugs to determine whether their use or distribution ought to be reserved for veterinarians. Serious thought should be given to how the general practice of lay administration of animal drugs (even those that, taken in isolation, may not be dangerous if given by nonveterinarians) affects the ability of veterinarians to protect animals and the public.

The AVMA argues that it must be made more difficult for farmers to obtain some animal drugs. Nevertheless, the AVMA maintains (57) that the sale of veterinary prescription drugs should not be restricted to veterinarians. ("Prescription" drugs can be made available to laymen by the marketing of a given drug under different brand names or with different label designs, depending upon whether it must be dispensed or prescribed by a veterinarian, or is available over-the-counter.) One problem with this approach is that it is a misuse of the language to speak of a "prescription" item that lawfully can be purchased without a doctor's prescription. Additionally, the existence of two parallel sets of identical drugs (some "prescription," and others "over-the-counter") surely hinders the efforts of authorities to prevent laymen from obtaining on their own drugs that should be available only from, or on the prescription of, a veterinarian. For as long as there is a wide range of "prescription" items that farmers can also obtain over-the-counter, many farmers will not attach any special significance to *prescription* labels. If they are permitted by law to obtain many so-called "prescription" drugs over-the-counter, some will try to obtain on their own "prescription" drugs that authorities declare should not be available over-the-counter.

The Extra-label Drug Use Issue

In 1983, the FDA announced its intention to prohibit the use of prescription veterinary drugs in food animals in ways not in accordance with accompanying labels. The FDA stated (58) that under its new policy

> "extra-label" use may be a basis for initiating regulatory action without a concurrent demonstration of illegal drug residues. This change is needed because experience has shown that our previous policy has not been adequate to control husbandry and veterinary practices relating to misuse or extra-label use and to assure the consuming public that it has available a wholesome food supply. Adequate tissue assay

procedures are often not available for certain drugs that are limited in their labeling to use in companion animals. Where assay procedures are available, personnel and funding limitations make surveillance and enforcement difficult.

The proposed policy was opposed quickly by the AVMA and many farm animal practitioners. They complained that strict adherence to label specifications would sometimes unnecessarily harm animals and producers without bringing verifiable benefits to the public. In early 1984, the FDA withdrew the proposed policy.

Another policy was soon announced (59). It defined "extra-label use" as "the actual or intended use of a new animal drug in a food-producing animal in a manner that is not in accordance with the drug labelling. This includes, but is not limited to, use in species or for indications (disease or other conditions) not listed in the labeling, use at dosage levels higher than those stated in the labeling, and failure to observe the stated withdrawal time." The FDA went on to declare that it

> will *consider* regulatory action when such use or intended use is found whether by a veterinarian, producer, or other person. ... Nevertheless, extra-label drug use may be considered by a veterinarian when the health of animals is immediately threatened and suffering or death would result from failure to treat the affected animals. In instances of this nature regulatory action would not *ordinarily* be considered provided all of the following criteria are met and precautions observed:
>
> 1. A careful medical diagnosis is made by an attending veterinarian within the context of a valid veterinarian-client-patient relationship;
> 2. A determination is made that, (a) there is no marketed drug specifically labelled to treat the condition diagnoses, or (b) drug therapy at the dosage recommended by the labelling has been found clinically ineffective in the animals to be treated;
> 3. Procedures are instituted to assure that the identity of the treated animals is carefully maintained; and
> 4. Significantly extended time period is assigned for drug withdrawal prior to marketing meat, milk, or eggs; steps are taken to assure that the assigned timeframes are met, and no illegal residues occur.

These rules, too, struck many practitioners as confusing and inconsistent. To some, the conditions made sense in principle, but were being applied incorrectly. For example, the FDA's proposal to prohibit the use of dimetridazole in swine seemed to many doctors to violate its stated intention to permit extra-label use required for effective disease control (60).

TWO KINDS OF OBJECTIONS TO FEDERAL EXTRA-LABEL USE REGULATION

One criticism of the FDA's attempts to regulate the extra-label use of drugs that seems justified is that the FDA sometimes has performed unconvincingly. Some of its proposals have been confusing, inconsistent, or premature. *When* will the FDA "consider" regulatory action? *When* will it deviate from the announced policy of "ordinarily" taking action if the specified conditions are violated? Does it make sense to require strict adherence to label specifications regarding species and dose and then demand "significantly" extended withdrawal times? Why is the FDA focused on regulating *labels* (some of which may be more accurate than others) when what is needed are hard facts about and perhaps better regulation of the drugs themselves? How are veterinarians to proceed under FDA policy when there are many animal diseases or veterinary procedures for which there is no effective FDA-approved drug? Is it reasonable to threaten veterinarians with criminal prosecution for presence of drug residues when, by the FDA's own admission, procedures for determining residues are often unavailable? Is the FDA's aggressive stance against veterinarian extra-label use justified when statistics show that no more than 9% of all drugs administered to food animals are given by or on the direction of veterinarians? Can the FDA's avowed desire to permit necessary drugs be taken seriously when it contradicts the experience of many food animal practitioners about a drug such as dimetridazole? Is the FDA justified in its apparent (and at the time of this writing unsuccessful) attempt to frighten veterinarians into acceptance of obscure or questionable rules by instituting criminal prosecutions of practitioners?[c]

Such questions seem reasonable. However, some of the criticisms made by veterinarians of current and proposed federal regulation of animal drug use go beyond the objection that the FDA sometimes has made mistakes. Some veterinarians believe that federal regulation of veterinarian drug use is inappropriate in principle. According to this objection, practitioners ought to be able to pursue good medical practice in their use of drugs, and any required governmental action must come from those bodies that are normally engaged in the regulation of practice, namely the state veterinary boards (61).

This more radical objection to federal regulation of veterinary drug use is unjustified. The supervision of food animal drug use must be a federal responsibility. State veterinary boards and public health departments have neither the legal authority, nor the ability, to assure the purity of products that pass in the stream of commerce far beyond their respective borders. Veterinarians who use drugs on food-producing animals are engaged in a vastly different activity than are physicians, whose extra-label use of drugs is not as closely monitored by federal authorities. Food animals and animal products are *eaten* by people. Most people cannot protect themselves against improper use of animal drugs. They need a governmental body powerful enough to protect them from abuse before it occurs. To ask that the federal government not regulate in this area is to propose that the public go unprotected.

SOLVING THE PROBLEM

The only way to address the medical, economic, and ethical issues posed by extra-label drug use is for the profession and government to cooperate in the

---

[c]Three lawsuits involving the FDA illustrate the difficulty it has had convincing some in the legal community of its effectiveness in this area. In 1987, the FDA instituted a criminal prosecution of two practitioners for dispensing liquid chloramphenicol. The case was dismissed by a federal court judge, who characterized the government's case as confused and a waste of the taxpayers' money (62). In that same year, several veterinarians brought suit in federal court challenging the FDA's authority to regulate extra-label use of drugs as violative of federal law and a usurpation of the legal right of the states to regulate the practice of veterinary medicine (63). This case was dismissed by a district court judge on the grounds that the plaintiffs' activities had not yet been challenged by the FDA. But the judge also appeared to support the claim of the plaintiffs that they ought to be free to use drugs as medical needs dictate. He held that the FDA extra-label policy guide was not a "binding legal requirement" precluding the plaintiffs from "practicing their profession within ethical boundaries" (63). In another case, the FDA confiscated 52 lots of bulk drugs destined for distribution to veterinarians. The distributor sued to regain possession of the drugs, and prevailed. The court criticized the FDA sharply, stating that the FDA does not have authority under present statutes "to meddle in the field of drug compounding done within the scope of the professional practice of medicine – be it veterinary or otherwise" (64). In 1988, this last decision was reversed by an appellate court (65).

development of rational regulatory standards. Such principles cannot result merely from good intentions of regulators, or from demands by impatient legislators who "want something done." There must be good-faith attempts to learn as much as possible about various kinds of extra-label use. Acceptable technical and ethical rules must take into account the legitimate interests of all relevant parties. The ability of the profession to take the lead in such deliberations is demonstrated convincingly by the Proceedings of the 1987 AVMA Symposium on the Case for Responsible Extra-Label Drug Use (66). These papers show an impressive attention to the wide range of relevant issues – including animal welfare. However, as Dr. D.W. Upson observes (67), the profession will not be able to establish its credibility in this area until doctors put aside "the philosophy that asks, 'What can I get away with?' versus the regulatory agency philosophy of 'Gotcha!'"

Ethical Issues in the Regulation of Drug Use in Food Animals

Many factual questions must be addressed regarding the use of therapeutic and subtherapeutic dosages of drugs in food animals. Although answering these questions is not the province of ethics, how they are answered will affect the resolution of moral issues. For example, there is sharp disagreement in the scientific community about whether the use of subtherapeutic levels of penicillin, tetracyclines, and other drugs in animal feed is already posing a threat to human heath by promoting the spread of drug-resistant bacteria (68). The extent to which the use of certain drugs is justified will depend in part on how these questions are answered.

There are also ethical issues regarding the appropriateness of drug use and regulation that no amount of factual investigation alone will resolve. The most important of these issues concerns the extent to which any verifiable risks associated with certain drug uses in food animals is *justified* by the benefits to society at large. In other words, if (as is generally conceded) the use of certain drugs promotes greater production at lower costs, and if such drugs are associated with risks to human health, how much risk is acceptable so that consumers may have a supply of safe and inexpensive products?

Lying beneath this general issue are difficult ethical questions that require sustained consideration by government, producers, veterinarians, and the public. In balancing risks against benefits, how important are the interests of those involved in the production process? To what extent does the government have the right, or obligation, to protect the public against its own desire for cheaper foodstuffs, if such products also carry health risks from drug use in feeds? When evidence regarding the risks of a drug is inconclusive, should the government err on the side of safety and prohibit its use, or on the side of productivity and allow it? To what extent does any individual citizen have a basic moral right to be free from risk from drug use, and thus to be protected from utilitarian analysis of total risks versus benefits? To what extent do government and producers have a moral obligation to inform consumers about the risks of drugs used in the production of foodstuffs?

There are also ethical issues regarding the effects of extra-label or subtherapeutic use of drugs on the animals themselves. One must consider the extent to which drugs substitute for good hygiene and management, mask underlying animal stress or discomfort, or threaten the development of uncontrollable animal diseases.

VETERINARIANS AND THE FEDERAL ACCREDITATION PROGRAM

In 1912, the USDA established its program of accreditation of veterinary practitioners to assist the federal government in performing a wide range of responsibilities in protecting animal and human health. The program is administered by the Animal and Plant Health Inspection Service (APHIS). Accreditation is limited to graduates of veterinary schools who hold a permanent license to practice in a state in which they wish to be accredited and who have passed an examination administered by APHIS. Accreditation permits the veterinarian to 1) "inspect animals and poultry and apply tests for intrastate, interstate or export shipment and to issue official certificates to accompany such animals in compliance with applicable State and Federal Regulations;" 2) "participate in cooperative State/Federal programs for the control and eradication of diseases of domestic animals, including, but not limited to, tuberculosis, brucellosis, hog cholera, and scabies;" and 3) "perform functions in accordance with regulations issued pursuant to the Horse Protection Act of 1970" (69).

In its "Standards for Accredited Veterinarians" APHIS sets forth technical and ethical requirements that accredited doctors are expected to follow. The Standards require, among other things, that "prior to completing and signing a certificate with respect to animals or poultry, the accredited veterinarian must individually inspect such animals" in accordance with professionally accepted procedures; and that an accredited veterinarian "shall be responsible for the proper use and prevent the misuse of all certificates, forms, records, tags, brands, bands, etc." (70). Although accredited veterinarians are subject to criminal prosecution for certain violations of the regulations, the strongest administrative remedy available to APHIS is revocation of accreditation (71). In many cases, the accused agrees to an administrative remedy such as revocation or suspension. There is no formal adjudication by a judicial officer on the merits, and the practitioner does not actually admit guilt.

The great majority of accredited veterinarians appear to comply with the technical and ethical standards of the program. Nevertheless, serious violations continue and remain a source of grave embarrassment to the profession. The following is a very small sampling of alleged violations for which penalties have been imposed in recent years:

• Permitting unlicensed technicians to conduct brucellosis calfhood vaccinations and to bleed cattle for testing while not being present, blood-testing underaged cattle and vaccinating others over the allowable age [6 months suspension of accreditation and termination of contract with cooperative state-federal brucellosis program] (72);
• Falsifying US-origin health certificates by reporting brucellosis test results of 12 bovine serum samples when all samples came from the same animal [1 year suspension] (73);
• Vaccinating cattle with outdated brucellosis vaccine over a 2-year period, falsifying brucellosis records, failing to complete vaccination records, failing to identify animals handled with an official tattoo [Revocation, with permission to restore accreditation by retaking the federal examination after 2 years] (74);
• Vaccinating cattle over the allowable age, misrepresenting the age and pregnancy status of a vaccinated heifer, falsely issuing certificates that cattle were tested for tuberculosis, certifying that blood samples were obtained from 105 hogs to test for brucellosis and pseudorabies when samples had been taken from 90 animals [Revocation, with permission to restore accreditation by retaking the federal examination after 2 years] (75);
• Leaving a signed but otherwise incomplete certificate with a livestock company, signing an improperly completed certificate, postdating a certificate to cover 43 cattle shipped interstate [3-month suspension] (74);
• Issuing an interstate health certificate for 12 cattle indicating that they had tested negative for brucellosis and tuberculosis, 2 days before blood samples were received for testing at the state-federal laboratory [1-month suspension] (76);

• Forwarding 66 specimens to a laboratory for brucellosis testing when 20 of the samples came from a single donor animal [Revocation of accreditation by a judicial officer after the veterinarian failed to answer the charges] (77).

The AVMA and APHIS attempt to educate accredited doctors about their technical and ethical responsibilities. The following approaches might add to the effectiveness of these efforts.

1. Imposition of more severe penalties (e.g., longer periods of revocation and suspension) for serious violations of ethical and technical standards;
2. Referral of cases of fraud and reckless endangerment of animal or public health to federal and state prosecutors for possible criminal proceedings;
3. Automatic reporting of the names of all violators (including those who agree to a penalty) to their state veterinary boards. In cases where a penalty is imposed by APHIS without admission or adjudication of guilt, the board should not impose disciplinary action without undertaking its own investigation of alleged technical or ethical violations;
4. Temporary suspension or permanent expulsion of violators from the AVMA, state and local VMAs, practice associations, and specialty boards;
5. Serious discussion of ethical and legal obligations of accredited practitioners in veterinary school courses. Meaningful courses in jurisprudence and ethics to promote students' general sensitivity to legal and moral issues in veterinary practice.

SPORT ANIMAL PRACTICE: GENERAL CONSIDERATIONS

Sport animal practice can be defined as veterinary practice upon animals that compete or are an integral part of competition in events requiring athletic or physical prowess by animals, human handlers, or both. The following discussion will focus upon ethical issues relevant to veterinary practice on the most common sport animals: thoroughbred, standardbred, and quarter horse racing horses; show horses (including participants in combined training events); greyhound racing dogs; and rodeo animals. There are important ethical issues regarding other kinds of sport animals (e.g., polo horses and competition sled dogs) and noncompetitive performance animals (e.g., circus animals), but these will not be considered here.

Sport animal practice presents many of the same ethical issues that arise out of food and farm animal practice. Like agricultural animals, many sport animals are on the one hand economic assets expected to yield income for owners, but on the other hand are also sentient beings with legitimate interests of their own. As is the case in agricultural practice, there are important unresolved conceptual, empirical, and ethical issues that must be addressed before a satisfactory approach to sport animal welfare can be fashioned. For example, as Dr. Reuben Rose observes, "in comparison with the extensive body of information available on human athletic performance, the scientific study of the equine athlete is still in its infancy" (78). Regarding the analysis of locomotion and gait, researchers still lack much needed data, standardized nomenclature and recording systems, and critical analyses of pain, fatigue, and the promotion of lameness (79).

There is one important difference between using animals for agricultural purposes and using them in competitive sporting events. Sport animals do not furnish sustenance or products used to satisfy basic human needs. They provide *entertainment*. Although people surely require entertainment for their well-being, it is difficult to maintain that they must have entertainment involving the use of animals.

Society provides innumerable opportunities for diversion, including many sports that do not utilize animals. As I have argued in this text, the more a given human use of animals has negative impact upon animal interests, the more weighty must be the legitimate human interests served by that use. Such sports as horse and dog racing provide many people enjoyment and profit. However, they (and other animal sports) are simply not, in the general scheme of things, nearly as important as feeding the population or conducting biomedical research aimed at the alleviation of disease and suffering. Some conditions that are acceptable for agricultural or research animals might be impermissible for sport animals, given the nature and weight of the human interests involved.

RACE AND SHOW HORSES

Precompetition Administration of Drugs

No issue regarding performance horses has aroused more controversy than the question of the appropriateness of administering certain drugs prior to competition. The disputes differ depending upon what drug is involved. In general, there is disagreement about whether medication 1) is "restorative," i.e., allows animals to perform more comfortably at their own levels, or is "additive," i.e., significantly affects performance; 2) permits the racing of animals that ought to be rested or retired by masking pain or other debilitating conditions; 3) leads in the long run to pain, debilitation, breakdown, or shortening of an animal's competitive career; 4) really increases the number of horses capable of competition; and 5) adversely affects the breed by permitting lower quality animals to continue to compete. The drugs that arouse the greatest controversy are phenylbutazone, furosemide, and corticosteroids. Precompetition administration of phenylbutazone, for example, is characterized by some as a mild analgesic similar to aspirin. Others see it as a heartless way of extracting more profits from animals, by permitting them to compete without feeling pain caused by underlying disease processes. Furosemide is believed by many to reduce bleeding from the nose. Others dispute this effect and see its real purpose as adding to performance by reducing weight, stimulating the animal, or preventing the detection of other performance-affecting drugs (80).

The controversies about these drugs and other medical treatments can be quite bitter. Opponents of premedication sometimes characterize veterinarians who administer drugs as not only ignorant, but cowardly and venal (81). There is also a good deal of broad generalization from both sides about "track veterinarians," "horses," "owners," "trainers," and "state racing commissions" – even though all these participants in the equine competitive world can vary greatly.

An outside observer cannot fail to be impressed by the fact that there are highly competent and respected veterinarians who have differing views regarding many of these issues. Such differences are also reflected in the variety of approaches that are taken by state governments, which regulate drug use in thoroughbred and standardbred racing horses. The following are among the matters about which states differ: restrictions on the ability of horses to race after bleeding episodes; criteria required for horses to be able to receive bleeder medication; detention requirements for horses receiving bleeder medication; maximum and minimum dose levels of furosemide; approved bleeder medications other than furosemide; the latest time of administration of nonsteroidal anti-inflammatory drugs (NSAID) prior to racing; criteria for the use of such drugs; NSAID postrace test level limits; whether urine and/or blood are tested for NSAID levels; which horses are tested for NSAID after a race; whether there must be public notification of horses receiving NSAID; and whether bleeder medication or NSAID may be used on 2-year-old horses (82).

It is beyond the scope of an ethics text to settle heated factual disputes regarding the effects of precompetition medication. The following thoughts are offered to facilitate consideration of some of the moral issues that are included within these controversies. Some of these suggestions are applicable to issues that relate to other means of influencing the performance of horses, such as neurectomies, ice-packing of legs, injection of corticosteroids into the joints, and removing blood from a horse for transfusion ("blood doping") prior to competition (83).

1. Ethical argument is not furthered by asking whether a drug merely permits a horse to do more comfortably what it is capable of doing anyway (and is therefore supposedly unobjectionable), or is improper because it "affects," "enhances," or "improves" performance. Many things, including good nutrition and training, affect, enhance, or improve performance. If trainers did not think that certain medications improved performance, they would not use these substances. Whether a certain drug use is morally acceptable will depend upon whether it is sufficiently respectful of the interests of the relevant parties – not on whether a cliché such as "affects" performance is attached to it (84).

2. If one accepts the legitimacy of animal athletics, one has already conceded that performance animals may be used for human ends. This, in turn, means that human interests also count, and may sometimes count enough to justify depriving some of these animals of optimal welfare. Regarding show and race horses, it seems obvious that there will sometimes be a departure from optimal welfare. Strenuous athletic activity is inherently associated with the possibility of pain and injury. We do not always prohibit human athletes from competing when they require medication to shield them from pain or discomfort, or when immediate resting would help an underlying problem. But they are not permitted to compete under such conditions indiscriminately. We do not want them to suffer unduly during competition. Nor do we want them to risk being seriously injured or shortening their careers. With horses, too, the question one must ask is whether performing in some discomfort or assisted by palliative measures is justified in light of the potential costs.

3. Intuitively, the following questions are among those that seem appropriate in evaluating the acceptability of a drug prior to competition: a) Will this drug lead the animal to experience significant pain or distress soon after competition? b) Will the drug permit the progression of underlying disease processes, thereby causing pain, debilitation, or breakdown in the long run? c) Does the drug give a horse an unfair competitive advantage? d) Does the drug tend to mask other substances whose use can result in pain, distress, debilitation, or breakdown, or that give the animal an unfair competitive advantage? e) Is the drug being used at least in part with the intention of assisting the animal in the short or long term or simply in order to permit it to compete? f) Are the effects of the drug sufficiently understood so that its impact on health and performance can be known by veterinarians and the public? g) Is the drug detectable on a routine and reliable basis?

4. Meaningful drug regulation requires that veterinarians cooperate with the letter and spirit of restrictions. Practitioners and trainers who constantly attempt to use new, as yet unregulated or undetectable substances to enhance performance seriously undermine the ability of authorities to protect the animals, owners, and the public. These tinkerers send the unmistakable message that they do not care about the animals, or the public at large. For they are willing to experiment with substances whose effects may not be known. The inevitable result of surreptitious use of ever newer drugs will be more stringent restrictions on *all* drug use. An additional effect may be the regulation of horse racing by the federal government, which might be forced to step in if the states appear unable to control abuses.

5. It is in the long-term economic and professional interests of veterinarians that horses be viewed as patients of value entitled to first-class, respectful medical care.

One thing that detracts from the value of patients is administering or selling drugs simply because trainers want them or a profit can be made. Another practice that undermines the value of equine patients is providing medications that allow horses to train or compete while permitting underlying disease processes to worsen so that proper treatment becomes more difficult, more painful, or impossible. Admittedly, there is sometimes strong controversy about when this point might in fact be reached.

6. The veterinary profession has a serious image problem. More than a few observers of the equine competitive world (including a fair number of veterinarians) believe that the chemical "quick fix" is coming to replace good management and good medicine. There are some practitioners who do shoot up horses with drugs because they can turn a profit doing so, because they do not have the time to attend to their patients' needs, because they share our society's irrational belief in chemical solutions to many of life's problems, or because they simply do not know enough about horses and the sports in which these animals compete (85; G.E. Fackelman, personal communication). The problem is not merely one of competence – some doctors who overmedicate know precisely what they are doing. The profession must support empirical and ethical studies that will protect not just the animals, but the profession's good name as well.

Moral Responsibilities of Attending Veterinarians

Administration of precompetition drugs is only one area in which attending veterinarians have important moral responsibilities. The following discussion highlights some other ethical issues in equine sport animal practice.

THE ATTENDING VETERINARIAN AS AN ADVOCATE OF THE PATIENT'S INTERESTS

There are many situations in which someone is needed to speak up on behalf of a horse. This can occur when an animal is worked very hard to earn money for its owner. An advocate for the horse may also be required when an owner lacks sufficient knowledge about how to care for his animal. The world of horse owners is varied, and generalizations are dangerous. But these two situations occur with significant frequency among the owners of performance animals. Many owners are in it for the money, and some who are not hand their animals over to trainers who view success in monetary terms. Other owners are new to the sport, or may be attracted more to its glamorous aspects than to the moral responsibilities it imposes regarding care of the animals.

The client hell-bent on winning can raise difficult problems for a practitioner. Clients who seek only profits may want something that is not in the animal's interests. They may request things that are not even in their own long-term economic interests. They may view the veterinarian as little more than a legal source of drugs and procedures already decided-upon. Some will go elsewhere if a demanded service is not provided. Veterinarians who will do whatever a client requests, even while knowing that doing it may harm the animal, make it more difficult for all doctors to speak up for horses' interests. Ultimately, the rationalization "If I don't do it, someone else will" can disappear only when enough doctors refuse to do it.

As Dr. M.D. Kingsbury observes (86), when clients do not have sufficient knowledge about how to care for their horses, it can become the veterinarian's task to provide basic instruction regarding general management and preventive medicine. From the purchase examination, to education about feeding, grooming, and sanitation, to instruction about first-aid, the doctor often may be able to best serve client and patient by assuming a role of general advisor. This, in turn, can enable him to prevent problems before they arise and to assure that he is called when his services are really required.

OBLIGATIONS TO OWNERS AND TRAINERS

Attending veterinarians have moral obligations to owners and trainers. Among these are the duties of honesty, loyalty and protection of confidences, trustworthiness, and respect (see Chapter 13). The primary foundation of an attending veterinarian's moral obligations to an owner or trainer is his agreement with them to provide professional services. Whether or not it is stated explicitly, part of this agreement is to assist the client in furthering the client's own goals. If the doctor disagrees with these goals, or if he believes that they are incompatible with his duties to the animal or to others (such as riders and the public), the doctor may attempt to convince the client to change his goals. The doctor may be justified in withdrawing from the professional relationship. But he may not surreptitiously substitute his own priorities for those of the owner, for then he is serving under false pretenses, which is a form of deception. True loyalty to a client sometimes requires declining to provide a service or product, even if the client wants it and it will not harm the animal. Some veterinarians sell drugs or special "home" remedies they know are useless because a trainer or owner wants them. Such an approach may be profitable in the short run, but it is deleterious to the image of the veterinarian as a healer and as a friend of the client.

Whom does one serve? Although veterinarians are obligated to serve clients loyally, it may sometimes seem unclear who the client really is. In the eyes of the law, the doctor almost always works for the owner, who ultimately pays the bills. But in actuality, it is often a trainer who engages one's services directly and requests treatments or procedures. Taking a course of action that displeases a trainer can result in loss of a patient (or many patients), even if it would benefit the owner. What should a doctor do when he finds something, or is asked to do something, that the trainer may be keeping from the owner or that the doctor believes is not in the interests of the owner or the animal? It is sometimes dangerous to presume that a trainer is not acting in accordance with the owner's instructions. I would argue that when a doctor is certain that the owner is not receiving important information or advice, he has a moral obligation to attempt to provide the owner with this information. This obligation flows from the fact that it is the owner who is paying for one's services, and that he is the person who owns the animal. This obligation is not always extinguished even if one has been told by the owner to deal exclusively with the trainer. Identifying and fulfilling one's ethical responsibilities to the "owner" can be especially difficult when one's patient is owned by a *group* of persons, many of whom may rarely come in contact with the animal or its trainer.

Purchase examinations. One of the most important areas in which the attending veterinarian's moral duties to the client come into play is in the conduct of purchase examinations. Because so much can turn on the results, a doctor must not only be thorough and honest but must also call relevant questions and issues to the client's attention even if the client does not raise them himself. As was discussed in Chapter 19, a doctor should not work for both a buyer and seller. Nor should his decision about a horse's suitability be affected by a desire to curry favor or economic gain from someone else (e.g., a trainer) who might have a stake in the sale.

OBLIGATIONS TO THIRD PARTIES AND THE PUBLIC

Attending veterinarians have moral obligations to some people who do not pay their fees. One who performs a procedure on a horse that can result in injury to riders or spectators commits a grave moral wrong. He also subjects himself to potential legal liability to those injured as a result of his wrongdoing. Practitioners who knowingly participate in attempts to gain an unfair competitive advantage for their clients by providing illegal substances or procedures also harm the betting public and owners and trainers who rely on general adherence to the rules of fair competition.

Insurance issues. It is immoral, and highly imprudent, for a doctor to be dishonest in completing documents relating to insurance applications or claims. One may think that it is helpful to a client to provide an incomplete or ambiguous statement about a horse's condition or history. One may think that the failure of an insurance company or client to pay adequately (or at all) for an insurance examination justifies a quicker, less careful approach. The result of dishonesty or carelessness may be denial of coverage by the insurer and legal action against the veterinarian by the company or client. Even when an insurance company can be fooled, others are victimized. "Successful" insurance fraud eventually leads to higher premiums for all. It is also profoundly immoral to help a client obtain an insurance payment by doing something to bring about or accelerate the illness or death of a horse. In addition to being fraudulent, such behavior can cause the animal unnecessary suffering.

One moral problem that seems to arise with some frequency concerns an attending veterinarian's obligations when a horse needs to be put out of its misery, but permission for euthanasia cannot be obtained quickly from the insurance company. I have heard credible stories about insurer representatives who delay returning telephone calls requesting permission, or who attempt to speak with younger, less experienced doctors in a practice in order to postpone euthanasia as long as possible. Insurers have a legitimate interest in avoiding making a payment on a mortality policy when euthanasia is medically premature or is motivated by fraud. But permitting a horse to suffer when there is no medical justification for doing so is intolerable. Several doctors have told me that the best way to avoid such a situation is to become known to insurance company representatives as someone who is honest, but who will not tolerate delay when euthanasia is necessary.

Moral Responsibilities of Official Veterinarians

An official veterinarian at a race or competition works for the institution or organization under whose control or auspices the competition is being held. He may be a full- or part-time employee or agent of the state or of a track or association.

Many of the legal and moral responsibilities of an official veterinarian flow from the regulations or rule books governing his actions. He must therefore know what his mandated responsibilities do and do not include.

An official veterinarian is called upon to serve many interests. He must attend to the interests of the horses and their riders. He also promotes the interests of owners, bettors, and spectators by assuring that rules upon which all rely are followed. The official veterinarian also serves to support the credibility of the state government or association in their roles as regulators. How an official veterinarian performs these functions can vary with the nature of the competition. As Drs. M. Mackay-Smith and M. Cohen observe, in combined training or distance riding events, "participation as a learning experience for the competitor is probably more stressed ... than is the case in more traditional horse sports. The veterinary officer stands, therefore, in the role of teacher as well as practitioner." These authors urge that in such events, the veterinarian's first moral obligation is "to protect the horse's interests and his or her second duty is to assist the rider in the competition" (87). The official veterinarian at a race track is typically forbidden by law to attend to routine, nonemergency matters.

An official veterinarian must apply the rules impartially and consistently. He must not permit himself to be influenced by his own economic interests. To preserve his ability to convince others that he is serving impartially, he should avoid any behavior that would give even the slightest appearance of impropriety. Therefore, whenever competition or money is a major element of an event (which is almost always the case), the same doctor ought not to serve as both the official veterinarian and an attending veterinarian to some or all competitors. Those using another veterinarian may wonder whether the official veterinarian will side with owners whose animals he is attending. Even when an official veterinarian will attend to the routine medical needs of all competitors, some owners may ask whether he will be most loyal to those from whom he can gain the most remuneration. The AVMA and the American Association of Equine Practitioners have adopted a policy critical of horse shows that permit the same person to serve as official and attending veterinarian. This policy recommends that a show select as official veterinarian a doctor from outside the local area, who is "not closely familiar with the horses being shown and who has no clients among the exhibitors" (88).

Moral Responsibilities of Government and Associations

Protection of the interests of horses, riders, owners, and the public requires vigorous activity by government and private groups charged with protecting these interests.

State governments. State racing commissions and veterinary boards have substantial authority to discipline attending and official veterinarians who violate these agencies' technical and ethical rules. Licenses to practice at tracks can be suspended or revoked by the racing commission. The state board can restrict the activities of a doctor who behaves incompetently or unethically at the track. Effective government supervision depends upon the willingness of those who encounter abuses to report them. Racing commissions and state boards must also have sufficient funding, personnel, and legal talent to make effective enforcement possible.

The fact that state racing commissions call for vigorous monitoring by official veterinarians does not necessarily make it so. A recent study of thoroughbred racing at a state fair in Massachusetts conducted by Dr. G. E. Fackelman found that 72% of the horses permitted to race exhibited orthopedic, respiratory or conformational unsoundness; 69% showed signs of previous injury or deformity of the musculoskeletal system; 6% were injured while racing; and 14 horses of the 296 entering the paddock could not complete the race because of already known orthopedic problems. The study documented injuries that worsened "as a direct result of the (sometimes successful) completion of a given competition." It was found that the mere presence of the veterinarians conducting the survey reduced the level of injury. "When owners came to realize that our undertaking was serious and steady, they showed the tendency to eliminate their animals [from competition] and not even present them in the paddock" (89). The study also revealed questionable adherence to state regulations prohibiting official veterinarians from treating horses except in cases of emergency.

State racing commissions must assure that official veterinarians have sufficient knowledge, experience, and courage to be able to stand up to owners, trainers, and attending veterinarians when necessary. Required prerace examinations must be conducted thoroughly and competently. Periodic investigations should be undertaken by racing commissions to evaluate the performance of official veterinarians. Racing commissions should consider including animal welfare experts among their full-time staff. Such persons might be able to assure that the interests of the animals, as well as those of owners, the public, and the state revenue department, are advocated in commission deliberations.

Another ethical issue that must be addressed more conscientiously by state racing commissions and veterinarians is the appropriateness of racing 2-year-old horses whose musculoskeletal systems have not yet matured (90).

Private associations. These associations, under whose auspices show events are held, have a moral obligation to monitor behavior by attending veterinarians. For example, the American Horse Shows Association has a drug testing program. However, I am told by practitioners that a very small proportion of competing horses may be tested at a show, and that some use of prohibited substances continues. Moreover, AHSA rules (91) do not allow for the disciplining of attending veterinarians who might knowingly administer drugs in violation of the rules; the entire burden is placed on owners and trainers. Associations must be able and willing to discipline attending veterinarians who knowingly participate in prohibited procedures with the purpose of enabling animals to compete in violation of requirements. It is unrealistic for associations, which are closer to the situation, to expect state veterinary boards or federal authorities to do the job.

The Federal Horse Protection Act of 1970 (92). This act gives the Animal and Plant Health Inspection Service responsibility for enforcing rules to protect the welfare of show horses. APHIS regulations provide that no "chain, boot, roller, collar, action device, method, practice, or substance shall be used with respect to any horse at any horse show, horse exhibition, or horse sale or auction if such use causes or can reasonably be expected to cause such horse to be sore" (93). The regulations define soreness, contain many specific prohibitions, and impose inspection, detainment, and reporting requirements. Private practitioners can participate in inspections and enforcement through licensing as a "designated qualified person" (DQP). Veterinarian-DQPs must have general APHIS accreditation. Additionally, they must be either members of the American Association of Equine Practitioners, large animal practitioners "with substantial equine experience," or "knowledgeable in the area of equine lameness as related to soring and soring practices" (94). DQPs are not licensed directly by APHIS, but by industry organizations or associations that have obtained general certification from APHIS for their DQP programs. Additional inspection and supervisory functions are carried out by APHIS veterinarians.

DOG RACING

Greyhound dog racing is an enormously popular sport. It attracts large numbers of spectators and generates tens of millions of dollars annually for state coffers.[d] Yet, many veterinarians will admit that they know very little about the sport or its impact on the animals. Few veterinary schools offer courses on the subject. Even state authorities empowered to regulate greyhound racing can lack a complete understanding of the sport. For example, in 1986, the Massachusetts Legislature

---

[d]In Massachusetts alone, which has a population of approximately 6 million people, attendance at greyhound racing meetings at the state's two dog tracks totalled 2,630,092 in 1986. Some $340 million was wagered, of which the state's share of the handle was almost $30 million (95). The State of Florida has over a dozen greyhound tracks.

appointed an advisory committee to determine what was happening to greyhounds "bred for racing who never qualify for pari-mutuel races or have reached the end of their racing career" (96). The Committee could not answer the question. It found "an abysmal lack of official or authoritative data concerning the number of greyhounds who race in Massachusetts, end their racing career in Massachusetts, are put to sleep in Massachusetts, are moved to other racing jurisdictions, are placed for adoption, or are given for medical research" (97).

Objections to the Sport

There is considerable opposition to greyhound racing among humane societies and animal welfare advocates. Objections typically are based on one or more of the following positions: 1) a belief in animal use abolitionism, which implies condemnation not just of dog racing, but of all animal sports; 2) the view that it is wrong to use *dogs* for sport and wagering; 3) opposition to the manner in which racing dogs are treated during breeding, training, or racing; and 4) opposition to the fact that the sport results in the killing of many surplus dogs or their use in research.

Animal use abolitionism is not a plausible position and need not be discussed again here. The view that it is disrespectful to use the beloved dog in a wagering sport does have intuitive appeal to some. However, I have found that when people who express a general opposition to dog racing are challenged to explain their feelings, they usually invoke the third objection listed above. For it seems unreasonable to single out dogs as inappropriate beings for sport and wagering events. It makes little sense to concede (as almost everyone will) that it is not inherently degrading or demeaning for human athletes to run around tracks or to compete in sporting events on which bets may be placed, but that it is so for dogs.

It is more plausible to try to object to dog racing on the grounds that the animals are not treated as well as they ought to be. Such an objection usually takes one of two forms. Some people believe that the dogs are subjected to bad conditions that cause them suffering or distress, such as poor living conditions, inadequate veterinary care, difficult training and racing schedules, inadequate opportunities for socialization, and so on. Other people assert that however well-cared for racing dogs may be, they will never be treated as they deserve to be treated because they cannot live the kind of life a valued family pet would enjoy.

The contention that some greyhounds live unpleasant lives is undoubtedly true. In any group of animal owners, there will be some who do not treat their animals properly. One hears stories of greyhound operations that do not have adequate heat or light or where animals are not given good care. But there are also greyhound breeding and training facilities in which the animals are well-cared for, and are genuinely liked by their owners and trainers. As I shall indicate below, there are a number of issues that must be explored regarding promotion of the welfare of these animals. However, the fact that some owners may not treat their animals properly or that more sometimes can be done to treat them better does not mean that all greyhounds are condemned to an unacceptable life.

It is more difficult to counter the objection that dogs used for racing, even when treated as well as can be expected within the context of the sport, simply do not live the kind of life that can be enjoyed by a typical family pet. As a statement of fact, this is surely correct. Racing dogs are kept in a kennel environment, they are trained and run in ways family dogs are not, and most do not experience the same measure of human companionship as do typical pet dogs. It would certainly be better for racing dogs if they had such a life. But this does not make the life they do lead morally intolerable – any more than it is wrong to race horses because these animals might have a better life as companion animals. Animals are not people. Therefore, most of us will accept treating different animals of the same species in varying ways. We believe this is sometimes appropriate because we do not regard all animals of a given species as entitled to the best life that can be provided to them. It is interesting to speculate whether dog racing would be as much the target of objections as it is today if dogs (like horses) were used primarily as working and sporting animals rather than as pets.

The Adoption Issue

In my view, the most difficult ethical issue in greyhound racing concerns what happens to the animals when they are no longer useful. This question cannot be addressed simply by improving racing dog welfare. The problem is generated by the sport itself and requires hard decisions by the industry and government.

The first source of the problem is the number of dogs needed to maintain the sport. In a state like Massachusetts, each greyhound race will have 8 animals. On average, a track will offer 12 races per racing performance, and on some calendar days, a track will have more than one performance. Some dogs are raced as often as twice a week. The number of dogs used in pari-mutuel races is therefore substantial. In 1986, there were in Massachusetts alone a total of 11,760 races involving some 95,000 entries (95). But the number of dogs that actually reach the betting races may represent only the tip of the iceberg. Dogs must first qualify in official schooling races. Not all make it, and some require so many attempts that they are not profitable for owners to keep. Moreover, the search by breeders for speedy animals results in the birth of many dogs that are not promising enough even to enter qualifying races. Dogs who do make it to the pari-mutuels may have brief careers if they do not do well, and few dogs race after they are 3½ to 4 years of age. Dogs weeded out of the process (and eventually all are) may be euthanized, sent to another state in which competition is less severe, adopted as pets, or sold or donated for medical research. Although the number of animals generated each year around the country is substantial, it is not yet possible to determine accurately how many there are or what becomes of them.

The second source of the problem is that in general, these animals are far from useless when their role in the sport ends. There is little doubt that most can make wonderful pets. The time required to acclimatize healthy, uninjured greyhounds to people and the life of a family pet can be quite brief, sometimes just a few days. Many of these animals are near the beginning of their natural life spans. They are no more expensive or burdensome to keep than most other breeds.

The present system discards countless animals that perform, or are an integral part of a system that performs, a profitable service. This is wrong. Greyhounds were all once valued companion animals. The species has been appropriated, bred, and trained for racing. This process earns millions of dollars for owners, trainers, tracks, associations, bettors, veterinarians, and state governments. In return, those who benefit – including states whose treasuries share the bounty – have a moral obligation to give something back to the animals.

WHAT CAN BE DONE?

The following approaches are suggested for consideration by the industry, government, and veterinarians. Some of these suggestions are already being tried or contemplated in several states.

1. Information should be gathered in each racing jurisdiction regarding the number of animals bred and their disposition, including transmittal out of state, adoption, euthanasia, and receipt by research facilities. Racing states must therefore require rigorous record-keeping of such occurrences by owners, tracks, track veterinarians, attending veterinarians, adoption services, animal shelters, and research facilities. Reliable information would enable state authorities to ascertain what is happening and would assist in the monitoring of programs to promote adoption or humane euthanasia.

2. Each racing jurisdiction should establish a fund to assist in the adoption of retired and surplus greyhounds. Moneys for such a fund should come from owner winnings and track and state shares of the racing handle. Proceeds from the fund would be distributed to greyhound adoption services (including individuals such as veterinarians) approved by the state. Consideration might also be given to providing rewards to owners who transmit animals to an adoption service or new owner.

3. Standards ought to be established for greyhound adoption services to assure that animals are properly socialized and placed in appropriate homes.

4. The industry ought to publicize the availability of greyhounds so that bettors and the general public become aware of adoption possibilities.

5. A concerted effort should be made by all beneficiaries of greyhound racing to counter the image of the breed as vicious and intractable. This view of greyhounds may make some people feel better about the fact that so many surplus dogs are killed. But the image is false and unnecessary. It also makes placing surplus animals more difficult.

6. Veterinarians might consider adopting surplus animals out of their practices. Dr. David Goodman, a Florida practitioner, regularly keeps one or two greyhounds in his hospital for acclimatization and adoption. He charges adopting clients a modest fee for sterilization and any required deworming and vaccinations. Goodman has found that he is performing an important service while at the same time gaining good public relations for his hospital (D. Goodman, personal communication).

7. State and local veterinary medical associations might encourage their members to publicize nonprofit greyhound adoption services in their waiting rooms. VMAs and individual doctors could provide or underwrite low-cost veterinary services for adoption agencies.

8. Veterinary hospitals ought to consider using surplus greyhounds as blood donors. Such use does not preclude attempts to adopt these animals.

9. States that promote greyhound breeding through cash prizes or other incentives for owners should require those who receive such subsidies to pay part of their rewards into the greyhound adoption fund. Additionally, state encouragement of breeding ought to be modified or withdrawn if it is determined that the state's policy is contributing to the destruction of an inappropriate number of unadoptable animals. It makes no sense for a state to promote adoption and at the same time encourage overbreeding that contributes to an increasing need for adoption programs.

10. Each racing state must place at least as much importance upon the adoption of retired and surplus greyhounds as it places on encouraging the breeding and racing of faster animals. In other words, if the quality of racing dogs bred or raced in the state must be compromised in order to control the number of animals euthanized, so be it. Owners and bettors should be able to live with somewhat slower dogs so that fewer animals have to be killed. A state policy refusing to tolerate increased euthanasias to improve dog "quality" might stimulate the search for breeding techniques that will not produce so many surplus dogs.

The Use of Surplus Greyhounds in Research

Some greyhounds whose racing careers have ended (or never began) find their way into scientific research facilities. Many animal welfare advocates find this aspect of the sport even more disturbing than the euthanasia of surplus animals.

I argue in Chapter 23 that it is preferable to use existing unwanted dogs in biomedical research (provided such research is scientifically justified and morally appropriate) than to kill existing animals and require the breeding of new animals that will be treated exactly as would those that are killed. I would apply the same general argument to surplus racing dogs. Indeed, using such animals in research might obviate one important complaint to the use of animals from pounds and shelters: the objection that former members of human-animal bonds ought not to be subjected to laboratory and experimental conditions. Nevertheless, because racing dogs have *already* been used for human purposes (many quite vigorously), I would argue that it is wrong to automatically and routinely use them in research. Given what they have already provided, no greyhound ought to be released for research until *serious* attempts have been made to adopt it.

There are several issues one might raise regarding greyhounds used in research. The Massachusetts Advisory Committee recommended permitting research use of retired dogs provided that they are 1) eventually scheduled for euthanasia; 2) used in approved kinds of nonsurvival projects; 3) donated and not sold for research; 4) "not used in safety evaluation or toxicity research projects, or in any medical research involving recovery from anesthesia or the consciousness of pain;" and 5) "disposed of humanely at the completion of any research exercise" (98). It is a legitimate ethical principle that retired greyhounds used in research be given special consideration for their previous service. However, several of the Massachusetts Committee's recommendations are not reasonable applications of this principle. Some research necessarily involves recovery from anesthesia, and some involves pain that is brief and trivial. Nor is it obvious why all greyhounds used in research are better off being killed than recovering from anesthesia or experiencing some pain or distress. Indeed, some relatively benign uses of research dogs (e.g., as long-term experimental blood donors) seem far better than automatic euthanasia. Killing all dogs would also preclude their being adopted after a research project is completed, a goal that I argue in Chapter 23 ought to be given more serious consideration by researchers.

Euthanasia

Rumors abound about owners and trainers who kill dogs in brutal and morally unacceptable ways. If racing dogs do have to be killed, they must be euthanized according to approved methods and by personnel (such as animal shelter technicians) who can assure a painless death. If there is inhumane killing of greyhounds, state authorities must make it a major priority to find, punish, and prevent it.

Other Moral Issues

Greyhound racing presents other important ethical issues, many of which are similar to those arising out of the use of horses in racing and show competitions. For example, there are legal restrictions on drugs that can be used on dogs prior to competition. These rules are not always followed. As is the case in horse racing, an attending veterinarian can play an important role in advocating the interests of the animal athlete. State laws require the presence of an official track veterinarian to protect the interests of the wagering public as well as the animals. As is the case in horse racing, some states expect more of dog track veterinarians than others, and some track veterinarians are more conscientious than others in protecting the welfare of the animals.

Research concerning race horses and their welfare has long been accepted as a legitimate part of the mission of the veterinary schools. Yet, few veterinary schools or academic institutions undertake serious scientific work on racing dogs. Substantial progress in improving welfare and performance requires acceptance of the racing dog as a subject of legitimate academic concern. The following are among the issues and challenges that research should prove helpful in addressing:

- Improvement in basic knowledge of racing greyhound kinetics, physiology, and biochemistry;
- Development of track materials and design that will enhance performance and provide greater protection against injury;
- Continuing development of training techniques to prevent and assist in the treatment of injuries;
- Systematic study of racing dog nutrition to enhance performance and welfare;
- Investigation of scientific breeding techniques to reduce scattershot searches for the "magic" dog and unnecessary surpluses of animals;
- Improved and more conscientiously applied measures for testing for prohibited substances; better training and state racing commission supervision of track veterinarians;
- Exploration of the use of Ivermectin for heart worm prevention. (Diethylcarbamazine citrate is prohibited by current regulations on the grounds that it masks the presence of other prohibited substances.)
- Exploration of the use of mechanical lures rather than live rabbits for the training of racing dogs. (The use of rabbits has already been abandoned in some areas.)

RODEO

There are over 1,000 rodeos held in the United States and Canada each year. The Professional Rodeo Cowboys Association (PRCA), the leading official organization for professional rodeos, sanctions over 600 performances each season, attracting an estimated 14 million paying spectators. Additionally, many communities, colleges, and local organizations sponsor their own rodeos (99).

Rodeo is much more than a source of entertainment or profit. As Dr. Elizabeth Lawrence observes (100), rodeo is

> a quintessential part of that complex (and perhaps indefinable) mystique which we call the American West. As the cowboy sport of rodeo developed out of frontier experience, so it also shaped and continues to shape our perceptions of all that the Western frontier has come to symbolize.

Rodeo proclaims and promotes such values as individualism, independence, egalitarianism, courage, toleration of pain and injury, and the desire to tame the wild. It provides "an opportunity for members of the contemporary society which support it to bring out and set forth for display and exploration the various themes still central to their occupation and ethos" (101).

Ethical deliberation about rodeo cannot underestimate the great importance the sport has to participants and observers. Nor should those for whom rodeo is unimportant forget that we are all enriched by the cultural diversity to which the sport contributes. On the other hand, the interests of rodeo animals do not disappear because these animals happen to be utilized in a culturally significant activity.

Welfare Issues: The Current Climate

Rodeo is anathema to many animal welfare advocates. The sport is regularly accused of offenses ranging from deliberate and willful cruelty to corruption of the nation's youth. In a joint statement, the Humane Society of the United States and the American Humane Society demanded complete abolition of rodeo. They claimed that rodeos

> result in torment, harassment, and stress being inflicted upon the participating animals and expose rodeo stock to the probability of pain, injury, or death ... [R]odeos are not an accurate or harmless portrayal of ranching skills; rather, they display and encourage an insensitivity to and acceptance of brutal treatment of animals in the name of sport (102).

The following are among the features of the sport that some animal welfare advocates find objectionable:

- The use of the flank strap to stimulate bucking in horses and bulls. The tightening of the strap around the animal's abdomen is frequently characterized as causing excruciating pain to the genitalia;
- Use of an electric prod ("hot shot") to stimulate bucking in bulls;
- Spurring of bucking horses and bulls;
- The fact that much of the animals' time is "spent in transit or in tiny enclosures behind the chutes [and that] ... these animals are not being 'saved' from anything, since the slaughterhouse is almost always their final destination after they have outlived their rodeo usefulness" (103);
- The calf-roping event, in which a rope is thrown by a mounted cowboy around the neck of a calf, which is then taken down to the ground and tied. This event has been called "a brutal mockery of western heritage" (103);
- The single cowboy steer-roping event, in which a rider ropes a steer around the horns, hits the steer with his rope as he turns, thereby taking it to the ground, and ties the animal's feet;
- The steer wrestling event, in which a mounted cowboy jumps from his horse, grabs one horn and the jaw of a running steer, and throws the animal on its side or back. This event has been characterized as pitting "man against animal in hand-to-hand combat" (103);
- The fact that spectators cheer for the cowboys to subdue the animals, which (with the exception of the cowboy's horse) are typically viewed as "the enemy."

As shall be discussed, many of these criticisms are mistaken. But far worse is the uncompromising assault by many humane societies upon the entire sport. This stance often makes it impossible for rodeo enthusiasts concerned about animal welfare to participate with humane societies in meaningful dialogue. It is not surprising that the rodeo community's response to demands that the entire sport be terminated is vigorous defense of rodeo as a whole. Humane societies might ask how they would react if they were told that their "'piece of Americana' should be relegated to the history books where it belongs" (103).

The following thoughts are offered to focus discussion.

1. Many criticisms of rodeo are incorrect or grossly exaggerated. For example, it is often alleged that the flank strap is impermissible because it induces horses and bulls to behave in ways they would not otherwise. Accordingly, rodeo people have been drawn into a debate about whether the strap enhances what these animals would do anyway or is an external, unnatural stimulation. But this is not the most

important issue. Sporting animals are often called upon to behave in ways that are not completely "natural" to their species. The issue is whether the strap is sufficiently invasive of the animals' interests to render it impermissible. As Dr. Frank Santos notes, the strap is not placed on the genitals, and horses or bulls do not behave as if tortured by pain for the 8 seconds or so during which the strap is tightened. If the animals were in significant pain, they would either "go into a wild frenzy, tearing up the chute, stampeding and crashing into fences, and throwing themselves down. Or they would simply lie down and sulk..." (104). The strap is undoubtedly irritating. However, it is hard to conclude that this short-lived stimulation is so horrendous as to make bucking events immoral. Indeed, such a conclusion can only appear reasonable to someone who has *already* decided that artificially inducing an animal to buck is enormously disrespectful and greatly invasive of its interests. Having made this judgment, one might then find the irritation caused by the flank strap sufficiently distressful to push its use over the line of what is permissible.

Likewise, several other objections to rodeo seem understandable only if one supposes that they reflect an already-reached condemnation of the sport. How, for example, can a humane society that would not denounce the use of animals for food, object to the eventual slaughter of rodeo animals, unless it believed that rodeo is inherently disrespectful to animals? (In fact, most rodeo animals have it much easier than their agricultural counterparts.) Similarly, those who find the spurring of horses or bulls offensive may not think it important that sharp spurs are prohibited and that injuries to animals from spurs are rare. To these people, it is still the *spurring* of a horse or bull. Likewise, those who object to the use of an electric prod to stimulate a bull to buck probably see this action as inherently disrespectful. They may not care that the prod is commonly used in ranching to move cattle into chutes. Characterizing steer wrestling as "hand-to-hand combat" seems more reflective of a conclusion about the appropriateness of such an event than of the facts. As Dr. Santos notes (104), such a characterization gives more equality to the participants than they really have. The human participant in a steer wrestling event is more likely to be the one injured. Indeed, most rodeo animals are far more dangerous to cowboys than the latter are to the animals.

2. Many rodeo enthusiasts do take animal welfare seriously. Participants who use their own horses in various events take great care of these animals, which are often the key to success and can require years of training. Stock contractors who provide animals to rodeos have a strong economic incentive to maintain them in good condition. Insistence upon proper treatment of the animals is a routine feature of instruction at organized rodeo schools. Rules of rodeo competition also address welfare considerations. For example, the Professional Rodeo Cowboys Association prohibits excessive use of the electric prod. Other practices that have been criticized by animal welfare activists, but are in fact prohibited or penalized by rodeo association rules, include abruptly "jerking" roped animals and holding a horse by the ears or nose during the wild horse race event.

Rodeo enthusiasts with whom I speak appear eager to reduce hardship or distress imposed on the animals. The PRCA, for example, worked with the legislature of one state to require the use of a padded flank strap after a law was passed prohibiting the strap (M. Etienne, personal communication). The Salinas, California rodeo found that it could reduce calf hind leg fractures significantly by making the footing in the arena firmer (G. Deter, personal communication). At many rodeos, veterinarians are present to provide medical care for animals and to assure that they are not being overworked or mistreated.

Nor does it follow from the fact that some rodeo events pit cowboys against animals that the sport inculcates cruelty to or dislike for animals. Most team sports invite spectators to oppose the "good" team against the "bad." This practice does not appear to promote general cruelty or disrespect toward people.

3. One cannot but be impressed by the spirit of professionalism many rodeo enthusiasts express. Stated time and again is the desire to maintain rodeo as a family sport that rejects inappropriate treatment of animals. Many in the rodeo world support efforts to train cowboys and cowgirls who are technically proficient and who take a serious view of their responsibilities to the animals.

4. The rodeo world is not monolithic. There exist significant differences regarding the appropriateness of certain activities and practices. Rodeo people readily admit that there are some in the sport who do not show enough respect for the animals. (This fact does not distinguish rodeo from any other animal sport or general use of animals.) Many cowboys criticize the traditional steer-roping event as inhumane, and it is allowed only in a few states (105). Some in the sport are urging shortening the distance calves in roping events are permitted to run before they can be chased, in order to reduce the potential for injury (G. Deter, personal communication). Female participation in some of the traditionally male-dominated events appears to be on the increase, although in general, rodeo still relegates women participants to an inferior role (106). The growing popularity of the sport may provide impetus for diversity and change. Rodeo has attracted participants and spectators who have geographic, cultural, and economic roots quite different from those of the traditional rodeo cowboy. For some of these people, athletic aspects of the sport might be more important than its cultural and economic underpinnings. They might take a different view of what the sport may demand of the animals.

5. It is clear that much more can be done to improve the welfare of rodeo animals. Such a statement could be made of any animal sport, so rodeo enthusiasts ought not to find it offensive. But there are more specific reasons why greater attention to animal welfare in rodeo is needed.

Rodeo differs from horse and dog racing in that the presence of an official veterinarian is not universally required. The argument is sometimes made that it would be impossible to require smaller rodeos to have a veterinarian, because there may be no veterinarian in the area who is sufficiently familiar with the medical problems of rodeo animals. Such an argument, however, only contributes to the shortage of practitioners who can serve at rodeos. If all rodeos were compelled to assure the presence of veterinary care, there eventually would be doctors able to do the job.

Some rodeo events, such as steer-roping, subject animals to a significant amount of violence and a high probability of injury. Lawrence reports that during one 9-day rodeo, more than 27 animals were lost, including 9 steers that had to be destroyed as a result of steer-roping, one of which suffered a broken neck (107). As the reduction in leg fractures achieved by the Salinas rodeo shows, steps can sometimes be taken to decrease the risk of injury and death while not materially altering an event. (Euthanasia or shipment for slaughter typically follows injuries such as leg fractures; decreasing the incidence of such problems would reduce markedly the number of animals lost.) Research can be conducted to find less dangerous ways of approaching some rodeo events and practices. However, if an event is inherently and irreparably dangerous to the animals, it ought to be eliminated. The fact that many states have already prohibited steer-roping proves that changes can be made without ruining the sport.

There is virtually no academic attention to rodeo animals or their welfare. There will be severe limitations on our ability to demand measures to improve rodeo animal welfare without serious understanding of what would in fact promote the welfare of these animals. If we are just beginning to accumulate reliable scientific knowledge regarding horse and dog athletes, can anyone doubt that there is an enormous amount that needs to be learned about rodeo animal welfare?

6. At present, the organized veterinary profession plays a minimal role in the promotion of rodeo animal welfare. There is no reason why this should be so. Leading conventions and conferences could include seminars in which practitioners serving at rodeos can share knowledge and suggestions with other veterinarians. Such information ought to be made available to veterinary students. The more veterinarians know about the sport, the greater will be the likelihood that the care and treatment of the animals can be improved.

REFERENCES

1. Fetrow J, Madison JB, and Galligan D: Economic decisions in veterinary practice: A method for field use. *J Am Vet Med Assoc* 186:792, 1985.
2. *Id.*, 794.
3. Van Saun R, Bartlett PC, and Morrow D: Monitoring the Effects of Postpartum Diseases on Milk Production in Dairy Cattle. *Compendium on Continuing Education for the Practicing Veterinarian* 9(6):F212-220, 1987.
4. *Id.*, F212.
5. E.g., Friend TH, Polan CE, *et al.*: Adreno gluticocorticoid response to exogenous adrenocorticotropin mediated by density and social disruption in lactating cows. *J Dairy Sci* 60:1958-1963, 1977.
6. Straw B and Friendship R: Expanding the role of the veterinarian on swine farms. *Compendium on Continuing Education for the Practicing Veterinarian* 8:F69, 1986.
7. Stein TE: Marketing Health Management to Food Animal Enterprises. Part II. *Compendium on Continuing Education for the Practicing Veterinarian* 8(7):S331, 1986.
8. Stein TE: Marketing Health Management to Food Animal Enterprises. Part II. *Compendium on Continuing Education for the Practicing Veterinarian* 8(7):S331, 1986, quoting Wilson MR, *et al.*: Computerized health monitoring in swine health management. *Proc Pig Vet Soc* 7:64-71, 1982.
9. Curtis SE: Animal Well-Being and Animal Care. *Vet Clin North Am Food Anim Pract* 3(2):373-374, 1987.
10. E.g., Husmann RJ: Dairy Cow Herd Health Management. In Howard JL (ed): *Current Veterinary Therapy: Food Animal Practice 2*. Philadelphia: W.B. Saunders Co., 1986, p 123; Erb HN: The Teaching of Animal Health Economics at the Undergraduate Level. In: *Third International Symposium on Veterinary Epidemiology and Economics*. Edwardsville, KS: Veterinary Medicine Publishing Co., 1983, p 343.
11. Brambell FWR, Chairman: *Report of the Technical Committee to Enquire Into the Welfare of Animals Kept Under Intensive Livestock Husbandry Systems*. London: Cmnd. 2836, Her Majesty's Stationery Office, 1965, quoted in Loew FM: The veterinarian and intensive livestock production: humane considerations. *Canadian Veterinary Journal* 13:230, 1972.
12. Jacobs FS: A perspective on animal rights and domestic animals. *J Am Vet Med Assoc* 184:1344-1345, 1984.
13. Beilharz RG and Zeeb K: Applied ethology and animal welfare. *Applied Animal Ethology* 7:3-10, 1981.
14. E.g., Hart BL: *Behavior of Domestic Animals*. New York, W.H. Freeman and Co., 1985, p 353 (stating that because of correlations between processes in human and non-human subcortical areas of the brain "in dealing with stimuli that we

relate to the production of pain or fear we feel somewhat justified in assuming that animals are experiencing some of the same emotions as we would"); Rowan AN: Animal Anxiety and Animal Suffering. *Appl Anim Behav Sci 20*, 1988, in press.

15. *J Am Vet Med Assoc* 191:1184-1298, 1987.
16. *J Am Vet Med Assoc* 191:1187, 1987.
17. Nielsen M, Braestrup C, and Squires RF: Evidence for a Late Evolutionary Appearance of Brain-Specific Benzodiazepine Receptors: An Investigation of 18 Vertebrate and 5 Invertebrate Species. *Brain Res* 141:342-346, 1978.
18. Gray JA: *The Neuropsychology of Anxiety: An Enquiry into Functions of the Septo-Hippocampal System*. Oxford: Oxford University Press, 1982.
19. Curtis, *op. cit.*, p 373.
20. *Id.*, 377.
21. *J Am Vet Med Assoc:* 191:1188, 1987.
22. *J Am Vet Med Assoc:* 191:1187, 1987.
23. Fox MW: *Farm Animals*. Baltimore: University Park Press, 1984, p 227.
24. Curtis, *op. cit.*, p 373.
25. Hughes BO: Behavior as an index of welfare. Vth Eur. Poult. Conf., pp 1005-1014, 1976, cited with approval by Wood-Gush DGM: Housing systems and animal welfare research requirements - a review. *Animal Regulation Studies* 2:275, 1979/1980.
26. Lorz A: *Tierschutzgesetz. Kommentar*. Munich: Verlag C.H. Beck, 1973, quoted in Fox, *op. cit.*, p 178.
27. Carpenter E: *Animals and Ethics*. London: Watkins, 1980, quoted by Duncan IH: Animal Rights - Animal Welfare: A Scientist's Assessment. *Poult Sci* 60:490, 1981.
28. Banks EM: Behavioral research to answer questions about animal welfare. *J Anim Sci* 54:435, 1982.
29. Beilharz RG and Zeeb K: Applied ethology and animal welfare. *Applied Animal Ethology* 7:3, 1981.
30. Dawkins MS: *Animal Suffering*. London: Chapman and Hall, 1980, p 10.
31. *Id.*, 25.
32. Simonsen HB: Role of applied ethology in international work on farm animal welfare. *Vet Rec* 111(15):341, 1982.
33. Curtis, *op. cit.*, pp 369-391.
34. *The Veterinarian's Role in Food Animal Welfare*. Schaumburg, IL: American Veterinary Medical Association, undated, unpaginated.
35. Loew FM: The Animal Welfare *Bête Noire* in Veterinary Medicine. *Canadian Veterinary Journal* 28:692, 1987.
36. See, e.g., Fox MW, *op. cit.*, pp 60-63; Curtis, *op. cit.*, pp 373-377.
37. Fox, *op. cit.*, p 94.
38. For more extensive descriptions of such husbandry methods and their effects on behavior see Fox, *op. cit.*, pp 95-103; Kiley-Worthington M: The Behavior of Confined Calves Raised for Veal: Are These Animals Distressed? *Int J Stud Anim Prob* 4(3):198-213, 1983.
39. Fox, *op. cit.*, p 102.
40. *AVMA Guide for Veal Calf Care and Production*, p 1 (stating that "about half the veal consumed goes to the kosher market").
41. Fox, *op. cit.*, pp 98-105.
42. USDA Food Safety and Inspection Service. 6200 Ante Mortem and Post Mortem Inspection Survey, 1987.
43. Fox, *op. cit.*, pp 99-101.

44. Scher G: Facts about Veal Production and the Economic Impact of H.R. 2859 on Veal Farmers, Dairy Farmers, Consumers. N. Manchester, IN: American Veal Association, undated, unpaginated.
45. *The Veterinarian's Role in Food Animal Welfare.* Schaumburg, IL: American Veterinary Medical Association, undated, unpaginated.
46. *AVMA Guide for Veal Calf Care and Production.* Schaumburg, IL: American Veterinary Medical Association, 1986.
47. E.g., Veal Crate Ban – We Are Still Waiting. *Agscene* Jun 1987:8 (reporting support by the Animal Welfare Committee of the British Veterinary Association for a government proposal to prohibit veal crates).
48. Fox, *op. cit.*, p 139.
49. Wise JK: *The US Market for Food Animal Veterinary Medical Services.* Schaumburg, IL: American Veterinary Medical Association, p 53.
50. *Id.*, 91-92.
51. *Id.*, 74-76.
52. *Id.*, 53.
53. *Id.*, 92, emphasis added.
54. *Id.*, vi.
55. *Id.*, 143-147.
56. Hooker TL and Brown AC: Letter to Maryland veterinarian licensees. March 18, 1987.
57. Prescription vs Over-the-Counter Labeling Is Focus of Veterinary Medicine Advisory Committee. *J Am Vet Med Assoc* 193:25, 1988 (also reporting that "80% of the approximately 700 drugs approved for use in companion animals are available only by prescription, while only 7% of the 700 approved food animal medications require a prescription").
58. FDA/BVA Release. July 17, 1983.
59. FDA Compliance Policy Guides. Guide 7125.06. Chapt. 25 – Animal Drugs. November 11, 1986, p 1.
60. E.g., Glock RD: Letter. *J Am Vet Med Assoc* 189:1260, 1986; Curran BJ: Letter. *J Am Vet Med Assoc* 189:1262, 1986; FDA Proposes to Withdraw Dimetridazole. *J Am Vet Med Assoc* 190:509, 1987.
61. Complaint, Cowdin *et al.* v. Young. US Dist. Ct., West. Dist. La., CV87-0912.
62. Walterscheid E: FDA vs. DVM: Profession Scores TKO Against Regulation. *Veterinary Economics* Apr 1987:34-42.
63. Cowdin *et al.* v. Young, 681 F. Supp. 366, 369 (W.D. La. 1987); see also, Extra-Label Use Drug Suit Dismissed. *J Am Vet Med Assoc* 192:145, 1987.
64. U.S. v 9/1 Kg. Containers, More or Less of an Article of Drug for Veterinary Use, *et al.*, 674 F. Supp 1344, 1348 (C.D. Ill. 1987); see also, US District Court Rules Bulk Drug Distribution is Legal. *J Am Vet Med Assoc* 192:145-146, 1988.
65. Court of Appeals Reverses Schuyler Decision and Rules in Favor of FDA. *J Am Vet Med Assoc* 193:529, 1988.
66. Symposium on the Case for Responsible Extra-Label Drug Use. *J Am Vet Med Assoc* 192:241-270, 1988.
67. Upson DW: Privileges and responsibilities relating to extra-label drug use. *J Am Vet Med Assoc* 192:246, 1988.
68. E.g., *Antibiotics in American Feed: A Threat to Human Health?* Summit, NJ: American Council on Science and Health, 1985, p 24 (stating that there is "no evidence of a current or imminent human health hazard from penicillin and the tetracyclines in animal feed"); cf., Spika JS, *et al.*: Chloramphenicol-resistant *Salmonella newport* traced through hamburger to dairy farms. *N Engl J Med* 316(10):565-570, 1987.

69. Application for Veterinary Accreditation. VS Form 1-36A (Mar 81). *See, A Guide for Accredited Veterinarians.* APHIS 91-18. Washington, DC: US Government Printing Office, 1981.

70. 9 C.F.R. § 161.3.

71. E.g., *APHIS News* Oct 23, 1987:3.

72. *APHIS News* October 23, 1987:3-4.

73. More Suspensions Imposed. *J Am Vet Med Assoc* 189:506, 1986.

74. Five Disciplined for Violations. *J Am Vet Med Assoc* 191:776, 1987.

75. Licenses Suspended or Revoked. *J Am Vet Med Assoc* 191: 510-511, 1987.

76. *APHIS News* January 13, 1988:5.

77. *APHIS News* January 22, 1988:1.

78. Rose RJ: Foreword, Symposium on Equine Physiology. *Vet Clin North Am Equine Pract* 1(3):437, 1985.

79. Dalin G and Jeffcott LB: Locomotion and Gait Analysis. *Vet Clin North Am Equine Pract* 1(3):568-569, 1985.

80. For an excellent discussion supporting "controlled" precompetition medication approaches see Tobin T and Heard R: *Drugs and the Performance Horse.* Springfield, IL: Charles C. Thomas, 1981; for a contrary approach see Baker RO: *The Misuse of Drugs in Horse Racing.* Barrington, IL: Illinois Hooved Animal Humane Society, 1978.

81. Baker RO, *op. cit.*, p xxv (stating that "undoubtedly, track veterinarians often find it difficult to follow the dictates of their own conscience and the ethics of their profession").

82. For summaries of prominent features of state rules with extended pari-mutuel meetings see, *State Racehorse Medication Rules: Drug Testing Programs. Penalty and Appeals Procedures.* Washington, DC: American Horse Council, 1986.

83. See, e.g., O'Connor JT: The untoward effects of the corticosteroids in equine practice. *J Am Vet Med Assoc* 153:1614-1617, 1968; Galley RH: The Use of Hyaluronic Acid in the Racehorse. *Proceedings of the 32nd Annual Convention of the Annual Convention of the American Association of Equine Practitioners*: 657-661, 1986.

84. For a critique of the usefulness of such terms as "restorative" versus "additive" in the use of drugs by human athletes, see Fost N: Banning Drugs in Sports: A Skeptical View. *Hastings Center Report* 16(4):5-10, 1986.

85. See, e.g., Baker R.O. *The Misuse of Drugs in Horse Racing.* Barrington, Il: Illinois Hooved Animal Humane Society, 1978, pp 63-66 and references cited therein; Gifford B: *A Day at the Races.* New York: Atlantic Monthly Press, 1988, pp 117-120.

86. Kingsbury MD: Pleasure and Show Horse Preventive Medicine. In Mansmann RA, McAllister ES, and Pratt PW (eds): *Equine Medicine and Surgery.* ed 3. Santa Barbara: American Veterinary Publications, 1982, pp 60-65.

87. Mackay-Smith M and Cohen M: Exercise Physiology and Diseases of Exertion. In Mansmann RA, McAllister ES and Pratt PW (eds): *Equine Medicine and Surgery.* ed 3. Santa Barbara: American Veterinary Publications, 1982, p 128.

88. AVMA Guidelines for Horse Show Veterinarians. *1988 AVMA Directory*, p 484.

89. In Deutschmann K: *Fairgrounds Thoroughbred Horse Racing in Massachusetts.* Boston: Massachusetts Society for the Prevention of Cruelty to Animals, 1986, App. B.

90. See, e.g., Baker, *op. cit.*, p 46.

91. *1987 Drugs & Medication Rule.* New York: American Horse Shows Association, 1987, Rule III, Part I, Sec. 3.

92. 15 U.S.C. § 1821, *et seq.*

93. 9 C.F.R. § 11.2(a).

94. 9 C.F.R. § 11.7.
95. *Report of the Advisory Committee on the Adoption and Humane Disposition of Greyhounds.* Boston: Commonwealth of Massachusetts Executive Office of Consumer Affairs and Business Regulation, 1987, pp 6-7.
96. *Id.,* 1.
97. *Id.,* 12.
98. *Id.,* 16.
99. Lawrence EA: *Rodeo.* Knoxville: University of Tennessee Press, 1982, pp 3-4.
100. *Id.,* 10.
101. *Id.,* 269.
102. Joint Statement of the HSUS and AHA. Quoted in Drennon C: Rodeo: Cruelty, Not Sport. *California Veterinarian* 37(1):65, 1983.
103. Drennon C: Rodeo: Cruelty, Not Sport. *California Veterinarian* 37(1):65, 1983.
104. Santos FK: Is Rodeo Really Cruel? *California Veterinarian* 37(1):66, 1983.
105. Lawrence, *op. cit.,* p 177.
106. *Id.,* 119-121.
107. *Id.,* 125.

Chapter

— 22 —

Employee Relations

Relations between practitioners and their employees is an important subject for veterinary ethics. If employees are mistreated or are unhappy, the interests of patients, clients, and practice owners can be harmed. Veterinary employees also have legitimate interests of their own. A veterinarian's professional moral obligations include his obligations to those who work for him.

This chapter considers some of the ethical issues that arise in relations between practitioners and their employees. The term "employee" will be used in its ordinary, nonlegal sense, in which an employee is any nonowner of a practice who works on a regular basis for and is paid by a practice owner or owners. In some contexts, the law defines an employee as any person who works for salary or wages. In this sense, owners of a veterinary professional corporation are also employees of the practice; and because all members of a professional partnership are legal agents of each other, there is a sense in which they, too, can be called "employees" of one another. There are many important ethical issues arising out of relations among practice owners, but they will not be discussed here. Nor does the chapter consider moral issues involving an owner's relations with uncompensated volunteers, or with practitioners (e.g., certain relief veterinarians) the law classifies as independent contractors.

LEGAL CONSIDERATIONS

Virtually every aspect of the employment relation is affected by law. Federal or state laws prohibit discrimination in hiring and firing on the basis of race, religion, color, national origin, sex or age; sexual harassment; and employment of undocumented aliens. Other statutes cover minimum wages, payment for overtime work, health insurance benefits, pension and profit sharing plans, and maternity leave. There are laws and regulations that protect employees from environmental work hazards such as x-rays, chemicals, and poisons. Words and deeds exchanged privately between employer and employee can themselves create legal rights and duties. For example, if an employer agrees with a worker, either verbally or in writing, to pay a certain salary or to extend certain benefits, that can create a contractual obligation on the doctor's part, a violation of which might support a legal action by the employee.

It is not possible to summarize here all laws relating to employer-employee relations. But in general, whenever one deals with an ethical issue involving employee relations, it is always advisable to ask whether the law has something to say about the matter (1).

THE VETERINARIAN EMPLOYEE

Compensation and Benefits

WHAT IS A FAIR SALARY?

A practitioner-owner is morally required to compensate his employees fairly. The following are among the relevant considerations in determining whether the salary paid by an owner to a veterinarian employee is fair:

1. **The extent of the doctor's training and experience.** Clearly, veterinarians have some moral entitlement regarding compensation because of the considerable time and expense they have invested in their skills. All other things being equal (and sometimes, there are considerations that make them unequal), a doctor with more or better education and practice experience deserves a higher level of compensation than one with less.

2. **The salary level of other professionals with comparable training, experience, and value to society.** Some new veterinary school graduates believe they are being paid unfairly because members of other professions with training, skill, and responsibility no more important than their own are sometimes paid much more than they. In the abstract, it does seem unfair that the typical new veterinarian is paid much less than a new lawyer, because the lawyer has had only 3 years of professional schooling to the veterinarian's 4, and is not likely to be as quickly entrusted with weighty matters of life and death. However, this argument does not show that all veterinarians must be paid as much as members of other valued professions. Veterinarians cannot earn more than their practices can pay them, and, as we shall see, there are other fair limitations on associates' salaries. What the argument shows is that there is *strong moral weight* in favor of a salary commensurate with a veterinarian's training and skills.

3. **The amount and difficulty of the doctor's work.** All other things being equal, a doctor who works 5 or 6 days a week merits more compensation than one who works 3 or 4. This is so not just because he probably is contributing more to practice revenues, but also because he deserves additional compensation for his greater effort.

4. **The quality of the doctor's work.** It is also fair to reward doctors for the quality of their work. A doctor who performs flawless surgeries that subject patients and clients to a minimum of complications may be rewarded for a job well done. This is so not just because he is likely to increase practice revenues, but because quality performance is a good in itself that can merit monetary reward.

5. **The ability of the practice to pay the doctor's salary, benefits, and support (including ancillary staff) required for his employment.** A doctor's actual compensation must conform to the economic limitations of his practice. There undoubtedly are many fine veterinarians who merit in the abstract a much higher salary than they are receiving but whose earnings are restricted by the financial capabilities of their clients. Other limitations on doctors' salaries that derive from the economic facts of life of their practices include the cost of labor for ancillary personnel such as receptionists and technicians, the indebtedness of the practice, and the costs of insurance and facility maintenance.

6. The right of the owner(s) to gain a fair profit from the practice. The moral right of a practice owner to gain a fair return on his investment must also be factored into the determination of the fairness of an employee doctor's compensation. Owners are obligated to share some of the fruits of an associate's labor with the associate. But in virtue of the fact that they have invested their time, efforts, and money in the practice, and are its legal owners, they usually are entitled to allocate the greater portion of revenues and profits to themselves.

7. The cost of living in the community. In determining an associate's compensation, owners must take into account the cost of living in their community, even if this sometimes means their receiving a smaller return on their investment. It might sometimes be necessary to adjust an associate's compensation for the cost of living so that he can remain an employee. But it is sometimes also a matter of fairness to make such adjustments. One of the legitimate rewards of working as a professional is being able to live decently in or near the community where one works. This is something veterinarians *deserve*, even though they bear little responsibility for the level of the cost of living in the communities in which they practice.

8. The compensation levels of other doctors in the practice. A particular doctor's compensation can be unfair if it is disproportionate to that of other doctors in the practice. A practice's existing compensation levels can place severe constraints on the weight the owners are able to give to other considerations relevant to fairness. For example, a practice with a large number of doctors might find it extremely difficult to adjust upward the salaries of all its doctors so that a newcomer can be given a salary that, considered by itself, might seem more fair.

9. The doctor's present contribution to the gross revenues of the practice. The more an associate contributes to gross revenues, the more he is paying his own way and that of personnel and facilities required for his support. He also is contributing more to the profits of the owners, and is therefore entitled to receive back some of the fruits of his labor. Nevertheless, a doctor's "productivity" is only one factor in determining the fairness of his compensation. New doctors typically need to be trained not just in the ways of a practice, but also how to practice veterinary medicine under real conditions. It can be unfair to new doctors to tie their compensation strictly to their contribution to revenues, because their need for an adequate income will exist before their capacity for significant productivity does. Tying compensation strictly to productivity can also be unfair to more experienced associates. A doctor can become ill, have personal problems or commitments (such as giving birth), or might, through no fault of his own, just not have a good run of profitable cases.

10. The doctor's potential contribution to practice revenues. It can be unfair to pay an associate a low salary during the time he is training to be able to make more substantial contributions to practice revenues. A novice doctor has legitimate economic requirements of his own. Moreover, he is training not just for his own benefit, but also for the benefit of the owner who hopes to profit from his employment in the future. Owners often must expect to invest considerable money and effort in a new doctor, patiently awaiting the time when the associate can pull his own weight. An owner's obligation to pay an associate more than he might be worth at the time gives rise to a moral duty on the part of the associate to try to return the owner's investment in him. To leave a practice soon after being trained at someone else's expense can be profoundly immoral. It can also strengthen any inclination owners might have to hold inexperienced associates to salaries tied strictly to their present productivity.

11. The extent to which the doctor is building equity in or is likely to become an owner of the practice. It can be appropriate to pay an associate doctor less than he might otherwise receive if he is working toward becoming an owner of the practice. If, for example, deferring an increase in an associate's salary is necessary to enable the practice to purchase equipment that will eventually inure to his benefit when he becomes an owner, it might be reasonable for the owners to ask him to agree to such a sacrifice – provided that they, too, share in the burdens. An owner and associate may decide that part of the latter's payment for progressive increments in ownership will be somewhat lower compensation in the short term.

SOME WARNINGS ABOUT FAIR COMPENSATION

Several important warnings emerge from these considerations.

First, fairness is not just a matter of what one can get an associate to accept. Accepting terms of employment can be a statement that one does regard them as adequate and fair. But the fact that an associate will work for a certain amount does not always settle the fairness issue, because in the real world, employees do not always have complete freedom of choice. A new graduate who must repay substantial educational loans and who wants to work in a certain community or kind of practice might find that he must accept a low salary, because this is what all employers of interest to him are offering. This does not necessarily make such a salary fair.

Second, fairness is rarely capable of exact mathematical quantification. There is no precise formula for determining, for example, how much a doctor's productivity should count in relation to his experience and the cost of living in the community. (And these are only three of the factors relevant to determining the fairness of compensation.) At best, one can attempt to come up with a figure that "feels" right. Moreover, there will often be many such figures. If a starting salary of $22,000 seems fair for a new graduate, it does not necessarily follow that a salary of $21,000 would be unfair or that one of $23,000 would be excessive. All these figures might fall comfortably within the boundaries of fairness, even though the differences among them could be significant to the employee.

Finally, it is impossible to reduce fairness to a single consideration or criterion, with or without accompanying mathematical formulae. Dr. Ross Clark recommends that employee doctors be paid a gross pretax income including fringe benefits of approximately 20% of their contribution to gross practice revenues. "Twenty percent of individual production," Dr. Clark states, "is fair" (2). There are doubtless many practices in which paying associates 20% of production would be fair. But there is no reason in principle why one should expect any percentage of "productivity" to be the *sole* measure of fairness. There is no guarantee – indeed, it seems highly unlikely – that such a figure will necessarily reflect some of the other factors identified above. For many of these factors have no intrinsic relationship to productivity. A new graduate who joins a sophisticated specialty practice in a city in which living expenses are extremely high might be treated unfairly if restricted at the start to 20% of his actual productivity. Moreover, even when considering an associate's contribution to gross practice income as a relevant factor, it is far from clear that one can settle on an appropriate percentage figure before looking at all the relevant factors bearing on fairness in the particular practice. For a practice earning minimal profits located in a community in which living expenses are low, 20% of an inexperienced associate's contribution to gross revenues could be excessive. On the other hand, it might be unfair for the same practice to pay 20% to an extraordinarily skilled surgeon who has the potential to generate substantial new revenues.

BONUSES AND FRINGE BENEFITS

In determining the fairness of benefits apart from straight salary, among the questions to be asked is whether a particular form of compensation inures as much to the benefit of the owner as it does to the employee, or is essential to the associate's continuing employment. In both of these kinds of cases, fairness can require the practice to extend such compensation. Among the things that benefit owners directly is malpractice insurance, which typically protects the owner or his corporation as well as the associate. Among employee benefits essential to maintaining morale and productivity are adequate health insurance and vacation time.

Some forms of compensation are better categorized as rewards rather than necessities. Such compensation may often be given differently (or not at all) to certain associates and still be fair. For example, it can be fair to give 3 rather than 2 weeks paid vacation only to associates who have worked for the practice for a certain number of years. Likewise, more senior associates may be afforded payment of professional association dues or continuing education fees as a token of appreciation for their time in the practice.

Certain kinds of compensation that are optional in one practice will be required as a matter of fairness in another. It is difficult to maintain that fairness requires all practices to pay professional association dues or continuing education fees for all associates. However, in a practice that does routinely cover such items, it would be unfair not to do so for a particular doctor who works as hard and well as the others.

Also relevant to whether a certain kind of compensation that might generally be regarded as a "fringe benefit" must, in fairness, be given to a particular doctor is whether that kind of compensation is really part of straight salary. Some owners prefer to protect their financial situation and encourage employee productivity by paying a somewhat lower than normal salary during the year and supplementing this amount with a large end-of-year bonus. In such a practice, a "bonus" is not entirely an optional payment whose availability and amount is contingent on performance or other factors; it is deferred salary. Likewise, if a practice decides to make up for a somewhat lower salary with generous contributions to a pension or profit sharing plan, such compensation, too, can become an entitlement of an associate doctor who has been working under the assumption that he will receive it.

ARE CURRENT STARTING SALARIES FAIR?

The average starting salary for 1986 graduates of U.S. veterinary schools was $20,478. The mean for private practice was $21,205. The 13.2% of graduates entering advanced study averaged $15,186, or over 25% less than their colleagues in private practice. The average educational debt of the 82% of graduates with debt was $23,420 (3). Female graduates, who comprised 51% of 1986 graduates, averaged $1,000, or 4.6% less, than their male counterparts entering private practice (4).

Many veterinary students tell me that current starting salaries for new graduates are profoundly unfair. They base this judgment on the fact that graduates of other kinds of professional schools begin at higher salaries, and on the assumption that because there is a substantial supply of new graduates, practice owners *must* be taking advantage of the market to unfairly depress starting salaries.

The facts do not seem to bear out such charges, at least as a general characterization of starting salaries nationwide. J. Karl Wise has determined that the 1985 mean salary of all private practitioners was $48,056 and that the mean return to practice owners (including return on investments) was $66,544 (5). Thus, even comparing the 1986 starting salaries (which were undoubtedly somewhat higher than those for 1985) to the 1985 private practitioner figures, beginning veterinarians have been earning on average somewhat less than half of what the average veterinarian is earning and almost one-third of what practice owners are earning. In contrast, although they were paid more in absolute terms than their veterinary school counterparts, 1985 law school graduates earned only one-quarter of what the average attorney was earning (6, 7). And figures for 1986 reveal (8) that nonowner attorneys working in small law firms (defined as those having 11 or fewer lawyers) earned, like associate veterinarians, approximately one-third as much as did owners of such practices. These comparisons indicate that although veterinarians are paid less (sometimes much less) than attorneys, in general, the problem with starting veterinary salaries does not appear to be greed on the part of practice owners, but the amount of money they have available to distribute in the first place.

This conclusion is also supported by estimates of the costs required to maintain a new veterinary associate. Dr. Clark calculates that a typical practice must gross three times a new associate's total compensation package to break even on his salary; he also estimates that the typical new graduate can contribute $108,000 to gross practice revenues (2). J. Karl Wise has determined that the 1985 mean gross practice incomes, for example, for small animal exclusive practices was $147,871 for a one-person practice, $283,359 for a two-person practice, and $458,694 for a three-person practice (5). It would appear that a one or two person practice that presently has a gross practice income at the national mean level might well be unable, at least in the short term, to maintain its gross revenues at or near the national mean when it adds a new associate doctor. The figures supplied by Drs. Clark and Wise support the view of other observers (9) that, at least initially, hiring a new graduate even at current typical salary levels can reduce the net income of practice owners.

That many practices pay starting doctors fairly does not, of course, mean that all practices are doing so. I receive credible accounts from job applicants about owners who have sufficient funds to operate satellite clinics or to finance impressive additions to present facilities – and who are paying no more, and sometimes a good deal less, than the national mean salary to new graduates. It is disgraceful for a practice to appeal to the national statistics and economic pressures on other doctors as an excuse for paying associates less than it can fairly afford to pay them.

THE RECORD OF THE VETERINARY SCHOOLS

In general, the veterinary schools have a terrible record regarding compensation for novice doctors. In 1987, a salary of $15,000 would not have been unusual for a first-year intern, and $16,000 would have been typical for a resident with one or more years of practice experience. Some institutions offer starting positions that pay nothing!

The low salaries are sometimes justified on the grounds that these doctors spend a great deal of time learning instead of producing revenue (10). But this can also be said of many new graduates in private practices who are paid substantially more. In fact, the typical intern or resident in a veterinary teaching hospital puts in extraordinarily long hours, many of them on income-producing cases. Moreover, veterinary schools are not supposed to be profit-making institutions. It is their job to train future practitioners. If they cannot accept the fact that their educational mission could cost them more than they earn, they might be in the wrong business. At the very least, they must be prepared to make choices regarding how many novice doctors, as well as experienced clinicians and support staff, they can hire so that all in the institution will receive a decent level of compensation.

There are two major reasons for the astonishingly low salaries offered to new doctors by academic institutions. First, they can get away with these salaries because there are many more applicants for the positions than openings. Second, some academic veterinarians believe that if low salaries were good enough for them when they were interns and residents, low salaries are good enough today. An academic institution would not accept such an argument for a certain method of medical care. It is no more acceptable as justification of unfair compensation.

THE ISSUE OF PROPORTIONAL OR COMMISSION SALARY

Serious ethical questions are raised by the apparently growing practice of basing all or part of employee doctors' compensation on a percentage of their contribution to gross revenues. This can be done either by offering a fixed base salary plus a certain percent of the doctor's contribution to gross revenues above a certain level (11), or by paying a straight percentage commission of contribution to gross revenues (12).

Such compensation plans are said to provide associates motivation to generate revenues. New doctors are supposed to learn much more quickly about the procedures of the practice and to waste less time in nonproductive activities. One owner believes that paying both doctors and support staff on a commission basis will prevent doctors from undercharging clients or reducing fees they regard as excessive (13).

However well-intentioned they might be, such methods of compensating doctors pose a grave moral threat to the profession. Associates paid in these ways might compete among themselves for higher dollar clients and cases, thus leading to difficult relations among doctors. Those who refuse to hustle clients for unnecessary services could find themselves working so many extra hours or packing so many extra patients into the work day that they risk premature burn-out.

Most important, tying compensation directly to "productivity" places enormous pressure on doctors to make recommendations and decisions based not on the needs of patients, but on their own pecuniary interests. Some doctors might be able to resist such pressures. But others will not, and there will often be a strong *potential* conflict of interest between a doctor's desire to earn more and his obligations to patients and clients. There will be pressure to recommend the most expensive procedures clients can afford, even if less expensive ones would do. There will be pressure to advise that a procedure be done immediately, even if time might prove it unnecessary. There will be pressure to recommend unnecessary procedures. There will be pressure to counsel longer and more expensive hospital stays. There will be pressure to dispense the most expensive drugs the client can afford, and to dispense as much of these drugs as possible. In practices with their own testing laboratory or that charge clients a mark-up on outside tests, there will be pressure to recommend as many tests as the traffic will bear. In practices that sell nonprofessional goods and services and credit such sales to a doctor's "account," there will be pressure on the doctor to move these items also, whether or not they are in the best interests of patients and clients. And all of these pressures will be greatest on the recent graduate, whose lower base salary and ability to generate revenues will act as still further inducement to sell, sell, and sell again.

In addition to threatening harm to the interests of patients and clients, proportional or commission salaries subject the entire profession to potentially irreparable damage. We are accustomed to the automobile or household appliance salesman who is paid on commission. We begin our dealings with such people with skepticism, and a firm grip on our wallets. Today, most people approach their veterinarian with precisely the opposite attitude: they *trust* that a veterinarian will recommend something because it is right medically, and not because it will earn him a larger salary. I submit that if the public learns that a significant number of veterinarians are being paid on commission, the entire profession will find it more difficult to persuade clients of the need for legitimate medical procedures. Once lost, the image of the trusted medical professional might be impossible to regain.

A doctor's contribution to practice revenues is one legitimate factor in determining a fair level of compensation for him. But the unavoidable link between economic productivity and compensation already places a heavy moral burden on doctors to assure themselves that they are working primarily for their patients and clients. The problem with proportional or commission compensation is that it makes every dollar brought into the practice a matter of direct benefit to a doctor. This, I submit, creates too great a risk that the veterinarian's interests will come before those of patients and clients.

Working Conditions and Environment

Just as owners have an obligation to provide fair salaries for their employees, so must they attempt to offer working conditions and a general practice environment that respects an associate doctor as a colleague and fellow professional. Among the complaints I hear most frequently from new doctors are that their employers do not give them enough time to have lunch, that they are always the ones who must endure weekend or night duty, and that their vacation plans can be canceled at a moment's notice. A number of novice doctors have also told me that they are restricted to tasks they can already perform and are not being trained to assume the duties of more senior doctors. New doctors must understand that they cannot be permitted to do certain procedures until they are ready, and that it is often fair to assign less pleasant jobs to more junior associates. However, owners must understand that many recent graduates are working at relatively low salaries precisely because they can convince themselves that they are investing in their own training. Some new doctors suspect that they are being relegated to routine tasks because their employer expects to turn them out when they can no longer stand the drudgery, and to hire another new graduate who is willing to do such jobs until he tires of them, and so on.

Understandings and Restrictions

Owners can promote satisfaction and good morale of associate doctors by reaching a clear understanding with them about their role in the practice.

EMPLOYMENT CONTRACTS

One way of doing this is to sign a written contract that sets out the most important understandings between the parties. Among the issues that can be addressed in such a document are hours of employment, salary, pension plan, vacation time, pregnancy or childrearing leave, and general and specific duties. With the exception of restrictive covenants of noncompetition (discussed below), employment contracts usually protect employees more than employers. (Courts will not, for example, force a doctor back to a practice if he quits during the term of his contract.) Nevertheless, an employment contract can be an important *moral* document. It can be a solemn expression by the parties of their understanding that they are entering into important ethical obligations to each other.

RESTRICTIVE COVENANTS OF NONCOMPETITION

Most states permit owners and an employee veterinarian to agree that the employee will not, after leaving employment, practice veterinary medicine for a specified period of time within a specified geographical area of the owner's practice. Such an agreement is typically contained in a more general employment contract. Its restrictions will be enforced if they are "reasonable." Commonly, added to the agreement of noncompetition is a clause stating that upon leaving the practice, the doctor will not take with him originals or copies of any patient or client records.

Such restrictions on the ability of an employee doctor to compete with a former employer are morally appropriate. In bringing a new doctor into his practice, an owner provides immediate access to his most valuable "asset:" his clients and their animals. He is entitled to some protection against an associate who might want to use this asset for his own benefit.

Because the law will not enforce restrictions of time and place that are unreasonable, associates usually need not worry about signing away more than what is morally fair. If they are asked to do so, the law will not hold them to the promise. (In some states, agreements deemed unreasonable will be voided altogether, and in others the courts will substitute reasonable geographic and time restrictions for those to which the parties agreed.) On the other hand, every employer should still exercise sensitivity in the presentation of restrictive covenants. It is wrong to try to induce an associate to accept restrictions that are not enforceable, hoping that he will not discover them to be invalid. A prospective associate should also be given the opportunity to consider any written agreement before he signs it and to consult an attorney so that he can understand his rights and responsibilities.

PROBATIONARY PERIODS OF EMPLOYMENT

One way of affording both the associate doctor and his employer time to determine whether they are right for each other is to have a probationary period of employment, a time in which the doctor works for the practice, but can leave upon the desire of either himself or the owner. This can be specified in a written document, or the signing of a complete employment contract can be delayed pending the end of the probationary period. Because probationary periods are entered into with the hope that the associate will remain, both parties are morally obligated not to terminate the relationship without adequate notice or in an otherwise unfair manner.

THE POSSIBILITY OF PROMOTION TO PRACTICE OWNERSHIP

Owners should be as clear as possible about the prospects of ownership for a new associate. If the owners are not now or ever likely to be interested in taking on another owner, that fact should be communicated to a potential employee, even if he does not raise the issue. Owners should be prepared to tell a prospective associate what percentage of employed doctors have become owners, as well as what criteria will be used to determine whether an associate will be offered, or will be permitted to purchase, a part of the practice. A prospective associate should be told if the possibility of ownership will depend on his contributing significant monetary assets to the practice. Because some associates accept a low salary with the hope that their efforts will someday translate into practice ownership, it can be profoundly unfair for an owner to be deceptive or misleading about the possibility and conditions of ownership. On the other hand, associates must understand that elevation to ownership is an extremely important step that rarely can be made quickly or promised definitively at the inception of employment.

PRACTICE PHILOSOPHY

The philosophy of a practice can be defined as its most central values, regarding both the goals of the practice as well as the procedures by which its day-to-day management is accomplished. Even when they are not adopted deliberately, practice philosophies tend to emerge from the values and personalities of owners. For example, some practices place great emphasis upon generating revenues and expect doctors to work aggressively at promoting services; in other practices, doctors place a higher value on leisure time and might be satisfied with less revenue. In some practices, veterinarians and support staff treat each other with formality, while in others, a looser camaraderie is accepted or expected.

It is in both an owner's and a prospective associate's interests that the latter be informed prior to employment about the owner's practice philosophy.

The following are among the questions relating to practice philosophy that veterinary students and recent graduates tell me are of greatest interest to them in approaching prospective employment:

- How many hours per week will I be expected to work? Will I often have to work nights or weekends? How flexible is the practice in excusing or rearranging work schedules for personal reasons?
- How vigorously must I sell services and products to clients? Will my economic productivity be monitored precisely? May I adjust fees to what seems fair or reasonable in particular circumstances?
- How often and under what circumstances will my performance be evaluated? Will I be given the opportunity to respond to criticisms or problems?
- What is the view of the practice concerning such procedures as ear-cropping, tail-docking, declawing, and euthanasia of healthy animals? If I object to any or all of these procedures, what should I do if they are requested by clients?
- Will I be expected to sell nonprofessional goods and services to clients?
- To what extent are important practice decisions made democratically, by all doctors in the practice? Am I expected to "grin and bear it," or will my opinions regarding problems be welcomed or accepted?
- Am I expected to become friendly with other doctors in the practice after work hours, or will my relationship with them be strictly professional?
- How long will I perform routine or menial jobs? To what extent does the practice believe in training new associates to handle difficult cases and to service more valued clients? If I believe I am not yet ready to handle certain kinds of cases, how will the practice respond?

The Woman Veterinary Associate

Few phenomena pose more important ethical issues for the profession than the fact that the majority of veterinary school students are now women (14). Because relatively few women doctors are yet practice owners, many of the ethical issues relating to women veterinarians involve their relations with employers.

THE UNCERTAINTIES

As Dr. Kathleen Smiler, president of the Association of Women Veterinarians, observes, one reason ethical issues involving female doctors are so difficult is that it is not yet clear what the profession (including its growing female component) wants for its women doctors. Nor is it clear how the profession might be able to accommodate these desires (K. Smiler, personal communication). Dr. Smiler points out, for example, that we simply do not know how many women doctors will want to work part-time during a substantial part of their careers. There are very few role models of the long-term successful female veterinarian that can be relied upon by either female associates or male practice owners. The profession does not know how easy it will be to arrange careers and practice economics around the various issues posed by pregnancy and childrearing. In short, although history appears to be in the making, it is still far too early to predict how the story will turn out.

THE NEED TO BE ABLE TO SPEAK OPENLY

Because so much is yet to be learned – because we do not even know all the questions that will need to be asked – it is extremely important that all who raise ethical issues relating to women veterinarians feel free to express their views openly. Many male practice owners tell me that they would like to discuss moral issues regarding women doctors with their colleagues and with prospective female associates, but are afraid to do so lest they be accused of "sexism."

The danger of substituting accusation for argument is illustrated by the reaction to a recent observation of that perspicacious observer of the profession, Dr. R. M. Miller. Miller reported that many male college students with whom he speaks have decided not to enter veterinary school because of the profession's low salaries. On the other hand, women veterinary students "often remark ... that they are willing to endure this because they want to work with animals and realize that what they earn will probably be a second income if they marry" (15). Miller concluded that the influx into the profession of women who might be able to tolerate lower salaries could be discouraging some qualified males from becoming veterinarians.

Miller's remarks evoked the outrage of some who saw in them a prejudice against women (16). In fact, there was nothing antifemale in Miller's observations. They raise several important points the profession cannot afford to ignore. First, the proportion of male veterinary school applicants is falling dramatically. (At Tufts University School of Veterinary Medicine, for example, 70% of the applicants and entrants for the class of 1991 were women.) Second, if veterinary medicine is to remain a first-rate profession, it must attract the most qualified people of both sexes. Anything that prevents the entrance of qualified males into the profession will lower the quality of the general body of practitioners. Third, some qualified males who would seek to become the major breadwinner of their family will not enter the profession if it cannot provide them with a reasonable income.

Dr. Miller did not claim to know how the profession should deal with these matters. But dealing with them (and other issues relating to the changing face of veterinary medicine) must not be hindered by accusations of antifemale prejudice. It is no better to treat a legitimate, good-faith question about the impact of women on the profession as evidence of an antifemale attitude, than it is to think that women veterinarians are inferior.

THE LAW OF SEX-BASED DISCRIMINATION

The task of normative veterinary ethics in considering sex-related issues is complicated enormously by federal, state, and local laws prohibiting discrimination on the basis of sex. Owners must know precisely what laws apply to their practices. This is not always an easy task because some of the federal laws do not apply to all practices, and state and local laws vary greatly. One must also be sensitive to the fact that some moral questions that seem perfectly reasonable might be prohibited by certain laws. The following discussion presents an overview of the most important laws that can affect consideration of moral issues regarding female veterinarian (or nonveterinarian) employees.

1. **The federal Equal Pay Act** (17) prohibits an employer from paying employees at a lesser rate than "he pays wages to employees of the opposite sex" for "equal work on jobs the performance of which requires equal skill, effort, and responsibility, and which are performed under similar working conditions." The law permits pay differentials based on "any other factor than sex," including seniority, merit, and quantity or quality of production.

2. **Title VII of the federal Civil Rights Act of 1964** (18) provides that employers may not hire, discharge, or otherwise discriminate against any individual (male or female) "because of" or "on the basis of" sex. (Title VII also prohibits discrimination on the basis of race, religion, national origin, and age.) All aspects of the employment relationship are covered, including advertising for employees, interviewing applicants, hiring, salaries, benefits, working conditions, reassignment, and discharge. Unlike the Equal Pay Act, which applies as long as there is more than one employee, Title VII only covers enterprises with at least 15 employees who work for at least 20 weeks a year. (The statute considers corporations to be employers and therefore includes owner-practitioners of professional veterinary corporations within its definition of "employees.") The statute is enforced by the federal Equal Employment Opportunity Commission (EEOC). The following aspects of the law are noteworthy:

(a) Pregnancy. One part of Title VII, called the Pregnancy Discrimination Act (19), prohibits discrimination based upon or because of "pregnancy, childbirth, or related medical conditions." A woman may not be denied employment, discharged, or compelled to take maternity leave simply because she is or might become pregnant. All decisions regarding pregnant or potentially pregnant employees must be based on a *bona fide* determination of whether prospective or present female employees can do the job.

The statute considers pregnancy to be a "disability," and all employers subject to the act must treat pregnancy as they would any other temporary disability. Thus, if an employer would reassign any employee to another task because of some temporary infirmity or disability, he must do so for a pregnant employee. An employer may ask a pregnant employee to stop work, or deny a leave to one who claims she can no longer work, but only if he uses the same procedures (e.g., acceptance of statements by an employee's personal physician) to settle such issues as he would use to determine whether an employee with another kind of disability must or may stop work. An employer must hold open a pregnant employee's job for her return "on the same basis as jobs are held open on sick or disability leave for other conditions" (20). If employers provide income maintenance for any worker with a temporary disability, they must do the same for a pregnant employee. Nor may employees absent due to a pregnancy-related disability be required to exhaust vacation benefits before receiving sick leave pay or disability benefits if such a requirement is not imposed upon all employees (21). Although Title VII does not specifically require post-pregnancy child care leave, the EEOC has stated that "if an employer allows its employees to take a leave without pay or accrued annual leave for travel or education which is not job-related, the same type of leave must be granted to those who wish to remain on leave for infant care, even though they are medically able to return to work" (22).

(b) Sexual harassment. Title VII also prohibits sexual harassment, which is defined by the EEOC as

> (u)nwelcome sexual advances, requests for sexual favors, and other verbal or physical conduct of a sexual nature ... when (1) submission to such conduct is made either

explicitly or implicitly a term or condition of an individual's employment, (2) submission to or rejection of such conduct by an individual is used as the basis for employment decisions affecting such individual, or (3) such conduct has the purpose or effect of unreasonably interfering with an individual's work performance or creating an intimidating, hostile, or offensive working environment (23).

(c) Reproductive and fetal hazards. EEOC regulations permit employers to exclude pregnant or nonpregnant women of childbearing age from "substances, physical agents, or conditions known or suspected to be hazardous to the reproductive health of employees and/or to the fetus through the employee" (24). However, such exclusion must be based on *bona fide* knowledge or suspicion of danger, cannot be a pretext for sex discrimination, and, whenever possible must be applied equally to employees of both sexes. As the regulations recognize, much remains to be discovered about the effects of various substances and working conditions on reproductive health. It therefore might sometimes be difficult to demonstrate whether an employer who asks a female employee to stop or continue work when a reproductive hazard might be present, is doing so for a medically defensible, nondiscriminatory reason (25).

(d) Pre-employment inquiries. Title VII permits employers to inquire about the sex of job applicants, unless such questions are asked for a discriminatory purpose. The EEOC has ruled that an employer may not ask a female job applicant about possible problems she might have with child care, at least if the same inquiries are not made of male applicants (26).

3. **State and local laws.** Forty-one states, Puerto Rico, and the District of Columbia, as well as some municipalities, have their own fair employment practice laws that prohibit sex-based discrimination. These laws apply in addition to federal statutes. When, as is sometimes the case, a state's law is stricter or more comprehensive than federal requirements, employees or potential employees covered by state as well as the federal laws are entitled to the greater protection of the state standards. The number of employees required before state laws apply varies greatly, ranging from just one to as many as 25. States also differ with respect to whether countable employees must have been employed for a minimum period of time for the statute to afford them protection. In addition to fair employment acts prohibiting sex discrimination, 36 states have equal pay acts analogous to the federal statute. Some states also have constitutional provisions (such as equal rights amendments) that prohibit sex-based discrimination (27).

THE EFFECT OF SEX DISCRIMINATION LAW ON MORAL DELIBERATION

Laws prohibiting sex-based discrimination can have significant impact on the ethical deliberations practice owners may prudently undertake among themselves or with prospective and current female doctors.

First, some issues regarding benefits for women doctors (as well as nonveterinarian female employees) are not as open for debate as some owners might think. For example, assuming that Title VII applies to a practice, if in their generosity the owners have already offered income maintenance during temporary physical disability to doctors, the owners will not be able to *consider* whether to provide income maintenance for a woman doctor while she is unable to work because of pregnancy. This benefit would be required by law. It is a consequence of Title VII that practice owners will sometimes be making decisions regarding women doctors even though there are as yet no women in the practice or a question concerning benefits for female doctors or nonveterinarian employees is not being raised explicitly.

Second, Title VII and similar state statutes sometimes can make it extremely dangerous to ask questions that seem reasonable. For example, one practice owner has told me that he asks his female associates whether they might consider planning their pregnancies so that they will be away from work at a time the practice is not busy. I submit that such a request, if made with flexibility and understanding, can make perfect sense; it need not be offensive if it is asked sincerely in an attempt to help both the practice and the woman doctor. But it is not clear that such a request is permissible under Title VII. The EEOC decision that male and female job applicants must be asked the same questions about childrearing can be interpreted to imply that an owner must also ask male doctors whether they would consider planning the birth of their children for a time the practice is not busy. However, it is unclear what the point of such a question would be in the case of some male doctors, who would not be expected to request more than a limited absence from duties immediately before and after the birth of a child. The requirements of Title VII probably would be met if owners offered both male and female doctors extended leaves of equal duration before and after the birth of their children. But this seems an unnecessarily expensive way of allowing oneself to ask a female associate whether she and her husband would consider planning the birth of a child for some time other than heartworm-testing season.

SOME PRINCIPLES REGARDING MATERNITY

The following general principles are suggested to assist in asking reasonable ethical questions regarding maternity issues, consistent with the demands of applicable laws:

1. At the outset, every practice should know what laws do apply to its situation. If, for example, there are too few employees to subject the practice to federal or state standards, owners as well as prospective and current women employees will have substantially more latitude to consider maternity and other sex-related issues.

2. All practices would do well to understand precisely what their policies regarding female employees are. This will enable them to inform female doctors and nonveterinarian employees honestly and clearly about their policies should issues regarding pregnancy and childrearing arise in a legally permissible manner. Because decisions taken without female employees in mind can have enormous ramifications regarding such employees, it might be wise for any practice that has not done so recently to undertake a general review of its compensation and benefit policies.

3. Where legally permissible, and relevant, employers need not shrink from good-faith, nondiscriminatory, noncoercive discussions with all associates, both male and female. For example, it is not unreasonable to ask all employees whether they plan to take advantage of any legally required maternity or parenting leave in the near future so that the practice can plan its affairs with the minimum amount of disruption. Nor is it illegal or unreasonable to inform all applicants for employment about the policies of the practice regarding disability leaves and the opportunities, if any, for part-time employment.

4. Many moral issues are left open by sex discrimination laws. If a practice governed by Title VII does not yet offer income maintenance during a temporary disability incurred by any doctor, it is still free to determine whether it wants to grant such a benefit to all doctors, including those disabled temporarily because of pregnancy. If a practice does not routinely allow doctors to work part-time during a significant part of their tenure, it may still determine whether any doctor, including women doctors with infant children, may do so. The law also allows employers some leeway to protect pregnant employees and their unborn from environmental hazards, such as x-rays, anesthesia materials, and excessive physical exertion.

5. It is in the interests of clients, patients, and the profession as a whole that each practice hire the most talented doctors available. Therefore, if the most qualified applicant is female, the practice should try, consistent with its economic needs and applicable legal requirements, to enable her to join the practice. For a prosperous practice with many doctors, this might mean a paid maternity leave even when this is not legally required. To be sure, a practice cannot make such a decision until it determines what effects the decision might have on benefits that must lawfully or as a matter of fairness be granted to other employees.

6. Given the sizable crop of talented young veterinarians seeking positions, it sometimes might possible to get away with legally prohibited sexual discrimination, because it can be difficult for the victim of such discrimination to prove that a decision was made because of her sex. A clever practice that wants to discriminate against women veterinarians might be able to protect itself, at least for a while, by making sure it interviews female applicants before choosing a qualified male. If charged with discrimination, the practice can argue that sex had nothing to do with the decision. Because the law can sometimes be circumvented, employers must keep in mind that discrimination on the basis of sex is profoundly immoral, even when sexual discrimination laws can be circumvented or do not apply. It is not just illegal, but morally wrong, to discriminate against women in hiring and firing, to pay them less than male doctors for equal work, or to subject them to sexual harassment or intimidation.

EVIDENCE OF IMMORAL BEHAVIOR AND ATTITUDES

There is statistical and anecdotal evidence that sex discrimination against women veterinarians does occur. As noted above, 1986 women graduates averaged 4.6% less in salary than their male counterparts in private practice. Moreover, although in mixed animal and small animal predominant practices the salaries of male and female graduates were nearly identical, in "large animal exclusive, small animal exclusive, and equine predominant practices ... men would earn higher salaries on average, by amounts ranging from about $1,200 in small animal exclusive to nearly $5,000 in equine exclusive practices" (28). The compiler of these statistics was unwilling to speculate about the reasons for the differences without further data about the duties of these doctors. But the inference that there was sexual discrimination seems reasonable. This inference is further supported by the finding of the same study that while 15% of 1986 male graduates received no job offers, the figure for female graduates was 30%.

Some veterinarians do have attitudes toward women doctors that are discriminatory or demeaning. Dr. Kathleen Smiler tells of a practitioner whose female associate had some teeth knocked out by a cow, and then vowed that he would never hire another woman doctor (K. Smiler, personal communication) – when, of course, many male veterinarian teeth have been removed by cows. Dr. Smiler also tells of male practice owners who treat their women associates more like daughters (who must be protected, for example, from crude or discourteous clients and neighbors) than as equal professional colleagues (13). Although the increasing number of women in the profession should eventually bury such attitudes forever, there is no reason why normative veterinary ethics cannot attempt to hasten this process.

THE NONVETERINARIAN EMPLOYEE

Many of the same considerations relating to the ethical treatment of associate doctors apply to nonveterinarian employees. However, because of the differences in training and duties between veterinarians and nonveterinarians, these considerations sometimes have different implications.

Salary and Benefits

Because they are less skilled than veterinarians and are not responsible for the great bulk of practice revenues, generally, nonveterinarian employees cannot expect to earn as much as doctors, even after years of service. Nevertheless, just as is the case with veterinarian employees, in establishing salaries and benefits for nonveterinarian workers, practice owners are obligated to consider such factors as the length and quality of their educational experience, the amount and difficulty of their work, the quality of their work, and the extent to which they participate in activities that contribute to revenue production.

All veterinarians have the obligation to hire nonveterinarian workers who are qualified and caring. However, because many owners face economic pressures (not the least of which is the need to pay their veterinarian employees fairly), there can be pressure to keep nonveterinarian compensation levels as low as possible. In many states, there is no government registration of technicians. Even where there is, someone without a technician's educational or practice experience is often permitted to engage in many of the same activities as a trained technician. The best technicians will have little bargaining power if they can be replaced with people with much less skill willing to work for less. The fact that the overwhelming majority of technicians and other nonveterinarian employees are women makes it still easier for those who think that women ought to earn less than men to rationalize depressed salaries for nonveterinarian workers. A crucial step in assuring fair compensation and treatment for nonveterinarian employees is a recognition by the profession that employee relations is a legitimate and necessary concern of official and normative veterinary ethics.

Proportional or Commission Compensation

If nonveterinarian employees work hard, and the practice prospers, it is fair that the owners share some of the bounty with them, and use such compensation as an incentive for further good work. However, paying nonveterinarian employees a direct percentage commission of the sales of goods or services for which they are responsible raises the same problems for clients and the long-term image of the profession as does paying doctors a percentage of their contribution to revenues. (Nonveterinarian employees must never be paid for recommending or inducing clients to purchase medical goods or services, because such recommendations may be made only by a veterinary medical doctor.) If veterinarians are to retain their image of trusted medical professionals, the public must remain confident that the primary goal of *everyone* who works in veterinary practices is first and foremost service to patients and clients.

Understandings and Restrictions

Like associate doctors, nonveterinarian employees have an interest in understanding the conditions of their employment, including vacations, health insurance, maternity leave, required notice for termination of employment, and severance pay. As is the case with doctors, probationary periods of employment may be used to permit employer and employee to judge their suitability for each other. The understandings of the parties may be set forth in a written contract or in an employment manual. Owners must be careful in composing such manuals, for they can sometimes constitute the terms of a contractual agreement between the practice and the employee, even if no formal document labelled "contract" is ever signed. Violations of the terms of the manual, or indeed of any employment policies in whatever form they are stated, might subject the owners to a lawsuit for breach of contract.

One issue about which practices must be especially sensitive is termination of employment. It is unfair to a prospective employee to state or imply a longer term of employment than the owners really intend. If the practice does intend what the law calls "employment at will" – employment that can be terminated by the employer or employee at any time and for any reason – this fact should be made clear to the prospective employee. Owners can find themselves subjected to legal action if they have indicated to an employee that his employment was not at will (whatever the employment manual might state), or fire him for a reason (such as age or sex) that the law does not recognize as a valid reason for termination even for employees at will.

Sex-related Issues

Sexual discrimination or harassment is no less illegal or immoral when directed at nonveterinarians than at licensed doctors. Veterinarians have no weaker a moral obligation to help pregnant nonveterinarian employees to protect themselves and their unborn from reproductive and fetal hazards than they have to female associates. Nor should male veterinarians think that they may treat their nonveterinarian women employees in demeaning or degrading ways because they are not veterinarians. (I know one veterinarian who speaks of female technicians, but not female veterinarian associates, as "girls.")

Maternity and childrearing issues can raise difficult problems. Ideally, all female employees with a good record and prospects for continuing contributions to the practice should be given paid maternity leave. But because paid leaves can drain a practice substantially, I would argue that as a general rule, if a practice can afford such a benefit for either a female doctor or a nonveterinarian employee, and is permitted by law to make a choice, it is preferable to extend this benefit to the doctor. Doctors deserve a higher level of compensation in virtue of their training and skills, they provide more valuable services, and they generate more revenue than nonveterinarian employees. However, it does not follow that, even when legally permitted to so, owners may ignore the needs of childbearing female nonveterinary employees. A valuable and devoted employee with a good record would seem to deserve at least the opportunity to return to work after some maternity time. (This opportunity, it must be reiterated, is sometimes required by law.) For a highly skilled and dedicated employee in a prosperous practice, such as an experienced anesthetist or intensive care nurse, a strong argument can be made that a paid maternity leave would be morally obligatory.

The Face of a Practice

Nonveterinarian employees have important obligations relating to clients and other visitors to the practice. A frequent observer of veterinary facilities, I am appalled by the number in which clients who sit in the waiting room are confronted by a loud radio, boisterous behavior behind the reception desk, or loud conversations of a personal nature among employees. Working in a veterinary facility need not, and should not, be a solemn and somber undertaking. But veterinary employees must understand that they play a vital role in presenting their practice's face to the world. Undignified and disrespectful behavior (including disheveled appearance) directed at or done in the presence of clients is offensive to clients, can harm the image and earning power of a practice, and ultimately makes it more difficult for the profession to maintain an elevated image.

Technicians

THE GREAT NOMENCLATURE CONTROVERSY

Many ethical issues involving nonveterinarian employees relate to technicians. One question that goes to the heart of the profession's most basic attitudes regarding technicians concerns what they should be called. The plurality of AVMA training programs use the term "veterinary technician," and most of the remainder "animal health technician." Nevertheless, the only designation that has been officially approved by the AVMA is one that is rarely used (at least by technicians): "animal technician." In 1987, the AVMA Council on Education requested that the official terminology be changed from "animal technician" to "animal health technician." But the term "veterinary technician" was disapproved by the Council on the grounds that it does "not indicate whether the staff person is a professional" (29). At the 1988 AVMA annual convention, a resolution was introduced in the House of Delegates recommending adoption of the "veterinary" technician designation. Although the resolution had the support of the AVMA Executive Board, it was defeated overwhelmingly by the House (30). Because the designation of "animal health technician" has not yet been officially approved by the House of Delegates, as of 1988, the only approved terminology remained "animal technician."

Dr. R. Leland West, the AVMA's former Director of Scientific Activities, presents the following argument against the "veterinary" technician designation. According to Dr. West, technicians are "minimally trained assistants." Calling them veterinary technicians "will encourage technicians and the animal-owning public to believe that in 2 years an individual has been trained to be a veterinarian," and will set "the stage for the next great cycle of fighting for our identity as professionally educated doctors of veterinary medicine" (31). Opponents of this view note that the public does not confuse medical technicians with physicians or dental technicians with dentists, and that the term "veterinary technician" is already widely used by technician training institutions and veterinarians, without apparent catastrophe (32).

If the term "veterinary" did not connote an elevated status, technicians would not be as interested as they are in using it. So, ultimately, the question of whether the term is appropriately applied to technicians is, as Dr. West recognizes, the issue of whether these nonveterinarian employees do have training that is substantial and do perform functions that are of great importance to patients, clients, and doctors.

It is difficult to look at veterinary technicians who have completed AVMA-approved degree programs and who assist surgeons in administering and monitoring anesthesia, nurse critically ill patients back to health, give medications, perform essential theriogenology services, assist in the humane care of laboratory animals, and instruct clients about nutrition and pet care, and not conclude that many are as valuable and deserving of the term "veterinary" as dental technicians or medical technicians are deserving of their titles. Indeed, some technicians are so highly skilled and perform such important tasks that it seems more accurate to analogize them to human medical nurses rather than to medical or dental technicians.

The battle to stop the designation of "veterinary technician" is one that the AVMA cannot, and should not, win. The term is already in use. The AVMA itself has been instrumental in assisting technicians to reach a level of sophistication and importance that makes the designation an appropriate one. Official approval of the designation would be a sign of generosity, and a token of respect for a group of dedicated people whose steadfast service is in the best interests not only of doctors, but of patients and clients as well.

SHOULD TECHNICIANS BE REGISTERED OR LICENSED?

A number of states register or license veterinary technicians. (The terms "registration" and "licensing" are sometimes used interchangeably, and neither has special significance in itself.) There are different possible kinds of registration, among them the following:

• *Option 1.* A nonveterinarian employee is prohibited from calling himself a "veterinary technician" or "animal health technician," unless registered as such with the state board of veterinary medicine. Such registration requires graduation from an educational program approved by the board and demonstration (e.g., by examination) of a level of knowledge or competence required by the board.

• *Option 2.* Option 1 plus continuing supervision of registered technicians (e.g., by requiring continuing education or through on-the-job inspections of technicians' work, conducted by the state board).

• *Option 3.* Option 2 plus prohibition of certain activities (e.g., assisting in surgeries or administration of anesthesia) by nonveterinarian employees who are not registered technicians.

All three of these options could benefit patients, clients, and doctors because they can all assist veterinarians to assure that qualified persons are hired as technicians. But all the options have potential drawbacks. Among such drawbacks is *not*, as some believe (33), that registration entails the authorization of technicians to provide services directly to the public. There is nothing inherent in "registration" or "licensing" that requires giving technicians permission to act other than in the employment and under the supervision of veterinarians.

A problem with Options 1 and 2 is that they would afford the public and its animals the benefits of more highly qualified registered technicians only if doctors *choose* to hire people who can call themselves registered technicians. Option 3 avoids this difficulty, and might give technicians greater bargaining power to obtain decent salaries.[a] On the other hand, Option 3 could harm those practices unable to afford higher technician salaries that might result from an Option 3 registration program. Ironically, Option 3 might also lead some practices to hire a new veterinarian rather than a registered technician, on the theory that if more must be paid to an employee, he might as well be a doctor.

---

[a]A 1983 AVMA survey of accredited animal technology programs found that average starting salaries for their graduates ranged from $8,583 to $12,500. Salaries of experienced graduates of these programs averaged from $9,133 to $17,735 per year (34).

Although Option 2 might appear to be a reasonable compromise, like Option 3, it would require resources in funds and personnel that many state veterinary boards do not yet have. Unless a state allocates sufficient funds to an Option 2 program, intolerable additional demands could be placed on the board. It might have difficulty adequately regulating veterinarians. More likely, the board would be unable to enforce the technician registration program or would not take it seriously.

ARE TECHNICIANS PROFESSIONALS?

The issue of whether technicians should be considered members of a profession is distinct from the question of whether they ought to be registered by state authorities. Some professionals (e.g., clergy and in some states psychotherapists) are not licensed and regulated by state authorities, and some persons who must have licenses (e.g., hairdressers and electricians) are not considered members of one of the professions.

Whether veterinary technology will be regarded as a profession will depend in large measure on whether technicians' educational attainments and tasks continue to improve in sophistication and importance, and whether technicians themselves take an active role in the self-regulation of technical competence and ethical behavior.

Veterinarians should take note that for many years physicians refused to call nurses professionals and spoke of them as the "handmaidens" of medicine. Today nursing is universally regarded as a profession. Yet, there remain strict limitations on what nurses are permitted to do. They are still under the supervision and control of physicians, and pose little threat to the earning power of the medical profession. As the public's regard for animals continues to rise, veterinarians should not be surprised if others who participate with them in providing sophisticated medical care for animals also come to be regarded by the public as professionals.

SOME BASIC ETHICAL PRINCIPLES REGARDING VETERINARY TECHNICIANS

In Table 22.1, I propose for further debate several general ethical principles regarding technicians. These suggestions are based upon considerable discussion with veterinarians and technicians and reflect many basic concerns of both. Some of the

Table 22.1

Ethical Principles Regarding the Veterinary Technician

1. *Technicians shall serve their employers loyally and faithfully.*
   A) A technician shall follow all orders and instructions given by doctors.
   B) A technician shall take no actions regarding any patient or client unless properly authorized to do so. When in doubt about the propriety of any action, the technician shall, whenever possible, ask for direction from a doctor or appropriate supervisory personnel.
   C) A technician shall not criticize any doctor or any employee of the practice to or in the presence of any client, but shall bring complaints or concerns to the attention of a doctor or other appropriate personnel.
   D) A technician shall not make any decisions or take any actions bearing upon the economic affairs of the practice unless authorized to do so. For example, the technician shall not change without permission the normal fee for a particular client or dispense gratuitous medications, goods, or services.

Table 22.1 – *continued*

E) A technician shall not take or use for any unauthorized purpose or in any unauthorized manner any patient or client records or any information contained in such records.

F) A technician shall work diligently, carefully, and competently, with the understanding that his employer can be held liable at law for the actions of employees.

G) A technician shall always act on the highest plane of honesty and integrity.

H) A technician shall treat all doctors and employees of the practice with courtesy and respect.

2. *Technicians shall serve clients loyally and respectfully.*
    A) A technician shall treat all clients courteously and respectfully.
    B) A technician shall comport himself in a dignified manner as befits an employee of a medical office.
    C) A technician shall respect the professional and personal confidences of clients. Nor shall he reveal to anyone, unless authorized by an appropriate member of the practice or required by law to do so, any information revealed to or in the possession of any doctor or employee of the practice regarding any patient or client.

3. *Technicians shall serve all patients with dignity and respect.*
    A) A technician shall treat all patients humanely and respectfully. The technician shall never inflict unnecessary pain or discomfort on any animal for the purpose of rendering that animal tractable or for any other purpose.
    B) A technician shall attend promptly to the needs of all patients and shall fulfill all orders and instructions regarding patients with the highest degree of diligence.

4. *Technicians shall strive to improve the knowledge, technical skills, and moral character of themselves and their fellow technicians.*
    A) A technician shall keep informed of developments in knowledge and techniques relating to his duties and shall fulfill all educational requirements of his technician association and state board of veterinary medicine.
    B) A technician shall strive to promote the entrance into employment as veterinary technicians persons of high competence and good moral character.
    C) A technician shall obey the veterinary practice act of his jurisdiction and all other laws governing or pertaining to his medical duties.

5. *Veterinarians shall treat technicians fairly and respectfully.*
    A) Veterinarians shall compensate all technicians in their employ fairly.
    B) Veterinarians shall strive to utilize technicians in their employ at tasks appropriate to their level of competence.
    C) Veterinarians shall encourage all technicians in their employ to maintain and improve their technical knowledge and skills.
    D) Veterinarians shall treat all technicians respectfully, as valuable members of the veterinary medical team.

principles are quite general, and are intended to permit further refinement or elaboration of appropriate subprinciples. For example, much more can be said about the ways in which technicians ought to be honest to their employers and about how veterinarians can exhibit respect toward technicians. Some of the principles follow from other of the standards, elaborating upon an ethical requirement in order to address more explicitly a concern of doctors or technicians. The principles are also general in the sense that some might admit of exceptions in extreme or special circumstances. For example, the principle that technicians ought not to criticize a doctor to clients might conceivably be overridden in a case in which the only way a technician could prevent heinous suffering by a patient would be to tell the client that something is amiss. But because such a case would be a highly unusual one, it is still possible to suggest a general rule prohibiting technicians from complaining about doctors to or in the presence of clients.

The suggested principles make two fundamental assumptions. First, the actions of technicians must be based on the best interests of patients and clients. This, in turn, implies the requirement that technicians must *always* be under the supervision and control of veterinarians and must *never* be permitted to engage in activities that for medical reasons ought to be reserved for a veterinary medical doctor.

Second, because technicians are legal agents of their veterinarian employers, these employers can often be held liable for, or as a result of, their actions. This not only requires technicians to act diligently and competently. It also explains the appropriateness of a general prohibition against their complaining about doctors or other employees to or in the presence of clients. An inadvertent, misinformed, or malicious comment by an employee can subject a practice and its doctors to undeserved legal problems.

INTERPERSONAL RELATIONS

Many difficult ethical issues can arise out of relations among owners and employees. Owners can face difficult choices when one or more of them cannot get along with or have a legitimate complaint about the performance of an associate doctor. Problems can also arise when any of the doctors in the practice have difficult relations with a nonveterinarian employee, or when employees, veterinarian or nonveterinarian, have difficulties in their relations with each other. Any of these kinds of problems can be exacerbated when a client complains about an employee. The owners can be faced with a dilemma between satisfying a client, for whom the practice works, and protecting the employee, in whom the owners might have invested a good deal of time and effort and whose continuing service is probably more important to the practice than any single client.

As is often the case in ethics, there is no simple rule that does justice to the variety and complexity of situations in which problems involving employees can arise. For example, regarding complaints against employees by clients, one cannot say that "the client is always right." Clients are sometimes wrong. And even if a client is correct that an associate or nonveterinarian employee acted incompetently or unethically, it does not follow that the owners must take some drastic action demanded by the client and thereby lose or seriously impair the effectiveness of a valuable employee. Likewise, when there are interpersonal difficulties within the practice, one cannot say that the owners should always favor the person with the greatest economic value to the practice, or should favor an associate doctor with greater seniority over one with less, or an associate over a technician, or a technician with greater seniority over one with less, and so on. Blaming or disciplining someone who is not at fault based on some pre-ordained hierarchical scheme is profoundly unfair. It can also have disastrous effects, if employees come to think that they are likely to receive certain kinds of treatment not because they deserve it, but on the basis of their status or importance.

Whoever in the practice is authorized to deal with a problem involving employees must consider his first order of business to ascertain the facts. If one allows devotion to, or economic interest in, a particular employee to cloud one's judgment about who is responsible for a problem, one risks all sorts of bad results. One might unfairly blame the wrong person. One might fail to discourage a tendency in an employee that will recur in the future, to the detriment of others in the practice as well as to clients and patients.

At the same time, owners have a legitimate interest in keeping their practices comfortable and profitable places in which to work. They are entitled to protect even those employees who deserve criticism from unreasonable demands of clients or other employees. If an employee treats a client or another employee improperly, and the situation must be addressed, the owners should strive to cause as little bad feeling or disruption as possible. There is no legal or moral principle requiring, for example, that an unhappy client participate in or observe the disciplining of an errant employee.

Finally, moral deliberation must pay due regard to legitimate hierarchies. The most important moral distinction in a veterinary practice is that between owners and nonowners. Owners should never permit their pre-eminent legal status to lead to self-deception about their own professionalism or ability to deal fairly with others; that can lead to as much harm to others in the practice, and to clients, and patients as blaming the wrong person for some problem. However, when an owner simply cannot get along with an associate or nonveterinarian employee, and someone must either change his ways or leave, it is the owner who has the right to prevail. He has this moral right in virtue of his legal position as owner as well as his investment in time and money that this legal status reflects.

A distinction that in my view is too often overdone in veterinary practices in approaching issues of an interpersonal nature is that between veterinarians and technicians. Many technicians tell me that when a problem arises between them and a doctor, they have little chance of getting their side of the story heard impartially and sympathetically. Indeed, a common complaint of technicians is that they are rarely treated with much respect, and that feelings of inferiority and subservience are almost a part of their job description. Anyone who spends a significant amount of time talking with technicians cannot help but be impressed by the deep-seated belief on the part of many that they are not treated with dignity and regard. For practical as well as moral reasons, technicians and other nonveterinarian workers must be respected by all doctors as important members of the veterinary medical team. This means respecting them both as valuable workers and as valued human beings.

REFERENCES

1. For helpful discussions of laws affecting veterinary employees see, What the Law Demands of You, the Boss. *Veterinary Economics* Jul 1987:62-72; Bancroft BR: Terminating Employees May Be Harder than You Think. *Trends* 3(1):36-37, 1987; and Beware of COBRA – A Snake in the Grass. *Trends* 3(4):28, 1987.
2. Clark R: What's a DVM Worth? *Veterinary Economics* Mar 1987:28.
3. Wise JK: Employment, starting salaries, and educational indebtedness of 1986 graduates of US veterinary medical colleges. *J Am Vet Med Assoc* 190:209-210, 1987.
4. Wise, JK: Employment of 1986 male and female graduates of US veterinary medical colleges. *J Am Vet Med Assoc* 190:449-450, 1987.
5. Wise JK: 1985 US veterinary practice income, expenses, and financial ratios. *J Am Vet Med Assoc* 190:1594-1598, 1987. These were the latest figures available at the time of this writing.

6. Thieberger J: More Graduates Turning to Law Firm Practice. *National Law Journal* 9(29):14-15, 1987 (reporting an average $29,224 salary for 1985 law graduates).
7. See How the Professionals Stack Up. *Veterinary Economics* Jul 1987:49 (citing figures from the American Bar Association reporting an average $114,331 for all attorneys in 1985).
8. Jensen RH: Partners Work Harder to Stay Even. *National Law Journal* 9(48):12, 1987 (reporting an average salary of $46,090 for associates and $119,944 for law practice owners).
9. Gallagher DP and Leininger TI: Considerations When Hiring an Associate. In Pratt PW (ed): *Veterinary Practice Management.* Santa Barbara: American Veterinary Publications, Inc., 1979, pp 268-281.
10. Incentives Speak Louder than Words. *Veterinary Economics* Jun 1987:48 (remarks attributed to Dr. D. McCurnin).
11. Clark R: What's a DVM Worth? *Veterinary Economics* Mar 1987:27.
12. Davis J: Discover the 15 Percent Solution. *Veterinary Economics* Jul 1987:77.
13. Incentives Speak Louder Than Words. *Veterinary Economics* Jun 1987:46 (remarks attributed to Dr. R. Ainslie).
14. Enrollment Declines in DVM-Degree Programs. *J Am Vet Med Assoc* 192:1028, 1988 (reporting that women comprised 50.8% of the total student body of U.S. veterinary colleges in 1985-1986; 53% in 1986-1987; and 55.03% in 1987-1988).
15. Miller RM: Response. *Veterinary Economics* Jun 1986:7.
16. Violante J: Letter. Free shovels to dig your own hole. *Veterinary Economics* Aug 1986:4.
17. 29 U.S.C. § 206(d)(1).
18. 42 U.S.C. § 2000e.
19. 42 U.S.C. § 2000e(k).
20. 29 C.F.R. Pt. 1604, App., Ans. 6. (1986).
21. 29 C.F.R. Pt. 1604, App., Ans. 17. (1986).
22. 29 C.F.R. Pt. 1604, App., Ans. 18. (1986).
23. 29 C.F.R. § 1604.11(a) (1986).
24. CCH EEOC Compliance Manual § 624.1 ¶ 4301 (1986).
25. CCH EEOC Compliance Manual § 624.8 ¶ 4308 (1986).
26. EEOC Dec. No. 72-0386 (Aug. 24, 1971), CCH EEOC Decisions ¶ 6295 (1973).
27. For an excellent guide to state sex discrimination laws, see Larson A and Larson LK: *Employment Discrimination.* New York: Matthew Bender, 1987, §§ 9, 38.60.
28. Wise JK: Employment of 1986 male and female graduates of US veterinary medical colleges. *J Am Vet Med Assoc* 190:449-450, 1987.
29. Council Bids Fairwell to Dr. West; CATAT Activities. *J Am Vet Med Assoc* 190:449-450, 1987.
30. Animal Technician – A Rose by Any Other Name. *AVMA Convention News.* Portland, OR: American Veterinary Medical Association, July 19, 1988, p 2.
31. West RL: The cycle syndrome. *J Am Vet Med Assoc* 191:298, 1987.
32. Tillman P: Letter. Prefers veterinary technician to animal technician. *J Am Vet Med Assoc* 191:5-6, 1987.
33. McCurnin DM: Utilizing the Animal Technician. *Trends* 1(2):52, 1985.
34. Animal Technology. *1988 AVMA Directory,* p 628.

Chapter

— 23 —

The Veterinarian and Animal Research

Relatively few veterinarians are engaged in animal research. Nor does biomedical and scientific research account for more than a very small fraction of all animals used by society.[a] Nevertheless, there are several reasons why a text on professional veterinary ethics must devote some discussion to moral issues arising out of the use of animals in research.

First, there already exists a sizable body of work addressing the morality of the use of animals in research. Many of the issues discussed in this literature bear upon animal welfare, which is a general concern of the veterinary profession.

Second, continued progress in preventing and alleviating animal and human disease depends upon the ability of veterinarians, physicians, and biomedical scientists to use animals in research. If the animal rights movement succeeds in curtailing animal research, it can threaten the ability of veterinary and human medical doctors to provide the kind of care patients require. Today, promoting the interests of their patients, clients, and the profession requires veterinarians to support animal research. This, in turn, necessitates that veterinarians know about current controversies and be able to participate in them persuasively.

Third, no other group of persons can speak more knowledgeably or convincingly than veterinarians about the legitimate needs of all those affected by animal research – including research animals. The deepest values of the profession include a recognition of the legitimacy of the human use of animals as well as a desire to treat animals fairly. The veterinary profession possesses great knowledge about animals, science, and human as well as animal disease. Adequate protection of both people and animals calls out for vigorous involvement by veterinarians in debates and policy-making relating to the use of animals in research.

This book focuses on ethical issues faced by veterinarians in private clinical practice. Therefore, no attempt will be made to discuss in great detail all the ethical questions that are posed by the use of animals in research. My aims here are to provide practitioners and students with useful information about some of the more important current issues and controversies, and to apply principles developed in the text to some of these issues.

---

[a]According to one estimate (1), "between 17 million to 22 million animals are used [annually] in the United States in research, testing, and teaching, while nearly 5 billion are killed and consumed for food." Another estimate (2) places the figure for research animals at 70 million.

WHAT IS ANIMAL RESEARCH?

Animal research can be defined as the search for or investigation of facts through scientific inquiry that utilizes animals. Research (whether or not it uses animals) can be "basic," in the sense of being motivated by a desire to obtain knowledge irrespective of any practical applications or benefits, or "applied," in the sense of being aimed at obtaining such results. One important justification for basic research is the desire to understand our universe and its components. But because making the world better almost always requires knowledge of it, basic research frequently stimulates, or eventually becomes of direct use to, applied research. The term "research" carries no implication of scientific or moral value. Research that is good from one of these standpoints may be questionable from the other.

There is enormous variety in activities that are properly called "animal research." This fact is not always appreciated or emphasized by opponents of the use of animals in research. Animal research does not necessarily involve manipulating animals or their environments; an ethologist or psychologist can sometimes do research on animals by observing them in their natural habitats. Animal research need not involve causing animals pain or distress; indeed, many research animals do better in a laboratory than they would in the wild. Animal research is not directed solely at benefiting human beings; much animal research helps animals. Animal research does not necessarily involve sacrificing the interests of a research animal for those of people or other animals; a great deal of animal research is conducted by veterinary clinicians and is directly beneficial to animals undergoing experimental procedures.

Moreover, in thinking about the morality of research on animals, it is important to understand that activities that, strictly speaking, might not be termed "research" are often important components of the general research enterprise – either because they can be involved in particular parts of research projects or because they provide training for those who do, or will eventually do, animal research. A complete account of the ethics of the use of animals in research will include consideration of the employment of animals in the extraction of products, production and standardization of biologicals, diagnosis of human and animal diseases, toxicity testing, and education.

DEFENDING ANIMAL RESEARCH: THE ARTICULATION OF STANDARDS

The contributions of animal research to the health, safety, and well-being of humans and animals have been enormous. There are countless people and animals alive and healthy today because of advances that would have been impossible but for the use of animals. To stop or seriously curtail animal research would wreak unspeakable and intolerable evil.

In my view, the major ethical task in the animal research area is not so much to document the benefits of animal research (although this is important) as it is to articulate standards by which various kinds of research can be justified. Thus far, defenders of research have been good at citing benefits of animal experimentation for human (3) and animal (4) health. But much more needs to be done in the articulation of *reasons* why such benefits justify particular kinds of animal uses.

This important process of articulating good reasons for animal research has been hindered by the fact that many proponents of animal research have become preoccupied with responding to attacks by abolitionists and other kinds of critics. Proponents of research often permit critics to choose the language and the premises around which argument turns.

For example, I speak often with animal researchers about their work. I would be happy to have a dollar every time I hear that a particular project is "necessary" for the attainment of some crucial advance in medical knowledge. The literature defending animal research is filled with statements about the indispensability of animal research to every medical advance known to man and animal alike (5).

Such claims seem to be in response to critics who charge that animal research is *not* "necessary" because, in their view, almost every important biomedical advance would have been or would be possible without it (6). There are, surely, some animal experiments that have been "necessary" in the sense that an important advance in medical knowledge could not have occurred without them. Such necessity, when it exists, would constitute a strong argument in favor of a research project. But why should defenders of research accept the premise that a given use of animals is unjustifiable unless it someday can be shown to have been "necessary?" We do not require farmers or meat-eaters to prove that hamburger or chicken is "necessary" for human well-being, health, or survival, or even for great esthetic pleasure.

The attainment of a modest piece of medically relevant knowledge or a moderately useful medical technique is surely far more important an achievement than the eating of even the most artfully prepared hamburger or pork chop. Indeed, the *attempt* to make advances in treating disease and illness, even when it fails altogether, is far more important an endeavor than the eating of any particular kind of food. Given the fact that science does not always succeed in producing significant or useful knowledge, and that the implications of scientific research are often unpredictable, animal researchers should not always feel compelled to demonstrate that their experiments are "necessary."

If proponents of animal research sometimes make their task overly difficult, they sometimes also make it too easy. The prime example of this is the widespread acceptance in the research community of the anticruelty position, and its implication that animal welfare consists entirely of freedom from unnecessary pain or other negative states. (See Chapters 11 and 21.) This view discounts the intuitively appealing notion that we sometimes are obligated to give animals we use for our own purposes some measure of happiness. The anticruelty position also implies that all animal experiments that do not cause *any* pain are justifiable (7). This is too simplistic an approach. I know very few researchers who believe that it is appropriate to experiment upon or kill an unlimited number of chimpanzees, for example, so long as this is done painlessly. With regard to some animals at least, there seems to be a higher burden of proof before even a completely painless experiment can be justified.

ANIMAL RESEARCH ETHICS: BASIC PREMISES

Moral issues relating to research animals are similar in important respects to those involving agricultural animals. Many laboratory animal veterinarians take a herd health approach to research animals. Like farm and food animals, animals used in research are usually kept in groups. Their usefulness typically derives from the role they play in relation to what can be gained from other animals. Because of similarities in laboratory and agricultural animal use, it is helpful for normative veterinary ethics to approach animal research with a basic set of premises similar to those it applies to agricultural animals. I therefore want to set out the 10 basic premises developed in Chapter 21, modified for the area of animal research, with some additional discussion.

1. *It is not inherently wrong to use animals in research.*

If some animals may be used in the production of food and clothing, some animals surely may be used for the important aim of preventing and curing disease and illness. At the same time, defenders of animal research should not be too hasty (as some are) to assume that direct benefit to people or animals is the only justifiable purpose of animal research. Understanding basic features of our world and taking pleasure in such understanding is, surely, no less worthy or valuable than taking pleasure from an animal food or clothing product. It follows that the search for basic knowledge – even when it does not present an immediate or clear prospect of applied benefits – can also be a legitimate use of animals. To be sure, there are additional considerations. I would argue that in general, a stronger showing of the importance of a piece of basic research must be made when that work would cause pain or discomfort to animals than when the research shows prospect of providing practical medical benefits. Considerations regarding other interests of the animals involved must also be taken into account. However, it is both inconsistent and anti-intellectual to accept ordinary uses of animals for food and other consumer conveniences and to require animal researchers to always show that their work must have some (usually *enormously* important) practical benefit.

2. Researchers may factor research and management considerations into decisions regarding the use, care, and treatment of their animals.

It follows from the fact that some animals may be used in research that optimal animal welfare sometimes may be compromised in animal experimentation. Otherwise, some legitimate research projects would be impossible. At the same time, one must ask whether any given level of welfare associated with an experiment is morally justified by the expected results (practical or theoretical) of the research.

3. The role of public needs and interests in the determination of how research animals are treated must not be underestimated.

Like farmers, animal researchers tend to be the targets of activist attacks, even though most research is done because of what is perceived to be in the public interest. Government and private agencies do not fund animal research on cancer, diabetes, heart disease, or AIDS in order to provide amusement for researchers. Ordinary citizens are not as actively involved in the choice of the employment of animals in research as they are in market forces that influence the use of agricultural and sport animals. Many people may not know why animal research is important for themselves and their loved ones. There is, I would argue, a general obligation on the part of the scientific community and government to inform the public about what is being done with their tax dollars to support animal research. The case for such education is even stronger today, when activists seek to persuade laymen that animal research is inherently cruel and useless. Ultimately, the most effective protection for animal research and research animal welfare may come from an informed public that will demand both.

4. Research animals have interests that must be taken into account.

Research animals, like those used for companionship and in agriculture and entertainment, have legitimate interests that must be taken into account in determining what may be done with them. Taking research animal interests seriously does not mean always giving their interests priority over the interests of others. But it does mean rejecting the notion that such other interests automatically must prevail. There is a variety of both human and animal interests, some of which are weightier than others. The avoidance of pain, for example, is clearly a very important interest of research animals. Overriding this interest will, in general, require the presence of important countervailing interests.

The concept of ethical costs (see Chapter 21) is important in the research animal area. As is generally the case, the need to consider ethical costs does not imply the legitimacy of a "cost-benefit" approach, i.e., utilitarianism. Utilitarianism is no more theoretically or practically satisfactory in dealing with laboratory animals than it is in deciding how to treat agricultural animals. It is no more possible to quantify with rigorous precision the mental states of research animals than it is to do so for other animals. Utilitarianism also refuses to recognize that research animals sometimes have the moral right not to be treated in certain ways, even if such treatment could be shown to maximize the total pleasure or happiness of all affected.

5. *Individual animals count.*

6. *Research animals have some basic moral rights.*

The fact that individual research animals can experience such states as pain and stress means that their interests must be taken into account. Moreover, like domesticated agricultural and sport animals, research animals are not without moral rights because they may have been bred for suitability for certain uses. They remain sentient beings with interests of their own, interests that sometimes cannot be overridden simply because doing so would be expedient.

In a recent defense of animal research, philosopher Carl Cohen maintains that animals "have, and can have, no rights against us on which research can infringe" (8). According to Cohen, rights by their very nature

> are in every case claims, or potential claims, within a community of moral agents. Rights arise, and can be intelligibly defended, only among beings who actually do, or can, make moral claims against one another (9).

Cohen concludes that because research animals (like other animals) cannot actually claim rights for themselves and are not "beings of a kind capable of exercising or responding to moral claims" (10), they can have no rights.

Cohen provides no argument for his assertion that only beings capable of exercising or responding to moral claims can have "rights," as speakers of the language ordinarily use the term. He offers the assertion as a truism. However, as I noted in Chapter 12, most people do ascribe moral rights to some beings (such as human infants and profoundly mentally deficient people) who cannot "exercise" or "respond" to moral claims. Cohen's response to this fact is to grant that deficient humans have moral rights. But animals, he says, "are of such a kind that it is impossible for them, in principle, to give or withhold voluntary consent or make a moral choice. What humans retain when disabled, animals never had" (10).

However, *what* is "retained" by a profoundly mentally deficient human, who (let us suppose for the purposes of discussion) cannot exercise voluntary consent or choice? It is not the ability to give or withhold consent or choice. Indeed, some such profoundly deficient humans who possess moral rights may never have had these abilities. Nor can one say that all deficient humans who have moral rights participate in a "community" of moral agents in any meaningful sense. Cohen seems to be suggesting that what disabled humans always "retain" is their inclusion in a general *class* of beings – humankind – most of whose members claim and exercise rights. But why, for the purposes of determining whether rights can be ascribed, should profoundly deficient humans incapable of making claims about their own rights be put in *this* class? Why should we not consider them part of a general class of beings (a class that includes nonhuman animals) whose members can never claim rights for themselves, from which it would presumably follow for Cohen that these humans can have no rights? Cohen does not say.

Cohen's definition of a moral "right" does not reflect how this concept is used in our language today. Our concept does not require that all right-holders be able, or be members of a biological species most of whose members are able, to make claims concerning their rights. Cohen offers no argument for supposing that our ordinary concept of rights is incoherent or ethically inappropriate. His approach seems to rest on a general position that human beings (whether normal or deficient) are simply of much greater value than animals. As I argued in Chapter 11, this view is defensible. But it does not imply that animals can have no moral rights.

There remains significant opposition to the concept of animal rights within the biomedical and scientific research community. This opposition stems largely from an identification of the concept of animal rights with certain particular claims of the animal rights movement.[b] However, as we saw in Chapter 12, *the concept of animal rights does not imply the anti-research platforms of the animal rights movement.* Recognition of the existence of *some* animal rights will be a necessary part of any satisfactory approach to the ethics of the use of animals in research.

7. Although assessment of mental states is an important component of determining research animal interests, one must avoid exaggerated claims about these mental states.

As is the case regarding other animals, identifying and assigning proper moral weight to the legitimate interests of research animals requires accuracy about what mental states they experience. As is the case generally, determining what mental states research animals have, either normally or in response to experimental environments, raises difficult conceptual and factual issues. Some of these issues are discussed later in this chapter.

8. All other things being equal, a research or husbandry method or course of veterinary care that causes a research animal less pain, suffering, distress, or discomfort is preferable to one that causes it more.

9. All other things being equal, a research or husbandry method or course of veterinary care that gives a research animal more positive mental states is preferable to one that gives it less.

These are intuitively appealing principles that will sometimes cut against certain current assumptions and positions. But they are minimal principles. They do not address the issues of when animals ought to be subjected to less pain or be allowed to experience greater pleasure when these options would impose extra costs on experimenters in terms of expense, inconvenience, or the prospects of success of a research project. Moreover, as we shall see, sometimes all other things are not equal;

---

[b]Consider, for example, the following statement of a well-known defender of animal research: "The animal rights position is not simply that animals and humans are equal. It is that man is less than animals. The animal rights advocate would in fact choose an animal over a human life. He sees human beings as morally unclean, and animals as innocent, and therefore more deserving of existence than evil man" (11). Here, an absurdly inaccurate claim about the animal rights movement is transformed into a preposterous characterization of the concept of animal rights.

there can be important ethical reasons why a given individual animal may have to experience more distress or less pleasure than might otherwise be required.

10. *It is often unhelpful to maintain that research animals should not be caused "unnecessary" pain, suffering, distress, or discomfort, or that they should be treated "humanely."*

As I observed in Chapter 21, typically to say that a certain treatment of animals is "necessary" or is "humane" is to claim that it is justified. But determining what treatment is justified is, of course, precisely the task of ethical argument.

The limited usefulness of the notions of "necessary" pain and "humane" treatment is illustrated by the following statements of two thinkers at distant poles in the research animal issue. According to Carl Cohen, "(i)n our dealings with animals, few will deny that we are at least obligated to act humanely – that is to treat them with the decency and concern that we owe, as sensitive human beings, to other sentient creatures. To treat animals humanely, however, is not to treat them as ... the holders of rights" (10). Dr. Michael W. Fox, who opposes much current animal research, disagrees. He insists that because animals, too, have "intrinsic value and thus rights within themselves," we must "if we are to be humane stewards judge [between competing human and animal rights] with caution and humility" (12). Clearly, the concept of "humaneness" is not doing argumentative work in these statements. Rather, the concept is being used to summarize positions about the proper treatment of animals that have already been reached for other reasons. Likewise, Cohen and Fox doubtless would disagree about whether certain animal research projects are "necessary," in part because they would disagree about whether any pain that might be associated with these projects is justified by their intended aims.

One should never permit the notions of "necessary" pain and "humane" animal treatment to substitute for the underlying empirical investigation and ethical argument that is required to assess the appropriateness of animal experiments.

THE ETHICS OF ANIMAL RESEARCH: POLITICAL CONSIDERATIONS

As we saw in Chapter 21, serious investigation of animal welfare requires attention to difficult conceptual, factual, and ethical issues. In the area of research animal welfare, there is another important consideration: politics. Government (and those who attempt to influence government) are exerting ever greater influence on how research animals are treated. The consequence is that investigations of research animal welfare can be affected and altered by political tests and demands. This happens in several ways.

1. Researchers are finding themselves compelled to explain their work and its effects on animals in terms understandable to laymen. My own experience serving as the nonscientist member of an animal care committee has been that researchers are perfectly capable of doing this. Indeed, they seem to be stimulated to think more clearly about scientific, practical, and welfare aspects of their experiments by having to explain these aspects to a layman.

2. The biomedical research community (as well as professional veterinary associations and veterinary schools) must devote resources to public relations and lobbying to support animal research. The consequence is that money and effort that might otherwise be spent on serious research animal welfare studies go into the political arena.

3. The necessity of addressing political issues can lead supporters of animal research to make decisions based not solely on rationality, empirical evidence, or

ethical argument, but also on political expediency. For example, there is currently a campaign to convince state legislatures and Congress to prohibit the release of abandoned dogs and cats to researchers by public pounds and animal shelters. As I shall argue below, grave questions can be raised about the wisdom of such laws. Nevertheless, some scientists and veterinarians appear to have concluded that they cannot prevail on this issue and that they only risk more general hostility to animal research if they try to raise the opposing arguments. This approach may or may not be justified on the grounds of expedience. But at the very least, some people who would like to be making certain arguments and developing certain positions are wary of doing so. Such a climate is not conducive to the search for truth.

4. The entry of politics into animal welfare investigations poses questions and imposes answers that may not always be entirely justified ethically or scientifically. Legislators and regulators are accustomed to ordering what they want done. However, progress in animal welfare science and ethics will not be a consequence of majority vote or administrative edict. For example, recent amendments to the federal Animal Welfare Act require that measures be taken to assure the "psychological well-being" of primates (13). But a great deal remains to be learned about what constitutes psychological well-being, for primates in general and various species of primates in particular. What mental states do these animals experience? How would one distinguish various *levels* of psychological well-being, and what moral weight might be assigned to these levels? Are certain practices (e.g., restraint for long periods of time) really required for certain experiments, and if they are not, what approaches would have less negative impact on the animals' psychological well-being while permitting important research to continue?

Legislation and regulation is a double-edged sword. It can promote animal welfare by requiring that necessary questions be asked and overdue steps be taken. It can also discourage continuing progress, by imposing answers before they may be justified. Premature regulation can stifle serious animal welfare research by allowing those who do not care about animal welfare to rest on minimal government standards when much additional work is required. For example, if regulators declare that larger cages and "enrichment toys" in which primates fit nuts or pieces of fruit into holes in a board, are sufficient to promote primate psychological well-being, will that be the end of serious research into primate psychological well-being? Will the requirement that primates enjoy psychological well-being discourage funding of research directed at improving psychological well-being for *non*primates?

RESEARCH ANIMAL WELFARE: GENERAL CONSIDERATIONS

The following are among the important factors relevant to research animal welfare.

Housing, General Care, Environment

The conditions under which research animals are kept is obviously critical to their welfare (14, 15). Among relevant issues are the size and construction materials of cages; temperature; ventilation; quantity and quality of food; lighting; the nature and quantity of bedding for nesting animals; density of animals within cages; ability of animals to come in contact with other animals; opportunities for adequate exercise; group housing of social species (16); segregation of controls from sick and distressed animals; and opportunities for contact with technicians and handlers (17).

Much more needs to be learned about all of these considerations. Researchers, ethicists, and regulators must be wary of approaches that seem intuitively appealing to someone who seeks to imagine what it would be like to be a laboratory animal, but may have little basis in fact. As is always the case in animal welfare science, assessing the effects of certain environmental conditions on welfare is rarely the end of the matter. The appropriateness of welfare-improving or lessening conditions cannot be evaluated without considering their impact on research protocols. But such deliberations must leave open the possibility that the interests of research animals require certain basic conditions irrespective of their cost, inconvenience, or impact upon a research project.

Pain and Other Negative Mental States

Although freedom from pain may not be a research animal's only interest, it is an important interest that must be given serious consideration. Among procedures that can cause pain and other negative mental states are surgical operations, induction of disease or illness, physical trauma, restraint, physical exertion, exposure to abnormal environments, and deprivation of food or water.

ETHICAL ISSUES

Although pain is a relevant moral variable, assessing its proper relevance is not always a simple matter. Some researchers appear to accept as obvious an obligation to minimize the *total* amount of pain experienced (18). This is a utilitarian approach. It is overly simplistic and does not recognize morally important factors. The utilitarian must favor an experiment that causes a very small number of animals extremely severe pain over one that might cause a larger number of animals much less pain if the former experiment would cause on balance less total pain than the latter. But such an approach ignores the intuitively appealing principle that animals have a much greater interest in avoiding very severe or prolonged pain than in avoiding trivial or fleeting pain. Therefore, it may be preferable to cause *more* total pain if doing so will cause less pain to each *individual* animal. Another morally relevant factor that cannot be recognized by a utilitarian is the issue of the *fairness* after a certain point of subjecting an animal to still more pain. The utilitarian must recommend continuing to cause pain to animals that have already been experimented upon, rather than using new animals, if the former approach will cause less total pain than the latter. However, at some point it simply may be unfair to subject an individual animal that has already undergone severe deprivations of its interests, to any more pain. The very plausible objection to repeated survival surgeries on individual animals is based upon this nonutilitarian principle.

CONCEPTUAL ISSUES: DEFINING PAIN AND NEGATIVE MENTAL STATES IN RESEARCH ANIMALS

Like their counterparts in farm animal welfare, some investigators in the research animal area appear to have an irresistible urge to set forth quickly definitions that may not always clarify or stimulate important empirical and ethical work.

The Proceedings of the recent AVMA Colloquium on Recognition and Alleviation of Animal Pain and Distress (19) contain examples of problematic definitions of exceedingly complex concepts relating to negative mental states in research animals. Kitchell offers the following "working definition" of pain in animals: "an aversive sensory and emotional experience (a perception), which elicits protective motor actions, results in learned avoidance, and may modify species-specific traits of behavior, including social behavior" (20). This definition seems to exclude one phenomenon that clearly has important applications for animal welfare: "learned helplessness," in which an animal responds to repeated or severe pain or distress by "giving up" and doing nothing (21). Kitchell's definition also appears to exclude, by definition, the contention of the AVMA Panel on Euthanasia (see below) that it is wrong to euthanize research animals by decapitation without prior anesthesia because brain waves in decapitated heads may provide evidence that pain is still being experienced.

A second paper in the Proceedings asserts that pain "is a perception or unpleasant sensation arising from noxious stimuli that are actually or potentially damaging to tissues and is a subjective perception that is accompanied by feelings of fear, anxiety, and panic" (22). As I argued in Chapter 21, it is far from obvious that all animals that feel pain can also be said to experience mental states such as anxiety or fear. Including such states within the definition of pain will either make of pain more than it need be or render such concepts as "anxiety," "fear", and "panic" far less descriptive and distinctive than they now are.

Another discussion in the AVMA Proceedings states that "suffering can be defined as a severe emotional state that is extremely unpleasant, that results from physical pain, emotional pain, and/or discomfort at a level not tolerated by the individual, and that results in some degree of physiologic distress" (23). Yet, people commonly speak of endurable suffering. Indeed, one of the most important ethical issues regarding suffering is how long an animal may be forced to tolerate it. Moreover, as we ordinarily speak of it, "suffering" does not require observable physiological distress. The proposed definition also ignores the fact that we do not always distinguish two mental states, pain and suffering, and say that the former *causes* the latter. Commonly, we regard an experience of pain as *itself* being sufficiently intense, lengthy, or bothersome to become an instance of suffering. This linguistic fact has great moral significance. As we use the term, "suffering" does seem to denote a mental state more intense and therefore worse to the individual than pain. Therefore, in general, the imposition of suffering upon an animal would appear to require greater justification than the imposition of pain alone. The fact that pain can itself *become* suffering means that sometimes nothing extra need be done to animals in addition to causing them pain in order to bring into play the stronger ethical requirements required for justification of suffering.

EMPIRICAL ISSUES

There are many unresolved factual issues relating to pain and other negative mental states experienced by research animals. Among these questions and challenges are the following:

• Learning more about the extent to which the degree of pain perception varies among species and individuals of the same species (24). Research already indicates that procedures that cause little or no pain in humans may cause significant pain in animals, and vice versa (25);
• Obtaining greater knowledge and appreciation of the effects of previous experiences of research animals upon their perception of pain and other negative states (26);
• Finding anesthetics, analgesics, and tranquilizers and methods of administration of these substances that will lessen pain, discomfort, or distress in research animals without interfering with experimental protocols or producing undesirable side-effects. It is already known that effectiveness and side-effects of anesthetics and analgesics can vary widely among different species (27);
• Developing new techniques to monitor pain and pain control in animals subjected to surgical and other procedures (28);

- Developing nondrug approaches (e.g., exercise, socialization, contact with human handlers) to the control of stress and other negative mental states (29);
- Learning more about behavioral indicia of pain and other negative mental states;
- Increasing our sophistication in distinguishing pain from other negative states. This is important, in part, because sedatives and tranquilizers, which lessen distress, might either have no effect on pain or might increase pain perception (25);
- Exploring environmental and behavioral measures (such as return to a familiar environment, and control of unpleasant visual, auditory, olfactory, and tactile stimuli) to minimize pain associated with surgical or other procedures (30);
- Developing restraint systems in primates and other animals that minimize pain, distress, or discomfort and maximize comfort while being consistent with important experimental aims (31);
- Minimizing pain and distress associated with the enhancement of antibody production through the use of adjuvants (32).

PRACTICAL ISSUES

Researchers, veterinarians, and animal care committees must be able to apply knowledge regarding animal pain and other negative mental states in the laboratory setting. To facilitate practical application of such knowledge, several pain categorization schemes have been proposed. These systems attempt to set forth the degree or severity of pain associated with experiments and procedures commonly utilized in animal research. The best known system has been adopted in Sweden. It divides research techniques into six categories: 1) those causing no pain or negligible pain (e.g., injections, blood sampling, some dietary experiments); 2) those involving anesthetized animals that are not permitted to revive or are killed painlessly; 3) those involving surgery under anesthesia from which the animal recovers and where the surgery or procedure causes minimal postoperative pain; 4) those involving surgery under anesthesia from which the animal recovers and where the surgery or procedure causes considerable postoperative pain (e.g., major surgeries, certain skin grafts); 5) experiments on conscious animals involving pain, or in which the animals are expected to become seriously ill or suffer pain (e.g., toxicity studies, tumor transplants); and 6) experiments on unanesthetized animals paralyzed by curariform agents (33). Another system, mandated by law in the United Kingdom, calls for "severity banding" of various procedures, with the aim of comparing their "cost" against their "benefits." "Severity is seen as a spectrum of adverse effects, but being broadly divisible into mild, moderate, substantial, and severe bands. If an animal is considered in the fourth category ... steps will have to be taken to alleviate the pain or distress or the animal will have to be euthanatized even though the experiment has not been completed" (34).

Such ways of categorizing procedures can stimulate researchers, veterinarians, and committee members to ask about what a given procedure is likely to do to the animals. But classifications are only as good as the factual evidence supporting them. Premature "scoring" can discourage further scientific research and can result in sloppy thinking regarding the degree of pain associated with already-categorized procedures. Categories can also be used as rationalizations for avoiding serious thought about particular cases. A researcher who is not inclined to worry about the welfare aspects of his work may find it convenient, and legally sufficient, to point to a category rather than ask about what he is doing to the animals. Finally, pain classification schemes must not lead to a simplistic, utilitarian approach that fails to consider *all* the ethical "costs" of a research project, including its effects upon the animals' interests or moral rights.

PAIN RESEARCH

Pain that is an unfortunate and necessary consequence of an experimental procedure is bad enough. Some animal research involves the intentional infliction of pain. This typically occurs when the object of research is to understand and facilitate the prevention of pain itself.

From the point of view of an animal, it cannot matter whether pain is an unfortunate by-product or is induced deliberately. But an investigator who intentionally inflicts pain knows that this is what he is doing. Therefore, he has a clear obligation to pay unswerving attention to signs of pain or distress and to try to assure that no more is being induced than is absolutely required for the conduct of a clearly justifiable research protocol. Dresser (35) suggests two general guidelines: 1) any painful stimulus should be kept well below the animals' pain tolerance threshold, and 2) animals should be given control over stimulus intensity and duration by enabling them to terminate or escape it. The International Association for the study of pain recommends that, where possible, the investigator first try out on himself any painful stimulus to be given to an animal (36).

Pleasure and Other Positive Mental States

Very little work has been done to explore pleasure and other positive mental states in research animals and methods of promoting such states. The difficulties of verifying the presence of positive states should not be underestimated. Nevertheless, it seems clear that the major reason for the paucity of serious thought about promoting pleasure and other positive mental states in research and other animals is the prevalence of the anticruelty position (see Chapter 11). As long as animal "well-being" is identified with the absence of unnecessary pain, suffering, or distress, animal welfare science will not find it relevant to investigate animal pleasure or happiness. Investigators will also continue to view such things as weight maintenance, reproductive success, freedom from disease, and normal behavior not as signs of the presence of something good, but of the absence of something bad.

Cancer and Immunology Studies

Research aimed at the prevention and cure of cancer and immunological disorders is of great importance and may therefore justify treatment of animals that would not be appropriate in other kinds of research. Nevertheless, researchers are obligated to reduce, as much as possible, pain or suffering that can be associated with cancer and immunological research (37). Tumors implanted in animals must be monitored carefully so as not to grow beyond a size that is required for the study. It is also important that such tumors be placed in areas where they are least likely to cause debilitation or discomfort, and that they not be permitted to grow too large. The use of adjuvants to stimulate antibody production also raises serious issues. Injection of Complete Freund's Adjuvant in the footpads of mice and small rodents and the feet of rabbits has been found to be distressing, and single rather than multiple injection techniques may also prove adequate and less problematic for the animals (32). Great care must also be taken in monitoring animals used in hybridoma antibody production (38).

Behavior and Psychology Research

Few areas of animal research have aroused more criticism than behavioral and psychological experiments. Part of this opposition stems from the fact that such work often employs stimuli that are painful or distressing, such as electric shock or deprivation of food or water. But some critics find the use of these techniques especially disturbing because they doubt the value of the research itself. Rollin, for example, states that

> it is difficult to defend such research on the grounds that it will help people or even help to understand such people. Few people would give much credence, for example, to the claim that blinding hamsters to see if it will increase their territorial aggression has positive implications for human welfare (39).

In fact, as Rowan notes, great benefits have come from behavioral experimentation on animals, including "major advances in the understanding and treatment of epilepsy, stroke, language disorders, and brain damage" (40). However, there has been behavioral research that does seem aimed at discovering what will happen if terrible things are done to animals (41). It is dangerous to jump from superficial descriptions of behavioral experiments without an appreciation of their underlying aims or justifications to condemnation of these projects, or of behavioral research in general. However, I submit that it is impossible for even a sympathetic supporter of animal research not to be deeply distressed by some of the things that are done to animals in the name of behavioral science. Theoretical foolishness and inattentiveness to animal interests in any area of animal research strengthens the hand of research abolitionists. For it helps them to argue that all animal experimentation is pointless and immoral.

As is generally the case, the articulation of appropriate standards for the use of animals in behavioral and psychological research will reflect a balancing of the potential results of research against the effects on the animals. Part of this task will be to consider how to apply the minimum amount of aversive or painful stimulation (including deprivation of food or water) and to substitute positive reinforcement or nonexperimental observation wherever possible (42). A strong argument can also be made that the most effective way of assuring morally appropriate animal research in the behavioral area will be to differentiate good from bad science (43).

Euthanasia

One of the most important ethical decisions researchers face concerns the appropriate time for euthanasia. Making morally correct decisions requires knowledge not just of what the animals may be experiencing, but also of when keeping them alive is no longer required by an experiment. An animal's interests may require euthanasia even if it would cause the researcher additional expense, inconvenience, or difficulty using other animals to achieve desired results.

The choice of a method of euthanasia often has ethical implications. Public Health Service policy (44) requires adherence to the AVMA Guidelines on Euthanasia (45), unless the institutional animal care and use committee is satisfied that departure from the guidelines is justifiable. As I discussed in Chapter 20, one issue arising from these guidelines concerns their approval of the use of T-61®. But the most heated controversy has arisen over the AVMA Panel's decision that decapitation should not be used unless animals are first sedated or lightly anesthetized or their heads are dropped immediately into liquid nitrogen (46). A number of scientists have disputed the studies cited in support of the contention that such methods are necessary to assure the cessation of pain perception in decapitated animals (47).

An important concern for researchers is the proper training and supervision of personnel who perform euthanasia. These people typically are not veterinarians. As the AVMA Panel Report on euthanasia emphasizes, a method of euthanasia that is ordinarily appropriate can cause pain if it is not performed properly.

One issue that seems to be considered rarely by researchers is whether animals whose usefulness has ended but are not terminally ill or diseased should be killed at all. Lack of further usefulness is typically viewed as sufficient justification for euthanasia. However, some animals used in research are capable of being rehabilitated and placed privately or in settings (such as zoos, science museums, schools, and nursing homes) in which they can lead relatively happy lives. The argument for at least *trying*, within reasonable economic limits, goes beyond the wastefulness of ending animal life with little attendant human benefit. An animal that has been used in a research project has (ideally) given something to the researcher. It is not too much, I submit, for the research community to think more creatively about how something might be given back, even if only a small proportion of research animals can be saved.

THE CONCEPT OF "ALTERNATIVES"

In recent years, much attention has been given to so-called "alternatives" to the use of animals in research and testing. As explained by Andrew Rowan, the concept refers to the "three Rs,"

> those techniques or methods that: *replace* the use of laboratory animals altogether, *reduce* the number of animals required, or *refine* an existing procedure or technique so as to minimize the level of stress endured by the animal. These three Rs provide a broad-based approach to reducing both laboratory animal numbers and laboratory animal suffering (48).

Among the alternatives that are often touted as replacements, reductions, or refinements are physiochemical testing techniques (e.g., gas-liquid chromatography and mass spectroscopy rather than animals for assay of substances), computer and mathematical models of biological organs or systems, use of microbiological systems (e.g., tests for detecting mutagens that utilize bacteria rather than animals), and tissue culture (49).

The concept of "alternatives" as defined above has some severe limitations.

First, the concept cannot be applied unless there are at least two options (one a so-called "alternative") that can be predicted to have identical or sufficiently similar theoretical results or practical benefits. This can be a major difficulty. The results of scientific research – whether or not animals are employed – are often unpredictable. An item of knowledge or a technique may find its way into unexpected areas of inquiry and application. Thus, it often is impossible to assert at a given time that an approach which does not use animals (or uses fewer animals or subjects those used to less distress than another) really will in the long run prove to be an "alternative." This is not to say that "alternatives" in Rowan's sense are never available. But they are likely to be available when 1) the researcher knows precisely what he wants or will obtain, or 2) he is close to an endpoint in some stage of a research project and can be sure that a nonanimal or reduced-animal approach would also be sufficient. For example, genetic engineering or tissue culture may sometimes provide a cost-effective non-animal "alternative" for the production of a specified substance. However, many research projects or general areas of inquiry in biomedical research are in their beginning stages. Precisely what will happen, and what questions will have to be asked down the line, are not yet known.

Second, because so much is yet to be done in biomedical research, it is scientifically and practically dangerous to now call for a drastic reduction in animal research. As Carl Cohen observes, biomedical research is constantly searching for better approaches to dreaded diseases. These approaches often must be tested before they can be utilized generally. But because it can be the case that "initial trials entail great risks, there may be no forward movement whatever without the use of live animal subjects" (50). It often would be immoral to attempt a trial, experiment, or technique on humans before doing it on animals.

Third, there are other ethical limitations on the use of reduced-animal alternatives, even when identical or sufficiently similar results can be expected. As we saw, it may sometimes be morally obligatory to use more animals in order to spare fewer individual animals a higher degree of stress or deprivation. Additionally, the expense of an alternative is a legitimate consideration in determining its advisability. Techniques that use fewer animals are often less costly than those using more, but this is not always the case.

Fourth, paradoxically, the vigorous search for "alternatives" might increase the number of animals used in research. It will sometimes be impossible, without using animals, to verify whether a nonanimal or reduced-animal approach is as good as some animal technique. For example, it might be impossible to determine whether computer modelling of an animal system can generate the same kinds of results as investigation of living systems without comparing the computer data against a large amount of animal-based data.

Finally, the concept of alternatives as it is explained by Rowan is typically employed in ways that do not square with other widely held attitudes regarding animals. The ultimate aim expressed by this concept is the replacement of animals, i.e., eventual cessation of their use in research. Rowan asserts that researchers

> readily admit that they would prefer not to use animals if it were not necessary. In other words, they would, in a perfect world, like to see the elimination of animal research. Therefore, their ultimate goal is the same as that of the most ardent [research animal use] abolitionist (51).

The eventual cessation of animal research – *all* animal research, of whatever kind – is stated as an intrinsically desirable goal, one that does not require any further justification. But why should cessation of the use animals in research be such a goal? Most of us do not regard termination of the use of animals for food, fiber, or entertainment as a fundamental, intrinsically desirable component of a perfect world. Why then should we regard cessation of the use of animals in all research a necessary component of such a world?

A proponent of this concept of "alternatives" appears to have two options. He can view his aversion to the use of animals in research as part of a general dissatisfaction with the use of animals for human purposes. Or, he can approve of at least some traditionally-accepted uses of animals but call for the eventual elimination of the use of animals in research. If he chooses the former option, he favors animal use abolitionism at least as an ideal and must be prepared to defend that position. If he chooses the latter option, he is being unreasonable. For it surely is unreasonable to consider the use of animals in the prevention and alleviation of disease less important than their use for such things as food, fiber, or entertainment.

The notion of "alternatives" does have intuitive appeal. The term can be used to express the following eminently reasonable principle: *If there is more than one way of using animals to attain a given legitimate goal, and one of these ways will achieve the very same goal while treating the animals better than would the other ways, we ought to choose the way that treats them better.* We can call this better way an "alternative." However, saying that we may sometimes be able to treat research animals better by not using them or using fewer of them or causing those we use less pain or distress is *not* the same thing as saying that we have a fundamental, independent obligation to try to eliminate or reduce their use in research. There are *reasons* researchers should *sometimes* seek replacement of animals, reduction in their numbers, or refinement in techniques so as to cause less distress. These reasons include the fact that some (but by no means all) research projects cause animals pain, suffering, distress, or discomfort. These reasons can also include (where appropriate) the cost-effectiveness or scientific advantages of not using animals or of using fewer animals.

The articulation and defense of good reasons for replacement, reduction, or refinement will be part of the general endeavor of exploring the ethics of the use of animals in research. This is an enterprise that must consider a wide range of interests and morally relevant considerations. It is an endeavor that at some points can be expected to conclude that some uses of animals in research simply are not objectionable, and that other uses with negative impact on the animals must be continued because of their potential benefits. Talking about "alternatives" can play a role in stimulating such ethical and scientific investigations – but only if the concept is purged of the implication that the use of animals in research is intrinsically evil and something to be tolerated only if absolutely "necessary."

WEIGHING THE POTENTIAL RESULTS OF RESEARCH AGAINST EFFECTS ON ANIMAL INTERESTS

The major ethical question that must be faced in the evaluation of animal research is whether the potential results of a given project justify its likely effects on the animals. As we saw in Chapter 21, animal welfare science and ethics have a long way to go in understanding how animals are affected in ways that are relevant to their welfare and interests. Neither should one underestimate the many difficult issues involved in assessing the likely value or importance of animal research projects.

For example, at first glance, it might seem plausible to think that an experiment that would benefit many people would have greater value than one that would benefit just a handful, and might therefore justify a greater amount of animal distress. But it is not always so simple. If these handful are suffering greatly, if there is no effective treatment for their condition, and if there are already ways of helping the many people who are suffering from another condition, a strong case can be made for concluding that animal research on the rarer condition has greater value and urgency than work on the more common one. However, this, too, may not be the end of the matter. If a proposed project on the illness suffered by the many might illuminate and eventually lead to the treatment of other conditions, that may provide stronger justification for it. And there are still other factors that might be relevant in determining the value of these proposals, including their expense, whether they promise a significant improvement of the lives of sufferers, and the likely ability of the researchers proposing the projects to achieve something of value.

Table 23.1 sets forth some of the factors that are relevant in assessing the value of an animal experiment for the purposes of determining whether that experiment justifies its likely effect on the animals. The table divides issues into questions relating to aims of research and the likelihood of success. Both kinds of considerations must be addressed in evaluating the relative weight or value of a research project. One must concede that the unpredictability of the results of scientific experiments is an important issue that raises problems in assessing the value of proposed animal research projects. Nevertheless, overblown exaggerations (52) about unexpected results of scientific investigation will not do. There are, as the table suggests, *clearly* some relevant questions that can be raised regarding the likelihood of potential theoretical or practical results. Because animal interests are often compromised in animal research, we need to try to think more critically about predictability of the results of various kinds of such research.

The table does not indicate who might bear the burden of proof regarding whether a proposal is morally justified, e.g., whether it is the task of a researcher to show that his use of animals is justified or that of someone with doubts (an animal care committee or granting agency, for example) to prove that it is not. Nor am I suggesting here who should make such determinations and by what procedures, or what general principles should be employed in making them.

I am not addressing these issues here because I do not think animal welfare science and ethics are yet capable of tackling them systematically. We need more conceptual and factual analysis of what promotes and hinders research animal welfare. We need more sustained ethical analysis of considerations such as those listed in the table. We will also need time to see how effectively institutional committees and facility veterinarians can monitor and assure animal welfare. The committees have been functioning under the present federal regulatory scheme only since 1986. We may not know for some time what kind of job they are doing. It will also take time for the committees to share with each other and government regulators different approaches they may be taking to various kinds of issues. Nor do we yet know whether greater involvement of regulators or others (such as more centralized study groups on animal welfare or present merit review committees) will prove advisable.

We are now just beginning to scratch the surface of theory and practice in the promotion of research animal welfare.

Table 23.1

Some Issues Relevant to Assessing the Value of a Proposed Animal Research Project

---

Aims of the Research

How many people or animals does the project aim to benefit?
How serious is the problem that is experienced by potential beneficiaries of the research?
To what extent is their problem presently treatable?
To what extent is their problem transmissible to other persons or animals?
What are the side-effects and dangers of present treatments?
What are the present or projected costs and burdens of the condition upon the economy or the health care system?
To what extent might a nonmedical or nonsurgical (e.g, an environmental, preventative, or public health) approach be a more effective or efficient way of dealing with the problem?
To what extent is the project aimed at understanding or treating several diseases or conditions?
To what extent is the project aimed at understanding a problem, condition, or area about which there is little good or useful knowledge?
To what extent is the research aimed at providing knowledge that could be relevant to several areas or fields of theoretical or practical importance?

Table 23.1 – *continued*

Is the research proposed as part of, or is it aimed at enabling, a progression toward experimentation, testing, or use upon the ultimate intended beneficiaries of a proposed treatment or technique?

Does the proposed project seem sound from a scientific point of view, or does it rest on questionable premises or assumptions? (For example, does it propose the use of too many or too few animals to achieve meaningful results? Is a proposed animal model scientifically sound?)

Is the proposed project aimed at confirming an important research result or resolving inconsistent or disputed results or conclusions of important experiments?

To what extent does the project have a clearly defined purpose and rationale, as distinguished from being a scattershot attempt to see "what will happen if" certain things are done to animals?

To what extent is the project aimed at providing a required educational exercise or funding for the person conducting the work?

Has the question posed by the researcher already been sufficiently settled or researched so that there may be insufficient scientific justification for the project, much less for its potential effect on the animals?

The Likelihood of Achieving Stated Aims

What are the general educational qualifications of the researcher proposing the project?

How knowledgeable in this area is the researcher?

Does he or his laboratory have a record of success or fruitful results?

To what extent does the researcher possess equipment and support personnel adequate for pursuing his stated aims?

Is funding likely to be sufficient to continue to support the work, so that animal use will be given a chance to achieve the desired aim or results?

To what extent have projects such as the one proposed provided good knowledge or useful techniques?

SOME CURRENT CONTROVERSIES

The "Pound Seizure" Debate

There are many controversies relating to animal research about which veterinarians should be aware. One of the most heated concerns so-called "pound seizure," the practice of allowing or requiring pounds and animal shelters to give or sell unadoptable animals to research facilities. (The general acceptance of the term "seizure" reflects the extent to which opponents of pound release have succeeded in framing the terms of the debate. "Seizure" conveys the false impression that all states in which pound animals can be released compel pounds to do so, and that all pounds would prefer not to release them.) Opponents of pound "seizure" have had some success in convincing state and local legislatures to prohibit the release of pound animals to researchers. As of this writing, 12 states and a number of counties and localities have prohibited pound release (53). The proponents of such laws often call them "pet protection" measures.

By all accounts, the use of pound animals in research (mostly dogs) always has accounted for a small fraction of the number euthanized. In 1974, before the advent of legislation prohibiting pound release, the Humane Society of the United States estimated that between 13 and 14 million dogs and cats were euthanized in pounds and shelters annually. About 6.5 million of these were dogs. Available figures indicate that in the late 1960s, approximately 105,000 dogs used in research came from pounds (54). Purpose-bred dogs are many times more expensive for research facilities to purchase than pound animals. In 1984, Rowan estimated that when institutions buy from pounds or shelters, the price ranges from $5 to $15, and that dealers sell conditioned dogs for $120 to $140, with 6-month-old beagles costing about $275 (55). In 1987, a cost of over $400 for a conditioned research dog would not have been unusual.

Opponents of pound release offer the following arguments:

1. *"Pound animals are inferior to purpose-bred animals for research purposes because they are genetically more variable and tend to have diseases and infirmities that compromise their usefulness."* This claim simply cannot be made about all pound animals used in research, especially those used in certain investigations of surgical techniques and cardiovascular disease. There may well be some use of pound animals that is scientifically questionable (55). But the most direct (and scientifically sound) way of preventing such situations would be for investigators not to use pound animals when such use is scientifically questionable – not an absolute ban on all use of pound animals.

2. *"Pound release discourages people from turning in strays they find."* As Rowan observes (56), there is little evidence supporting this claim.

3. *"Pound release subjects animals to torture and abuse."* This assertion is, first of all, false as a general characterization. Second, if a researcher does abuse or perform unjustified experiments on animals, the fact that they might come from a pound would appear to be irrelevant. Abuse of research animals is wrong because it is wrong, not because some animals that might be abused come from pounds. The most direct way of preventing such abuse would be to prevent it, not to cut off the supply of pound animals.

4. *"Pound release is inconsistent with the primary task of humane societies as 'effective promoters of animal welfare'"* (56). It is difficult to understand how the killing of millions of unwanted animals each year (and the vast majority of pound animals are unwanted) constitutes an effective way of promoting animal welfare. It might prevent some unnecessary suffering, but so might using abandoned animals to benefit people and other animals.

In my view, the strongest argument against pound release is that it may well be unfair to subject animals that have been part of a human-animal bond to the kinds of treatment research animals receive. Such treatment sometimes involves distress and almost always greater confinement and a less pleasurable life than that to which a valued pet has been accustomed. This argument can be made with or without the premise that a former beloved pet appreciates the change in its condition; if true, the latter premise would add to the forcefulness of the argument. One problem with this argument is that many, perhaps most, pound animals did not "enjoy" a rich human-animal bond; many are strays or were abused, neglected, or abandoned by their owners. Nevertheless, I think there is some plausibility to the desire to protect animals that have participated in a meaningful human-animal bond or that did lead a relatively pleasant life from conditions that are likely to be far less enjoyable.

However, what follows from this argument is that every reasonable attempt ought to be made to enable owners to locate lost animals, or to place them with other owners. In contrast, total prohibition of pound release is illogical and wrong.

First, many of the animals that would be released by pounds are not significantly different from purpose-bred animals. Many have led no better a life prior to use in research, and they are just as capable of feeling pain or distress and of enjoying human companionship. It simply makes no sense to "protect" such animals by killing them and replacing them with other animals that will be used exactly as the "protected" (dead) animals would have been.

Second, although permitting some pound release is bound to result in the release of some members of human-animal bonds,[c] and this is unfortunate, absolutely precluding such situations through total prohibition of pound release is not preferable to the wastefulness of total prohibition. It is costly to euthanize and dispose of pound animals, which are of use to no one as a result of the process. The effect of a total prohibition of pound release would be to make much animal research more expensive than it need be. Even though total abolition of pound release might benefit some former beloved pets, this benefit would not be so important as to outweigh the horrendous waste of total prohibition. For purpose-bred animals are not drastically different from even the most beloved of pets. There does not seem to be such a chasm of difference between these two kinds of animals to justify concluding that it is right to use one but not the other, if the consequence of this is that one group of animals will be substituted (at great cost) for another.

Third, protection of beloved pets is not the aim of many who oppose pound release. Many of these people hope that the increased cost associated with purpose breeding will reduce the number of animals used in research. Indeed, for many activists, "pet protection" laws are just the first step toward ending *all* animal research. As one animal rights organization has declared (57), "when the supply of dogs and cats from pounds and dealers is finally cut off, the animal rights field will then be able to address cutting off the supply of all purpose-bred species of animals for scientific purposes."

The only straightforward and effective way to address abuses in animal research is to openly identify and prevent them. It is folly to suppose that increasing the cost will stop research that uses dogs or cats. A few relatively poor institutions may be forced to reduce their use of such animals; but even so, there is no assurance that the least valuable or most distressful experiments will be the ones sacrificed. In the most prestigious and best-endowed institutions, general animal research will continue – as it should. Increased expenses will be borne by taxpayers or others who ultimately pay for the costs of research (such as health insurance companies, medical patients, and veterinary clients). Imposing additional costs on biomedical research by forcing all unadoptable animals to be killed will not give pet owners sufficient time or means to locate their animals from shelters. It will not reduce society's enormous burden of dealing with our millions of unwanted animals. It will not eliminate unjustifiable animal research, or protect research animals from neglect or abuse. These worthy goals can be promoted only if they are addressed directly.

Toxicity Testing

An issue that has connections with research and that has aroused significant controversy concerns the use of live animals in toxicity testing of drugs, pesticides, chemicals, and various consumer products (58). The two main targets of criticism have been the LD50 test, which determines the dose of a substance that will kill 50% of test organisms, and the Draize test, in which a substance is placed in one eye of

---

[c]But more creative thought should also be given to lessening the possibility of this happening. Because it would be worse to release a pet accustomed to a human-animal bond than one not so accustomed, rules might be considered to prohibit, e.g., the release of older dogs and cats.

several rabbits (the other eye serving as an untreated control) to determine its irritating effects. These tests can cause substantial pain and distress.

An important ethical question that must be asked about any test that can cause distress is whether, even if the test provides satisfactory evidence regarding the safety of a substance, the distress of the animals is justified by the importance of the substance being tested. This question is especially significant with regard to nonmedical household or personal items. The marketing of a new consumer product may be important to those who might profit from it. However, it is extremely difficult to maintain that yet another shade of makeup or a new toilet bowl cleaner is of sufficient general importance to require any significant amount of animal suffering or distress.

It seems clear, however, that compelling objections to the LD50 and Draize tests can sometimes be made without judging the worth of a particular substance or product to be tested. There is substantial scientific evidence that these tests do not establish the safety of certain substances, or make determinations with a degree of precision that is unnecessary for an assurance of safety. Rowan has estimated that if regulatory bodies required the submission of LD50 figures only when there is scientific justification for the test, the number of animals used in determining lethal doses would be reduced by between 80 and 90% worldwide. This would represent an annual saving of between 2 and 4 million animals (59).

Because toxicity testing can involve distress, and because consumers have a legitimate interest in safe products even when such products are not essential for life or happiness, the search for nonanimal alternatives seems especially important in this area. Such work is proceeding. Largely as the result of a campaign against the Draize test led by animal activist Henry Spira, the Revlon Corporation donated $750,000 for research into alternatives to the Rockefeller University. Additional industry support for alternative ways of testing cosmetics and consumer products has followed, but much more, clearly, needs to be done.

The Use of Animals in Education

One research-related issue that has received some attention in veterinary publications concerns the appropriateness of the use of live animals in education. Among the targets of critics have been the use of animals in elementary and high school courses, science fairs and competitions; college biology courses; the training of graduate biology and psychology students; medical school courses; and continuing education courses for physicians. There is also controversy about the use and euthanasia of healthy animals in veterinary school student surgery exercises. Some argue that this practice is inconsistent with the veterinarian's commitment to alleviate animal pain and suffering (60).

At least two very different questions can be raised about a given educational animal use: 1) whether it is permissible at all, and 2) whether a student in a given educational setting may be compelled to participate in the animal exercise on pain of a reduced or failing grade. Addressing each of these issues requires consideration of the educational importance of a given animal experience. Nevertheless, the two issues should not be confused. There may well be certain educational uses of animals that are not sufficiently objectionable to render them impermissible, but are at the same time not sufficiently important to justify compulsory student participation.

Disputes about the educational necessity or value of various animal educational experiences are long-standing (61) and cannot be resolved here. However, it is worth pointing out that progress sometimes appears to be hindered by a highly charged atmosphere in which opposing parties approach the situation with an uncompromising general attitude that leaves no room for examination of relevant *facts*. This sometimes seems to be the case when veterinary educators and students argue about required third-year surgery exercises on live animals. Some educators refuse to entertain any suggestions regarding different ways of doing things on the grounds that they are the teachers and therefore know what is best. On the other hand, some veterinary students base their opposition to surgery laboratory on the principle that it is always morally wrong for a veterinarian to kill or perform procedures upon healthy animals. Neither of these uncompromising positions permits careful examination of the factual issues regarding the usefulness of educational exercises for the variety of students a veterinary school must train.

Issues Regarding Laws Affecting Animal Research

STATE AND LOCAL LAWS

Anticruelty statutes. At the state level, an interesting current controversy concerns whether anticruelty statutes should be capable of being applied to animal research. Such application would permit criminal prosecution of researchers who neglect or abuse their animals, or whose experiments cause unjustifiable pain or suffering. As of this writing, 22 states and the District of Columbia specifically exempt activities by researchers from the application of their anticruelty laws. In most other states, neglect, abuse, or unjustified distress caused by a researcher is a prosecutable criminal offense.

Realistically, inclusion of animal research within the purview of a state's anticruelty statute is unlikely to have much general effect on the conduct of research. Even in states without research exemptions, prosecutions of researchers are rare. This is so not only because most prosecutors' offices do not attach a high priority to animal cases, but also because it usually is extremely difficult to convict a researcher of cruelty. Although most states do not require willful animal abuse for a conviction of cruelty, the government must still prove, beyond a reasonable doubt, that the manner in which a researcher treated an animal was unjustified. In many cases, investigators will be able to be sufficiently persuasive about justification to cast some doubt in the minds of a jury or appellate court. Cruelty convictions of researchers are likely only in cases of extreme neglect or malicious abuse.

An argument can, nevertheless, be made for including animal research within the potential application of cruelty statutes. This would permit criminal prosecutions when appropriate and feasible. Including research within the scope of a state cruelty statute also makes a symbolic statement that it is part of the official public policy of the state that researchers, like other people, must not subject animals to unjustified pain, distress, abuse, or neglect.

State and local licensing and regulation programs. As of this writing, 21 states and the District of Columbia had laws imposing some kind of licensing or regulation upon animal research facilities. These laws, and the extent to which they are enforced, vary. (For example, two jurisdictions require licenses for the use of dogs or cats, and eight others require licenses only for facilities receiving impounded animals.) Several localities have also debated instituting regulation schemes for licensing and inspecting research facilities.

State regulation of animal research might supplement the federal program, which many supporters of animal research concede has been underfunded (62). Time will tell whether states can implement programs that promote animal welfare without infringing unduly upon research. It also remains to be seen whether the courts will invalidate state or local regulation schemes that might attempt to restrict certain kinds of animal research permitted under federal law, on the grounds that these schemes are pre-empted by federal law.

FEDERAL LAW

Robust debate is likely to continue for some time regarding the proper extent of federal regulation of animal research. The federal Animal Welfare Act applies to all research facilities using laboratory animals in basic or biomedical research, education, and product safety testing. In 1985, the following important amendments were added to the Act (63). Researchers must consult with a veterinarian to assure that pain and distress will be minimized. Tranquilizers, anesthesia, analgesia, or euthanasia of animals in pain or distress may be withheld only when "scientifically necessary," and any unavoidable pain or distress may be permitted to continue "only for the necessary period of time." Multiple surgeries on animals are to be done only when "scientifically necessary." The "psychological well-being" of primates and appropriate exercise for dogs is to be assured. Each facility governed by the Act must have an institutional animal care and use committee. At least one member of the committee must be a doctor of veterinary medicine. At least one member must not be affiliated with the institution and must represent "general community interests" in the proper care and treatment of animals. It is the responsibility of this committee to assure compliance with the provisions of the Act, to "minimize pain and distress to animals," and to "represent society's concerns regarding the welfare of animal subjects used" at the facility. Facilities must train researchers and support personnel in "the humane practice of animal maintenance and experimentation" as well as in "research or testing methods that minimize or eliminate the use of animals or limit animal pain or distress."[d]

In early 1987, the USDA published proposed new regulations to implement the amended Animal Welfare Act (64). These proposals elicited so much comment and criticism that they were withheld by the Department for further consideration. (As of this writing, some 18 months after the initial proposals were first published and 3 years after enactment of the amendments to the Animal Welfare Act requiring new regulations, the regulations still had not been adopted.) The following are among the questions raised generally by the Animal Welfare Act as well as by the 1987 proposed regulations. These questions are likely to remain controversial whatever the precise content of future regulations.

1. *Should mice and rats be included within the scope of the Animal Welfare Act?* Although these species constitute at least 80% of all animals used in research, the statute permits the USDA to determine whether they should be brought within the

---

[d]Among other federal statutes and regulations relating to animal research (65) are the following: The Health Research Extension Act of 1985 (66), which requires a committee system similar to that imposed by the Animal Welfare Act and mandates use of the Public Health Service Policy on the Humane Care and Use of Laboratory Animals for facilities doing research funded by the PHS; the Good Laboratory Practice Standards (GLPs) promulgated by the Environmental Protection Agency pursuant to the Toxic Substances Control Act (67); GLPs of the EPA pursuant to the Federal Insecticide, Fungicide, and Rodenticide Act for conducting studies to support application for research or marketing permits (68); and GLPs of the Food and Drug Administration for conducting studies pursuant to the Federal Food, Drug, and Cosmetic Act (69).

scope of the Act and its regulations. The Department has thus far decided not to include them on the grounds that it would be impossible for it to enforce compliance with rules extending to so many animals.

2. *How should institutions decide who should serve as a representative of "community interests?"* Should these persons have some background in research animal welfare? Should they be "advocates" for the animals? Can institutions be trusted to appoint appropriate persons, without some government oversight of their choices?

3. *To what extent should nonaffiliated persons be full, coequal members of animal care committees?* In general, how should nonaffiliated members function in their assessment of research proposals? How much weight should their comments and concerns be given by institutional members?

4. *Should the facility veterinarian or animal care committee report directly to the USDA, or should reporting be by the institution, which would bear full responsibility for compliance?* The AVMA argued that the 1987 proposed regulations improperly shifted the burden of reporting and compliance to veterinarians and committee members (70).

5. *What qualifications should be required of veterinarians who serve in research facilities governed by the Act?* Is licensure to practice veterinary medicine in any state sufficient, or must the veterinarian be licensed in the state in which he functions? Should he be required to demonstrate competence in the area of laboratory animal medicine, and if so, how might this be done? The AVMA has opposed accreditation of facility veterinarians by the USDA (71).

6. *To what extent should animal care committees, research proposals, and decisions by committees be open to observation or discovery by members of the public?* Several states require that animal care committee meetings at state-owned research institutions (such as state universities and medical schools) be open to the public. Many researchers believe that permitting public attendance of committee meetings or access to research protocols would stifle committee debate and discussion.

7. *Should members of the public have legal standing to sue institutions for alleged violations of the Animal Welfare Act, or should legal action be restricted, as it is presently, to the USDA?* Many researchers believe that standing for private citizens will result in harassment of institutions, committees, and researchers by animal activists.

8. *To what extent should animal care committees review the scientific merit of research proposals?* Some contend that merit review is improper, on the grounds that the task of the committee is only to assure adequate animal welfare. But this position seems untenable. The committees must sometimes ask whether animals are being subjected to *justifiable* pain or distress. It sometimes is impossible to make such a determination without considering whether proposals are sufficiently strong scientifically to provide such justification. It is not altogether clear, however, what kinds of merit review would be appropriate by animal care committees. For these committees are not intended, and are typically not qualified, to provide another forum for full merit review.

9. *To what extent may government regulation be permitted to increase the costs of running a research facility?* Where, if at all, should compromises be made in regulation or assurance of animal welfare on the grounds of cost? How much paperwork may reasonably be imposed upon researchers and animal care committees? Should costs attributable to federally required animal welfare measures be paid by individual grant recipients, their academic departments, the institution, the animal care committee budget, granting agencies, or the federal government?

Illegal Activities

Any discussion of contemporary issues must mention the extent to which some animal activists have been engaging in unlawful behavior. In 1987, the NIH reported a total of 26 incidents in which animals had been stolen from research facilities (72). The following are but four recent examples of an apparent trend.

In 1984, members of the Animal Liberation Front broke into the Experimental Head Injury Laboratory at the University of Pennsylvania. They stole videotaped records of experiments showing the induction of head trauma upon restrained baboons. The Pennsylvania break-in eventually led to the suspension of NIH funding for the laboratory and a $4,000 fine by USDA for violations of the Animal Welfare Act (73).

In 1986, activists broke into a facility at the University of Oregon, stole over 150 animals, and caused more than $50,000 in property damage. Animal activist groups held a news conference at which they distributed several hundred photographs allegedly taken during the break-in. These photographs were in fact from another university and did not clearly show any abuses (74).

In 1987, an animal rights group calling itself the Band of Mercy stole 37 cats from the USDA Animal Parasitology Institute in Beltsville, Maryland. Eleven of the cats were infected with *Toxoplasma gondii*. The "liberators" of these highly infectious animals stated that their purpose was to obtain veterinary care for the cats and to place them in "caring, permanent homes." The theft caused the loss of 3 years of research on the transmissibility of toxoplasmosis after cessation of immunity (72).

In 1987, activists broke into and set on fire the veterinary diagnostic laboratory under construction at the University of California at Davis. The fire caused over $3.5 million in damage. The facility was to have been part of a reorganization of the California diagnostic laboratory system for the control of animal disease (75).

Although advocates of law-breaking and violence may prefer to cite their success at the University of Pennsylvania, the other incidents related above are more indicative of what happens when true believers consider themselves above the law. Innocent people and animals can be harmed. Property is mindlessly destroyed. What may have been motivated at first by high ideals begins to resemble common thuggery.

Not all members of the animal rights movement condone such behavior. But law-abiding activists will find it increasingly difficult to convince the public that theft and violence is not an integral part of the program of the animal rights movement (76). Eventually, some people may come to associate such tactics with the concept of animal rights itself. This could well be the most destructive and tragic legacy of the lawbreakers.

THE ROLE OF THE LABORATORY ANIMAL VETERINARIAN

Not all laboratory veterinarians have been successful in promoting animal welfare in their facilities. As the Animal and Plant Health Inspection Service has observed,

> Some facilities have not provided required veterinary care and others have switched veterinarians every few months causing confusing situations that are difficult to trace....
>
> Many other veterinarians ... indicated [to APHIS] that they felt their efforts were a waste of time as their recommendations concerning the health care of the animals were ignored, and they had no authority to see that such recommendations were carried out.

Veterinarians at many research facilities indicated that often they did not have the authority to enter the animal facilities of certain Departments or investigators and thus could not certify what conditions might be at those animal sites. Many of these veterinarians also indicated that due to various local political or managerial systems, their jobs would be in serious jeopardy if they tried to force adequate veterinary care in certain instances or if they refused to certify that all was in compliance at the facility when they, in fact, had no such knowledge (77).

My own conversations with laboratory animal veterinarians confirm the accuracy of these observations. I am told repeatedly that there are two main reasons why some laboratory animal veterinarians find it difficult to function effectively. First, some investigators do not want anyone to interfere with their work. Second, some investigators do not have great respect for veterinarians and use this attitude to ignore or belittle the laboratory animal doctor's efforts to improve the treatment of research animals.

The problems some laboratory animal veterinarians have in assuring adequate animal welfare will not disappear overnight. The veterinary profession can help by promoting the expertise of laboratory animal doctors. This must be done not only through public relations, but by encouraging the training of specialists in this area, and supporting laboratory animal welfare research that will enable veterinarians to play a pre-eminent role in the protection of research animal welfare. Yet, history already shows that laboratory animal veterinarians will not achieve the respect and influence they deserve, and that the animals require, without the vigorous assistance of government.

WHAT THE PROFESSION CAN DO

This is an exciting time in laboratory animal medicine. Many important scientific and practical breakthroughs are being made. Continuing progress will require the efforts of the entire profession, including veterinarians on the front line who utilize the products of research for the benefit of their patients.

First and foremost, the profession must encourage, promote, and fund first-class research in the area of laboratory animal welfare. The biomedical research community cannot be counted on to do this work by itself. Animal welfare studies conducted by or with the active participation of veterinarians will also enable the development of techniques that can be applied by laboratory animal doctors in the research setting.

Second, conceptual and ethical investigations must be made an important component of research into laboratory animal welfare conducted by veterinarians. These investigations must include participation by ethicists committed to the study of animal- and veterinarian-related moral issues.

Third, the veterinary schools must make it a major priority to encourage students to consider a career in laboratory animal medicine. Training in this area must include substantial exposure to animal welfare science and to animal and normative veterinary ethics.

Finally, veterinarians must be active in discussions regarding laboratory animal welfare. Front-line practitioners should be able to discuss with clients, community leaders, and politicians the benefits and justifications of animal research. Veterinarians with a special interest in research animal welfare can join or support organizations that represent their points of view in continuing discussions. Among such groups are the National Association for Biomedical Research of Washington, DC and the Scientists Center for Animal Welfare of Bethesda, Maryland. These (and other) groups may not share the same perspectives or conclusions. However, progress in complex moral issues is rarely benefited by unanimity of opinion.

REFERENCES

1. Loew FM: The challenge of balancing experimental variables: Pain, distress, analgesia, and anesthesia. *J Am Vet Med Assoc* 191:1193, 1987.
2. Rowan, A: *Of Mice, Models, and Men.* Albany: State University of New York Press, 1984, p 70.
3. Gay WI (ed): *Health Benefits of Animal Research.* Washington, DC: National Association for Biomedical Research, undated.
4. AVMA Council on Research: Contributions and Needs of Animal Health and Disease Research. *Am J Vet Res* 42:1093-1108, 1981.
5. E.g., Raub W: Foreword. In Gay WI (ed): *Health Benefits of Animal Research.* Washington, DC: National Association for Biomedical Research, undated, p i (stating that "(v)irtually *every* medical innovation of the last century – and especially of the last four decades – has been based to a significant extent upon the results of animal experimentation").
6. E.g., Kuker-Reines B: *Psychology Experiments on Animals.* Boston: New England Anti-Vivisection Society, 1982, p 67 (stating that "the animal modelling technique has proved virtually useless against the bona fide noninfectious diseases including cancer..."); Ryder R: Experiments on Animals. In Godlovitch S, Godlovitch R, and Harris J (eds): *Animals, Men, and Morals.* London: Victor Gollancz, 1971, p 78 ("The probability of unequivocal benefits arising out of any individual experiment is so small as to be negligible. ... We can far better benefit our species, as well as the others, by effectively disseminating the enormous technology and materials we already possess rather than by striving cruelly to extend our knowledge a little further.").
7. E.g., Hewitt HB: The Use of Animals in Experimental Cancer Research. In Sperlinger D (ed): *Animals in Research.* Chichester, England: John Wiley & Sons, 1981, p 170 ("The question the prospective animal experimenter has to ask himself is whether he considers that the painless taking of animal life is itself an immoral act. For me it is not...").
8. Cohen C: The case for the use of animals in biomedical research. *N Engl J Med* 315(14):869, 1986.
9. *Id.*, 865. For a similar analysis of the concept of rights see, McCloskey HJ: Moral Rights and Animals. *Inquiry* 22:23-54, 1978.
10. Cohen, *op. cit.*, p 866.
11. Compton C: Defending Animal Research. In: *The Biomedical Investigator's Handbook.* Washington, DC: Foundation for Biomedical Research, 1987, p 80.
12. Fox MW: What Future for Man and Earth? Toward a Biospiritual Ethic. In Morris RK and Fox MW (eds): *On the Fifth Day.* Washington, DC: Acropolis Books, 1978, p 226.
13. 7 U.S.C.A. § 2143(a)(2)(B).
14. For useful discussions and references regarding these and other welfare considerations see, *Guide to the Care and Use of Experimental Animals.* 2 vols. Ottawa: Canadian Council on Animal Care, 1984; *Syllabus of the Basic Principles of Laboratory Animal Science.* Ottawa: Canadian Council on Animal Care, 1985; *Guide for the Care and Use of Laboratory Animals.* Washington, DC: U.S. Government Printing Office, 1980.
15. See, *Comfortable Quarters for Laboratory Animals.* Washington, DC: Animal Welfare Institute, 1979.
16. E.g., Reinhardt V: Advantage of Housing Rhesus Monkeys in Compatible Pairs. *Scientists Center for Animal Welfare Newsletter* 9(3):3-6, 1987.

17. E.g., Wolfle T: Laboratory Animal Technicians: Their Role in Stress Reduction and Human-Companion Animal Bonding. *Vet Clin North Am Small Anim Pract* 15:449-454, 1985.
18. E.g., Morton DB: Epilogue: Summarization of Colloquium highlights from an international perspective. *J Am Vet Med Assoc* 191:1292, 1987 (calling for "the minimum amount of pain consistent with a scientific objective").
19. *J Am Vet Med Assoc* 191:1184-1298, 1987.
20. Kitchell RL: Problems in defining pain and peripheral mechanisms of pain. *J Am Vet Med Assoc* 191:1195, 1987.
21. Seligman MEP: *Helplessness. On Depression, Development and Death.* San Francisco: W.H. Freeman, 1975; Fox MW: *Farm Animals.* Baltimore: University Park Press, 1984, pp 237-249.
22. Benson GJ and Thurmon JC: Species difference as a consideration in alleviation of animal pain and distress. *J Am Vet Med Assoc* 191:1227, 1987.
23. Spinelli JS and Markowitz H: Clinical recognition and anticipation of situations likely to induce suffering in animals. *J Am Vet Med Assoc* 191:1216, 1987.
24. Benson GJ and Thurmon JC: Species difference as a consideration in alleviation of animal pain and distress. *J Am Vet Med Assoc* 191:1227-1230, 1987.
25. *The Biomedical Investigator's Handbook.* Washington, DC: Foundation for Biomedical Research, 1987, p 4 and references cited therein.
26. Loew FM: The challenge of balancing experimental variables: Pain, distress, analgesia, and anesthesia. *J Am Vet Med Assoc* 191:1193, 1987.
27. E.g., Thurmon JC and Benson GJ: Pharmacologic consideration in selection of anesthetics for animals. *J Am Vet Med Assoc* 191:1245-1251, 1987; Stanley TH: New developments in opioid drug research for the alleviation of animal pain. *J Am Vet Med Assoc* 191:1252-1253, 1987; Crane SW: Perioperative analgesia: A surgeon's perspective. *J Am Vet Med Assoc* 191:1254-1257, 1987.
28. Smith NT: New developments in monitoring animals for evidence of pain control. *J Am Vet Med Assoc* 191:1269-1272, 1987.
29. Wolfle TL: Control of stress using non-drug approaches. *J Am Vet Med Assoc* 191:1219-1221, 1987.
30. *The Biomedical Investigator's Handbook.* Washington, DC: Foundation for Biomedical Research, 1987, pp 5-6 and references cited therein.
31. Morton WR, *et al.*: Alternatives to chronic restraint of non-human primates. *J Am Vet Med Assoc* 191:1282-1286, 1987.
32. Amyx HL: Control of animal pain and distress in antibody production and infectious disease studies. *J Am Vet Med Assoc* 191:1287-1289, 1987, and references cited therein.
33. Rowan A: *Of Mice, Models, and Men.* Albany: State University of New York Press, 1984, p 282.
34. Morton DB: Epilogue: Summarization of Colloquium highlights from an international perspective. *J Am Vet Med Assoc* 191:1295, 1987.
35. Dresser R: Assessing Harm and Justification in Animal Research: Federal Policy Opens the Laboratory Door. *Rutgers Law Review* 40:795, 1988.
36. Rowan, *op. cit.*, pp 281-282.
37. See generally, Hewitt HB: The Use of Animals in Experimental Cancer Research. In Sperlinger D (ed): *Animals in Research.* Chichester, England: John Wiley & Sons, 1981, pp 141-174.
38. Dresser, *op. cit.*, pp 792-793 and references cited therein.
39. Rollin BE: The Moral Status of Research Animals in Psychology. *American Psychologist* Aug 1985:925.
40. Rowan, *op. cit..*, p 135. See also, Gallup G and Suarez S: On the Use of Animals in Psychological Research. *Psychol Rec* 30:212, 1980.

41. For a description of some of these experiments that is balanced by acknowledgment of important psychological animal research see, Drewett R and Kani W: Animal Experimentation in the Behavioural Sciences. In Sperlinger D (ed): *Animals in Research*. Chichester, England: John Wiley & Sons, 1981, pp 175-201 (summarizing an experiment in which conscious rats were taped to a restraining board and driven to epileptic fits with a combination of a convulsive drug and a 90 dB sound).
42. Rowan, *op. cit.*, pp 147-148.
43. See, Drewett and Kani, *op. cit.*, pp 175-201.
44. *Public Health Service Policy on Humane Care and Use of Laboratory Animals*. Washington, DC, 1986.
45. Report of the AVMA Panel on Euthanasia. *J Am Vet Med Assoc* 188:252-268, 1986.
46. *Id.*, 265.
47. See, e.g., *The Biomedical Investigator's Handbook*. Washington, DC: Foundation for Biomedical Research, 1987, pp 33-34 and references cited therein.
48. Rowan, *op. cit.*, pp 261-262. The terms "replacement," "reduction," and "refinement" were first proposed in Russell WMS and Burch RL: *The Principles of Humane Experimental Technique*. London: Methuen, 1959, p 64.
49. Rowan, *op. cit.*, pp 262-264.
50. Cohen, *op. cit.*, p 868.
51. Rowan, *op. cit.*, p 3.
52. E.g., Thomas L: Hubris in Science. *Science* 200:1461, 1978 (stating that "committees cannot formulate the ideas or lay out the plans; this is work that can only be done in the mind of the investigator himself. ... Sometimes an idea emerges from what can only be called intuition, and when the mind producing the idea is very imaginative, and very lucky, the whole field moves forward in a quantum jump."). What might be true regarding a Lewis Thomas does not necessarily apply to a more typical scientist or graduate student.
53. For a summary of state laws affecting the use of research animals see, *State Laws Concerning the Use of Animals in Research* ed. 2 Washington, DC: National Association for Biomedical Research, 1987.
54. Rowan, *op. cit.*, pp 155-156.
55. Rowan, *op. cit.*, pp 157-159.
56. Rowan, *op. cit.*, p 161.
57. Two-Fold Effect in Stopping Use of Pound Animals for Labs. *International Society for Animal Rights Report* May 1986:6.
58. For a thorough discussion of these issues, see Rowan, *op. cit.*, pp 189-248.
59. Rowan AN: The LD50 – The Beginning of the End. *Int J Stud Anim Prob* 4(1):6, 1983.
60. E.g., Dodds WJ: Letter. Use of animals in the education of veterinary students. *J Am Vet Med Assoc* 190:1372, 1987.
61. See Rowan A: *Of Mice, Models, and Men*. Albany: State University of New York Press, 1984, pp 93-108.
62. *1987 Annual Report*. Washington, DC: National Association for Biomedical Research, p 5.
63. U.S.C. § 2143.
64. *Federal Register* 52(61):10292-10392, 1987.
65. For an excellent summary of federal laws and regulations see, *The Biomedical Investigator's Handbook*. Washington, DC: Foundation for Biomedical Research, 1987, pp 45-64.
66. Pub. L. No. 99-158; 42 U.S.C. § 290aa-10.

67. 15 U.S.C. § 2603 *et seq.*; 40 C.F.R. § 792.1 *et seq.*
68. 7 U.S.C. § 136 *et seq.*,; 40 C.F.R. § 160.1 *et seq.*
69. 21 U.S.C. § 321 *et seq.*, 21 C.F.R. § 58.1
70. AVMA Comments on Animal Welfare Act Amendments. *J Am Vet Med Assoc* 191:506, 1987.
71. AVMA Comments on Animal Welfare Act Amendments. *J Am Vet Med Assoc* 191:510, 1987.
72. Infected Laboratory Cats Stolen by Activists. *J Am Vet Med Assoc* 191:1536, 1987.
73. Sun M: USDA Fines Pennsylvania Animal Laboratory. *Science* 230:423, 1985.
74. *1987 Annual Report.* Washington, DC: National Association for Biomedical Research, p 11.
75. Terrorist Group Suspected in Fire That Ravages UC-Davis Laboratory. *J Am Vet Med Assoc* 191:174, 1987.
76. See, e.g., *1987 Annual Report.* Washington DC: National Association for Biomedical Research, p 10 (stating that "as anticipated the animal rights movement became even more bold this year. Lawless acts of violence escalated.").
77. *Federal Register* 52(61):10303, 1987.

CONCLUSION

High Ideals, Charting a Middle Course

Veterinary ethics as a distinct field of study will be a rich and complex endeavor, but it is still in its formative stages. Investigation of the moral views of the profession (descriptive veterinary ethics) is just beginning. The governmental application of ethical standards to practitioners (administrative veterinary ethics) is too often a matter of unexercised legal authority, and has sometimes been inspired more by good intentions than rigorous investigation and argument. Ethical self-regulation by the organized profession (official veterinary ethics) is necessary and valuable. However, official veterinary ethics must be tempered with the understanding that matters of right and wrong cannot be settled by vote, and are not the property of any profession or group. Consideration of moral issues relating to veterinarians should not be restricted to veterinarians alone. The search for right answers to these issues (normative veterinary ethics) needs to be developed into a systematic and useful discipline.

This book attempts to break the ice, to offer a structure that will help get things moving. The text has addressed questions involving complex interactions among the interests of veterinary patients, clients, practitioners, employees, and the public. There are many issues that could not be treated here. The wide range of ethical questions facing veterinarians is itself a measure of the profession's influence and importance.

The central message of this book is that all in the profession should participate in the consideration of moral questions relating to veterinary practice in particular and animals in general. Veterinarians must include a serious discipline of ethics within their professional mandate. Failure to do so could be dangerous not only to doctors, but to patients, clients, and the public.

Although I have urged first and foremost cultivation of a *process* of ethical deliberation, two general substantive conclusions emerge from the discussion.

First, veterinarians ought to maintain the high ideal of dignified and respectful service. Animals, clients, and doctors will all benefit from the image of the veterinary patient as a being of value, and of the client as an autonomous person worthy of respect and concern. The status of the veterinarian as a medical professional should be treasured, not cast aside for the sake of short-term economic gain. In a commercialistic and competitive world, holding to high ideals is not easy. But veterinarians have always been special, and if anyone can do it, they can.

Second, the profession must maintain a firm, middle course as it charts its way through sometimes turbulent waters. Veterinarians should resist the blandishments and pressures of those who belittle human obligations to animals, and of those who condemn the human use of animals. Ours is a time accustomed to confrontation, polarization, and quick answers. The animal area has more than its share of extremists and bullies. Some thunder with such certitude and self-righteousness that those located somewhere in the middle who still have *questions* can wonder whether they themselves are worthy of the task. The serious study of ethical issues relating to animals is new, its questions are complex. Much remains to be learned. There is need for patience, moderation, and more than a bit of humility. In this process of discovery, veterinarians – armed with a serious discipline of professional ethics – will play a pre-eminent role.

SUGGESTIONS FOR FURTHER READING

The following is not a complete bibliography of all works useful in the study of professional veterinary ethics. Its purpose is to offer a basic core "library" of sources. These are not the only publications one might include in such a list. Many of these sources do not focus directly upon ethical issues faced by practicing veterinarians. Some do not mention veterinarians at all, and most are not, strictly speaking, works of moral theory. The publications differ widely in their general points of view and specific arguments, some of which are criticized in this book. For additional sources, the reader should consult references cited in the text.

Original Texts

American Veterinary Medical Association: *Marketing and Practice Strategies for the Companion Animal Practice*. Schaumburg, IL: American Veterinary Medical Association, 1987.

Canadian Council on Animal Care: *Guide to the Care and Use of Experimental Animals*. 2 vols. Ottawa: Canadian Council on Animal Care, 1984.

Dawkins MS: *Animal Suffering: The Science of Animal Welfare*. London: Chapman and Hall, 1980.

Fox MW: *Farm Animals: Husbandry, Behavior, and Veterinary Practice*. Baltimore: University Park Press, 1984.

Griffin DR: *Animal Thinking*. Cambridge, MA: Harvard University Press, 1984.

_____ *The Question of Animal Awareness*. New York: Rockefeller University Press, 1976.

Harrison R: *Animal Machines*. London: Vincent Stuart Ltd., 1964.

Herriot J: *All Creatures Great and Small*. New York: St. Martin's Press, 1972.

Midgley M: *Animals and Why They Matter*. New York: Penguin Books, 1983.

_____ *Beast and Man: The Roots of Human Nature*. Ithaca, NY: Cornell University Press, 1978.

Regan T: *The Case for Animal Rights*. Berkeley: University of California Press, 1983.

Rollin BE: *Animal Rights and Human Morality*. Buffalo: Prometheus Books, 1981.

Rowan AN: *Of Mice, Models, and Men: A Critical Evaluation of Animal Research*. Albany: State University of New York Press, 1984.

Singer P: *Animal Liberation*. New York: Avon Books, 1975.

Turner J: *Reckoning with the Beast: Animals, Pain and Humanity in the Victorian Mind*. Baltimore: Johns Hopkins University Press, 1980.

Anthologies and Collections

Animal Welfare and Animal Rights. Is There a Choice? Special Issue. *California Veterinarian* 37(1): 3-104, January 1983.

Proceedings of the AVMA Colloquium on Recognition and Alleviation of Animal Pain and Distress. *J Am Vet Med Assoc* 191:1184-1298, 1987.

Proceedings of the 8th Symposium on Veterinary Medical Education: Exploring Ethical and Value Issues in Veterinary Medicine. *Journal of Veterinary Medical Education* 9:71-143, 1983.

Symposium on the Case for Responsible Extra-Label Drug Use. *J Am Vet Med Assoc* 192:241-270, 1988.

Godlovitch S, Godlovitch R, and Harris J (eds): *Animals, Men, and Morals*. New York: Taplinger, 1971.

Katcher AH and Beck AM (eds): *New Perspectives on our Lives with Companion Animals*. Philadelphia: University of Pennsylvania Press, 1983.

McCullough LB and Morris JP (eds): *Implications of History and Ethics to Medicine – Veterinary and Human*. College Station: Texas A&M University Press, 1978.

Magel CR: *A Bibliography on Animal Rights and Related Matters*. Washington, DC: University Press of America, 1981.

Miller HB and Williams WH (eds): *Ethics and Animals*. Clifton, NJ: Humana Press, 1983.

Morris RK and Fox MW (eds): *On the Fifth Day: Animal Rights and Human Ethics*. Washington, DC: Acropolis Books, 1978.

Price EO (ed): *Farm Animal Behavior. Vet Clin North Am Food Anim Pract* 3(2), July 1987.

Quackenbush J and Voith VL (eds): *Symposium on the Human-Companion Animal Bond. Vet Clin North Am Small Anim Pract* 15(2), March 1985.

Regan T (ed): *Animal Sacrifices: Religious Perspectives on the Use of Animals in Science.* Philadelphia: Temple University Press, 1986.

_____ *All that Dwell Therein.* Berkeley: University of California Press, 1982.

Schroeder RJ (ed): Veterinary Services in Disasters and Emergencies. *J Am Vet Med Assoc* 190:701-799, 1987.

Sechzer J (ed): *The Role of Animals in Biomedical Research. Annals of the New York Academy of Sciences.* Vol 406, 1983.

Sperlinger D (ed): *Animals in Research.* Chichester, UK: John Wiley & Sons, 1981.

U.S. Congress, Office of Technology Assessment: *Alternatives to Animal Use in Research, Testing, and Education.* OTA-BA-273. Washington, DC: U.S. Government Printing Office, 1986.

Papers and Shorter Discussions

Farm animal wefare in Canada: Issues and priorities. Report of the Expert Committee on Farm Animal Welfare and Behaviour. Ottawa: Agriculture Canada, 1987.

Principles of Veterinary Medical Ethics. Schaumburg, IL: American Veterinary Medical Association, 1988.

Report of the AVMA Panel on Euthanasia. *J Am Vet Med Assoc* 188:252-268, 1986.

Scientific Aspects of the Welfare of Food Animals - Excerpts from Report 91, dated November 1981, published by the Council for Agricultural Science and Technology (CAST). *California Veterinarian* 37(1): 45-60, 1983.

The Veterinarian's Role in Companion Animal Welfare. Schaumburg, IL: American Veterinary Medical Association, undated.

The Veterinarian's Role in Food Animal Welfare. Schaumburg, IL: American Veterinary Medical Association, undated.

Antelyes J: The *Human* Side of Veterinary Medicine. [A monthly series of articles on the subject of relations with clients appearing in *J Am Vet Med Assoc* beginning in Vol. 190, No. 10, 1987.]

Armistead WW: Soul search. *J Am Vet Med Assoc* 188:338-339, 1986.

Bustad LK: Dean's Responsibilities and Bioethics. In Proceedings of the 8th Symposium on Veterinary Medical Education: Exploring Ethical and Value Issues in Veterinary Medicine. *Journal of Veterinary Medical Education* 9:97-98, 1983.

Caplan AL: Beastly Conduct: Ethical Issues in Animal Experimentation. *Ann NY Acad Sci* 406:159-169, 1983.

Caras R: Public Viewpoint of Veterinary Medicine. In Proceedings of the 8th Symposium on Veterinary Medical Education: Exploring Ethical and Value Issues in Veterinary Medicine. *Journal of Veterinary Medical Education* 9:110-112, 1983.

Cohen C: The case for the use of animals in biomedical research. *N Engl J Med* 315(14):865-870, 1986.

Curtis SE: Animal Well-Being and Animal Care. *Vet Clin North Am Food Anim Pract* 3(2):369-382, 1987.

Dresser, R: Assessing Harm and Justification in Animal Research: Federal Policy Opens the Laboratory Door. *Rutgers Law Review* 40:723-795, 1988.

Feinberg J: Human Duties and Animal Rights. In Morris RK and Fox MW (eds): *On the Fifth Day: Animal Rights and Human Ethics*. Washington, DC: Acropolis Books, 1978, pp 45-69.

_____ The Rights of Animals and Unborn Generations. In Feinberg J: *Rights, Justice, and the Bounds of Liberty*. Princeton: Princeton University Press, 1980, pp 159-184.

Goodall J: A Plea for the Chimpanzees. *American Scientist* 75:125-128, 1987.

Hart BL: Contributions of Behavioral Science to Issues in Animal Welfare. In Hart BL: *Behavior of Domestic Animals*. New York, W.H. Freeman and Co., 1985, pp 344-369.

Jacobs F: A perspective on animal rights and domestic animals. *J Am Vet Med Assoc* 184:1345-1346, 1984.

Kay WJ: Euthanasia. *Trends* 1(5):52-54, December 1985.

Kronfeld DS and Parr CP: Ecologic and symbiotic approaches to animal welfare, animal rights, and human responsibility. *J Am Vet Med Assoc* 191:660-664, 1987.

Loew FM: The Animal Welfare *Bête Noire* in Veterinary Medicine. *Canadian Veterinary Journal* 28:689-692, 1987.

Passmore J: The Treatment of Animals. *Journal of the History of Ideas* 36:195-218, 1975.

Rollin BE: The concept of illness in veterinary medicine. *J Am Vet Med Assoc* 182:1222-1225, 1983.

_____ Updating veterinary medical ethics. *J Am Vet Med Assoc* 173: 1015-1018, 1978.

Tannenbaum J: Ethics and Human-Companion Animal Interaction: A Plea for a Veterinary Ethics of the Human-Companion Animal Bond. *Vet Clin North Am Small Anim Pract* 15:431-447, 1985.

Tannenbaum J and Rowan AN: Rethinking the Morality of Animal Research. *Hastings Center Report* 15(5):32-43, 1985.

Index

Page numbers followed by "t" denote tables.